Phototherapy in the 21st Century

Editor

ELIZABETH A. BUZNEY

DERMATOLOGIC CLINICS

www.derm.theclinics.com

Consulting Editor
BRUCE H. THIERS

January 2020 • Volume 38 • Number 1

ELSEVIER

1600 John F. Kennedy Boulevard ● Suite 1800 ● Philadelphia, Pennsylvania, 19103-2899

http://www.theclinics.com

DERMATOLOGIC CLINICS Volume 38, Number 1
January 2020 ISSN 0733-8635, ISBN-13: 978-0-323-71058-9

Editor: Lauren Boyle
Developmental Editor: Laura Kavanaugh

Dermatologic Clinics (ISSN 0733-8635) is published quarterly by Elsevier Inc., 360 Park Avenue South, New York, NY 10010-1710. Months of publication are January, April, July, and October. Business and editorial offices: 1600 John F. Kennedy Blvd., Suite 1800, Philadelphia, PA 19103-2899. Customer service office: 11830 Westline Drive, St. Louis, MO 63146. Periodicals postage paid at New York, NY, and additional mailing offices. Subscription prices are USD 408.00 per year for US individuals, USD 780.00 per year for US institutions, USD 456.00 per year for Canadian individuals, USD 952.00 per year for Canadian institutions, USD 510.00 per year for international individuals, USD 952.00 per year for international institutions, USD 100.00 per year for US students/residents, USD 100.00 per year for Canadian students/residents, and USD 240 per year for international students/residents. International air speed delivery is included in all *Clinics* subscription prices. All prices are subject to change without notice. **POSTMASTER:** Send address changes to *Dermatologic Clinics*, Elsevier Health Sciences Division, Subscription Customer Service, 3251 Riverport Lane, Maryland Heights, MO 63043. **Customer Service: 1-800-654-2452 (U.S. and Canada); 314-447-8871 (outside U.S. and Canada). Fax: 314-447-8029. E-mail: journalscustomerservice-usa@elsevier.com (for print support); journalsonlinesupport-usa@elsevier.com (for online support).**

Reprints. For copies of 100 or more, of articles in this publication, please contact the Commercial Reprints Department, Elsevier Inc., 360 Park Avenue South, New York, New York 10010-1710. Tel.: 212-633-3874; Fax: 212-633-3820; Email: reprints@elsevier.com.

The *Dermatologic Clinics* is covered in *MEDLINE/PubMed (Index Medicus)*, *Current Contents/Clinical Medicine*, *Excerpta Medica*, *Chemical Abstracts,* and *ISI/BIOMED*.

Contributors

CONSULTING EDITOR

BRUCE H. THIERS, MD
Professor and Chairman Emeritus, Department of Dermatology and Dermatologic Surgery, Medical University of South Carolina, Charleston, South Carolina, USA

EDITOR

ELIZABETH A. BUZNEY, MD
Assistant Professor, Department of Dermatology, Brigham and Women's Hospital, Harvard Medical School, Associate Vice Chair of Clinical Affairs, Brigham Dermatology Associates, Boston, Massachusetts, USA

AUTHORS

KRISTEN M. BECK, MD
Department of Dermatology, University of California, San Francisco, San Francisco, California, USA

TINA BHUTANI, MD
Department of Dermatology, University of California, San Francisco, San Francisco, California, USA

ELIZABETH A. BUZNEY, MD
Assistant Professor, Department of Dermatology, Brigham and Women's Hospital, Harvard Medical School, Associate Vice Chair of Clinical Affairs, Brigham Dermatology Associates, Boston, Massachusetts, USA

JOI B. CARTER, MD
Assistant Professor, Dartmouth Geisel School of Medicine, Section of Dermatology, Department of Surgery, Dartmouth-Hitchcock Medical Center, Lebanon, New Hampshire, USA

HENRY W. CHEN, BS
The University of Texas Southwestern Medical Center, Dallas, Texas, USA

ABIGAIL CLINE, MD, PhD
Research Fellow, Center for Dermatology Research, Wake Forest School of Medicine, Winston-Salem, North Carolina, USA

JENNIFER COIAS, BA
The University of Texas Southwestern Medical Center, Dallas, Texas, USA

SARINA B. ELMARIAH, MD, PhD
Assistant Professor, Harvard Medical School, Department of Dermatology, Massachusetts General Hospital, Boston, Massachusetts, USA

STEVEN FELDMAN, MD, PhD
Professor, Department of Dermatology, Pathology, Social Science and Health Policy, Wake Forest School of Medicine, Winston-Salem, North Carolina, USA

ARI M. GOLDMINZ, MD
Instructor, Harvard Medical School, Associate Physician, Department of Dermatology, Brigham and Women's Hospital, Boston, Massachusetts, USA

ANNA L. GROSSBERG, MD
Assistant Professor of Dermatology and Pediatrics Interim Director of Pediatric Dermatology, Department of Dermatology, Division of Pediatric Dermatology, Johns Hopkins School of Medicine, Baltimore, Maryland, USA

JONATHAN GUIYAB, BSN, RN
Department of Dermatology, Johns Hopkins School of Medicine, Baltimore, Maryland, USA

ILTEFAT H. HAMZAVI, MD
Department of Dermatology, Henry Ford Health System, Detroit, Michigan, USA

ANDREA N. HINTON, BS
Harvard Medical School, Boston, Massachusetts, USA

KATHIE P. HUANG, MD
Assistant Professor, Department of Dermatology, Brigham and Women's Hospital, Harvard Medical School, Boston, Massachusetts, USA

JASON JACOB, MD
Attending Physician and Site Director for Inpatient Undergraduate Medical Education, Department of Medicine, Hartford Hospital, Hartford, Connecticut, USA; Clinical Instructor and Associate Clinical Faculty, University of Connecticut School of Medicine and Internal Medicine Residency, Farmington, Connecticut, USA

HEIDI JACOBE, MD, MSCS
The University of Texas Southwestern Medical Center, Dallas, Texas, USA

ANGELA J. JIANG, MD
Department of Dermatology, Henry Ford Health System, Detroit, Michigan, USA

MICHELLE C. JUAREZ, BS
Johns Hopkins School of Medicine, Baltimore, Maryland, USA

NOORI KIM, MD
Assistant Professor, Department of Dermatology, Johns Hopkins School of Medicine, Baltimore, Maryland, USA

WILSON LIAO, MD
Department of Dermatology, University of California, San Francisco, San Francisco, California, USA

HENRY W. LIM, MD
Department of Dermatology, Henry Ford Health System, Detroit, Michigan, USA

KAREN LY, BA
Department of Dermatology, University of California, San Francisco, San Francisco, California, USA

ARTHUR MARKA, BS
Dartmouth Geisel School of Medicine, Hanover, New Hampshire, USA

GINETTE A. OKOYE, MD
Department of Dermatology, Howard University Hospital, Washington, DC, USA

ADRIAN PONA, MD
Research Fellow, Center for Dermatology Research, Wake Forest School of Medicine, Winston-Salem, North Carolina, USA

SMRITI PRASAD, BSA
The University of Texas Southwestern Medical Center, Dallas, Texas, USA

ELISABETH G. RICHARD, MD
Assistant Professor of Dermatology, Johns Hopkins School of Medicine, Baltimore, Maryland, USA

MARY P. SMITH, BS
Department of Dermatology, University of California, San Francisco, San Francisco, California, USA

QUINN G. THIBODEAUX, MD
Department of Dermatology, University of California, San Francisco, San Francisco, California, USA

KATHERINE G. THOMPSON, BS
Research Trainee, Department of Dermatology, Johns Hopkins School of Medicine, Baltimore, Maryland, USA

OLIVIA R. WARE, BA
Howard University College of Medicine, Washington, DC, USA

PETER WOLF, MD
Department of Dermatology, Research Unit for Photodermatology, Medical University of Graz, Graz, Austria

REBECCA L. YANOVSKY, BS
Medical Student, Tufts University School of Medicine, Boston, Massachusetts, USA

ZIZI YU, BA
Medical Student, Harvard Medical School, Boston, Massachusetts, USA

CONNIE S. ZHONG, MSc
Harvard Medical School, Boston, Massachusetts, USA

RAHEEL ZUBAIR, MD, MHS
Department of Dermatology, Broward Health Medical Center, Fort Lauderdale, Florida, USA

Contents

Psoriasis is a chronic, autoimmune condition characterized by abnormal epidermal hyperproliferation affecting about 3.2% of adults in the United States. Narrowband UVB (NBUVB) is a commonly used phototherapy option for patients with psoriasis and is an effective first-line therapy for generalized plaque psoriasis. This article covers fundamental considerations for physicians using NBUVB and highlights changes in the newest guideline recommendations for phototherapy treatment. Protocols for treatment initiation, maintenance, dose increases, and maintenance are compared and discussed. Readers will achieve a greater understanding of the fundamentals of NBUVB phototherapy and promising advances in the field, including home phototherapy and combination treatment.

PUVA phototherapy is the therapeutic use of psoralens and UVA light to treat inflammatory skin diseases, with psoriasis the prototype disease. Naturally occurring phototoxic compounds, psoralens interact with UVA to suppress DNA synthesis and cell proliferation and induce apoptosis of inflammatory cells. Well-developed therapeutic protocols for psoriasis guide psoralen and UVA doses, treatment frequency, and safety measures, and these protocols also may be used to treat other inflammatory dermatoses.

Ultraviolet (UV) radiation contributes to the development of skin cancer through direct and indirect DNA damage, production of reactive oxygen species, and local immunomodulation. The association between UV radiation and skin cancer has raised concern for the risk of carcinogenesis following phototherapy. The photocarcinogenic impact of psoralen and UVA radiation (PUVA) has been extensively studied, whereas limited safety studies exist for other phototherapy modalities, such as broadband and narrowband UVB and UVA1. Because of the as of yet unclear risk, patients who have undergone any type of phototherapy should be followed for age-appropriate skin cancer screening.

Phototherapeutic modalities induce apoptosis of keratinocytes and immune cells, impact cytokine production, downregulate the IL-23/Th17 axis, and induce regulatory T cells. As in anti-IL-17 or anti-IL-23 antibody treatment, the dual action of phototherapy on skin and the immune system is likely responsible for sustained resolution of lesions in diseases such as psoriasis. In cutaneous T cell lymphoma, phototherapy may function by causing tumor cell apoptosis and eliminating the neoplastic and inflammatory infiltrate. Further research on phototherapeutic mechanisms will help advance, optimize, and refine dermatologic treatments and may open up novel avenues for treatment strategies in dermatology and beyond.

Phototherapy is an effective treatment modality for many types of pruritus. Although the exact mechanisms by which phototherapy reduces itch vary across pruritic conditions, its effects may result from immune suppression and/or neural modulation. In this article, the authors review the efficacy of different types of phototherapy for common inflammatory and noninflammatory pruritic conditions and discuss common side effects, such as erythema and exacerbation of pruritus. Although phototherapy may be an effective and relatively safe option for skin-directed treatment of chronic itch, barriers may exist for individual patients.

The excimer laser has emerged as an efficacious treatment modality for many dermatologic diseases. The excimer laser is an alternative to standard narrowband ultraviolet B (NBUVB) phototherapy treatment in patients with limited disease. In comparison to standard NBUVB, the excimer laser requires fewer treatment sessions, has reduced treatment duration, requires a lower cumulative UVB dose, and limits UVB exposure to lesional skin. This review addresses the mechanism, safety, application, and efficacy of the excimer laser for the treatment of these conditions.

An interaction between light's radiation and certain exogenous and endogenous substances can lead to the development of photoallergic and/or phototoxic dermatoses. Clinically, reactions may range from acute and self-limited to chronic and recurrent. Delays in diagnosis are not uncommon due to complex clinical presentations, broad differentials, and limited number of specialists who perform phototesting. Therefore, a critical understanding of these dermatoses is essential for accurate diagnosis and appropriate management. The epidemiology, light sources, mechanisms, clinical presentations, evaluation protocols, common culprits, treatments, key challenges, and future directions related to photoallergy and phototoxicity are reviewed herein.

DERMATOLOGIC CLINICS

SERIES OF RELATED INTEREST

Facial Plastic Surgery Clinics
Available at: http://www.facialplastic.theclinics.com/
Surgical Oncology Clinics
Available at: https://www.surgonc.theclinics.com/

THE CLINICS ARE AVAILABLE ONLINE!
Access your subscription at:
www.theclinics.com

Preface
Shedding Light on Phototherapy

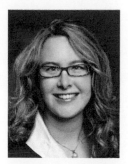

Elizabeth A. Buzney, MD
Editor

Phototherapy remains an essential tool in the dermatologist's treatment armamentarium, and yet, we find that as less time is spent teaching phototherapy to our dermatology trainees, that more dermatologists view what happens in the phototherapy center as an unknown, a literal and figurative "black box." The goal of this issue is to bridge that gap and to give dermatologists the tools to both learn and teach the standards and pearls of phototherapy.

I am excited to present this issue of *Dermatologic Clinics* on phototherapy, which intends to be as practical as possible while answering some of the questions that arise most frequently with regards to phototherapy. To name a few: What are the new, recent guidelines on how to treat psoriasis, vitiligo, and cutaneous T-cell lymphoma? What is the latest understanding of how phototherapy works on cutaneous inflammation? What are the challenges that face patients of color as they are treated with phototherapy? And last, before we assume that narrowband UVB has made psoralen with UVA (PUVA) irrelevant, pearls from the master clinician show us that PUVA very much still has a role.

New and exciting treatments for psoriasis and atopic dermatitis are available, but not for everyone. Light remains a relatively inexpensive and effective immunotherapy, which is ours as dermatologists, and we must remember the art of how to use it and the importance of continued innovation in this space. Thanks to all our writers for their hard work and continued passion in this area. I hope that your reading will only stimulate more questions, which our specialty will answer together. Enjoy!

Elizabeth A. Buzney, MD
Harvard Medical School
Boston, MA 02115, USA

Brigham Dermatology Associates
221 Longwood Avenue
Boston, MA 02115, USA

E-mail address:
ebuzney@bics.bwh.harvard.edu

Dermatol Clin 38 (2020) xiii
https://doi.org/10.1016/j.det.2019.09.002
0733-8635/20/© 2019 Published by Elsevier Inc.

Optimizing Narrowband UVB Phototherapy Regimens for Psoriasis

Rebecca L. Yanovsky, BS[a], Kathie P. Huang, MD[b],
Elizabeth A. Buzney, MD[b],*

KEYWORDS

- Psoriasis • Phototherapy • Narrowband UVB • Protocol optimization

KEY POINTS

- Narrowband UVB phototherapy (NBUVB) is a safe and effective first-line therapy for generalized plaque psoriasis.
- New data and guidelines have resulted in updated considerations for the main aspects of NBUVB phototherapy protocols: therapy initiation, dose escalation, treatment frequency, dose maximums, and maintenance regimens.
- Home phototherapy increases accessibility to phototherapy treatment of patients.

INTRODUCTION
Psoriasis

Psoriasis is a chronic, autoimmune condition characterized by abnormal hyperproliferation of the epidermis that affects up to 3.2% of adults in the United States.[1] The autoimmune component of psoriasis is thought to be driven by T-helper cells that are inappropriately activated, leading to the overproduction of inflammatory cytokines, such as tumor necrosis factor-alpha, interferon-gamma, and interleukin-17, as well as the characteristic hyperproliferation of keratinocytes leading to silvery plaques on body surfaces.[2] Apart from skin and nail manifestations, patients can have systemic symptoms, including cardiovascular disease, metabolic syndrome, depression, and joint involvement with psoriatic arthritis. There have also been numerous studies that elucidate the significant impact that psoriasis has on quality of life.[3]

The range of therapeutic options for psoriasis is broad and varies depending on geography, cost, and associated side effects. Treatment options include topical and oral therapies as well as phototherapy and newer biologic medications. Despite a wide range of treatments, many patients are dissatisfied with their therapy and continue to suffer decreased quality of life and work productivity owing to the disease.[4]

Narrowband UVB

Narrowband UVB (NBUVB), which uses wavelengths of 311- to 313-nm light, is one the most commonly used types of phototherapy for patients with psoriasis and is an effective first-line therapy for generalized plaque psoriasis. The direct effect of UV light on Langerhans cells in the epidermis has an immunomodulatory effect, which inhibits their antigen-presenting capability to the T cell.

Disclosure Statement: Dr. K.P. Huang has received royalty payments from Pfizer for licensing ALTO and consulting fees from Pfizer. She has also participated in clinical trials related to alopecia from Incyte, Aclaris, Concert, and Lily. The other authors have nothing to disclose.
[a] Tufts University School of Medicine, 145 Harrison Avenue, Boston, MA 02111, USA; [b] Department of Dermatology, Brigham and Women's Hospital, Harvard Medical School, 221 Longwood Avenue, Boston, MA 02115, USA
* Corresponding author. Department of Dermatology, Brigham and Women's Hospital, 221 Longwood Avenue, Boston, MA 02115.
E-mail address: EBuzney@BICS.BWH.harvard.edu

Dermatol Clin 38 (2020) 1–10
https://doi.org/10.1016/j.det.2019.08.001
0733-8635/20/© 2019 Elsevier Inc. All rights reserved.

Other proposed mechanisms include downregulation of cytokine expression and the inhibition of epidermal hyperproliferation via interference with protein and nucleic acid synthesis.[2]

Broadband UVB (BBUVB) and psoralen UVA (PUVA) phototherapy are no longer used as commonly for treatment of psoriasis. Although a Cochrane Review including 13 randomized controlled trials[5] was inconclusive in a comparison of NBUVB, BBUVB, and PUVA, for plaque psoriasis, NBUVB has emerged as the preferred therapy for moderate to severe psoriasis in adults[6] and is considered first line for plaque psoriasis according to both the American Academy of Dermatology (AAD) and the European S-3 guidelines because of its favored safety profile, convenience, and cost-efficacy.[7,8] A systematic review of the literature covering the period from 1980 to 2010 found that PUVA and NBUVB are both effective therapies; although PUVA can clear psoriasis more reliably and in fewer sessions (average of 17 vs 25), it has higher known carcinogenic risk and more difficult administration because of the need for exogenous photosensitizer use before therapy and increased burn risk.[9,10] Reviews have shown that NBUVB is more effective than BBUVB and safer than PUVA. No increased risk of skin cancer has been shown in several studies assessing the carcinogenic risk of NBUVB.[10,11] NBUVB is also a convenient therapeutic option because it can be administered in a variety of treatment environments, including patients' homes, with similar efficacy and higher patient satisfaction compared with in-office treatment.[5,12] Although NBUVB is currently the most widely used treatment worldwide,[2] a review of the literature highlights the significant heterogeneity among proposed NBUVB treatment regimens for psoriasis.[4,11]

NBUVB has the potential to achieve high clearance rates and vastly improve quality of life for psoriasis patients when administered appropriately. A systematic review of 2416 patients across 41 randomized controlled trials using a Psoriasis Area and Severity Index (PASI)-75 calculated an average of 68% (95% confidence interval [CI] 57–78) improvement for NBUVB across PASI-75 monotherapy trials.[13] The optimal NBUVB treatment protocol for psoriasis patients aims to maximize efficacy and minimize recurrence and side effects.

INITIATING THERAPY
Considerations and Contraindications

Before initiating NBUVB phototherapy, it is important to conduct a baseline evaluation of disease using objective measures. Although standardized tools, such as the PASI-75 or Physician Global Assessment (PGA), are typically used within the context of clinical trials, estimation of body surface area coverage should be used routinely in the practice setting. In the authors' practice, they encourage photodocumentation before starting phototherapy as a means of following patients' progress during treatment. It is also important to assess for the presence of associated symptoms, such as psoriatic arthritis, not only when starting phototherapy but also during follow-up visits.

Despite the general safety and efficacy of NBUVB, there are 2 absolute contraindications: xeroderma pigmentosum and photodermatoses in the UVB spectrum, such as solar urticaria or chronic actinic dermatitis.[2] Although previously contraindicated in lupus erythematosus, expert opinion from the most recent 2019 AAD guidelines advises that NBUVB can be used with caution in these patients as long as there is no history of photosensitivity, and testing shows anti-Ro/SSA negativity. These guidelines also recommend that it is safe to administer NBUVB to patients on photosensitizing medications, because NBUVB light sources emit negligible UVA radiation.[14] Although NBUVB is generally safe and well tolerated, expert recommendations include precautions, such as eye goggles and genital shields, for all patients undergoing NBUVB to protect against ocular toxicities, such as cataracts, keratitis, and corneal burns, and the development of genital skin cancers.[14] Data regarding risk of developing genital cancer are largely applied from studies of PUVA; 1 study of 892 men treated with PUVA demonstrated a 4.6 times relative risk (95% CI 1.4–15.1) of genital tumors in patients treated with high versus low doses of UVB phototherapy after controlling for PUVA exposure.[15] No known studies to date have looked at incidence or prevention of genital cancer in NBUVB phototherapy patients.

Before NBUVB phototherapy, a thin emollient layer can enhance efficacy and minimize erythema; a study of 40 patients comparing pretreatment with crude coal tar, petrolatum, and phototherapy alone found significantly higher improvement in PASI and PGA scores for tar compared with placebo, and petrolatum pretreatment had higher PGA increases than tar.[16] In the authors' practice, they use mineral oil for patients with significant amounts of scale on larger plaques, which may interfere with phototherapy absorption. Pretreatment medications should also be practical for patients; certain distributions of disease or subtypes, such as guttate psoriasis, are diffuse and therefore less well suited for this option.

Relative contraindications include unfavorable patient-centered logistics (ie, inability to regularly travel to therapy site), a history of poor compliance, physical or emotional inability to tolerate therapy (ie, claustrophobia), as well as epilepsy, skin type I, and a history of melanoma or multiple nonmelanoma skin cancers.[4] Home-based therapy, an attractive option for many patients, may be used on an individual basis to alleviate some of these patient-centered barriers to treatment. NBUVB is considered safe in pregnancy and has been recommended as first line for pregnant women with moderate to severe disease.[7] It is recommended that all women of childbearing age supplement with 0.8 mg folate daily to decrease risk of neural tube defects in planned or unplanned pregnancies while undergoing NBUVB phototherapy; a recent review has concluded that NBUVB exposure is associated with a dose-dependent degradation of folate by 19% to 27% at cumulative exposure greater than 40 J/cm^2 or average >2 J/cm^2 per treatment.[14,17] Performing a thorough history and physical examination can identify these absolute and relative contraindications, enabling the appropriate treatment approach, counseling, and preparation.

Starting Dose

Starting dose is most often chosen based on a standard dose recommended by skin type or by using a percentage of the minimal erythema dose (MED), defined as the lowest dose that produces clinically perceptible erythema with distinct borders at 24 hours after exposure. According to the AAD 2010 guidelines, skin type is associated with significant variation in MED for NBUVB, and therefore, MED testing is generally recommended, although it can cause discomfort and be inconvenient for the patient.[7] Of note, skin type–based standard doses may be conservatively low to minimize unexpected side effects, and therefore, MED-based dosing may achieve a more rapid result.[18] The 2019 AAD guidelines now outline both methods of initiating without a firm recommendation favoring either.

Indeed, there is currently no strong evidence demonstrating increased efficacy in 1 protocol over the other. A study of 51 psoriasis patients, half of whom initiated therapy at 50% of the MED and followed MED dosing standards, and half who followed a fixed dose schedule of therapy initiated based on skin type, found no significant difference based on PASI, cumulative NBUVB dose, total number of treatment sessions, or side-effect profiles between the 2 regimens.[19] One hypothesis is that this is due to skin color

being well correlated with MED, implying either could be used to initiate a phototherapy protocol.[20] However, this may not be true for darker skin types. Youn and colleagues[21] have suggested a weak relationship between Fitzpatrick skin type and MED in Korean and brown skin. Baron and colleagues[22] similarly found low correlation between skin type and MED, suggesting that basing dosing solely off of skin type can lead to underdosing or overdosing, given the wide range of MED within each skin type.

Although not standard of care, other options are being explored. One example is the use of colorimeters, an instrument designed to measure color intensity, to assign a value to a patient's skin color, which is subsequently used to determine starting dose. Colorimetric values of unaffected skin were shown to be noninferior to MED dosing when comparing response rate, mean number of treatments, duration of treatment, maximum and cumulative doses in 27 patients with skin phototype III to V, while offering increased convenience to patients and physicians.[18]

If using MED, choosing a starting dose of NBUVB has generally reached consensus at a starting rate of roughly 50% of the MED, although some protocols, including the most recent European guidelines,[8] initiate at as high as 70% of MED, and 50% to 80% is generally acceptable.[2,4] Initial dosing based on Fitzpatrick skin type has demonstrated a wide range of protocol-dependent proposed starting doses.[23] For example, in 2004 and 2005 alone, 3 protocols were published, one with a starting dose of 400 mJ/cm^2, one with a starting dose of 800 mJ/cm^2, and one with a starting dose of 1500 mJ/cm^2 for skin type VI patients.[24–26] This variation may have been in large part owing to metering differences between booths used at different treatment centers. Furthermore, initial dosing based on skin type can be subjective, because assessment of skin type depends on both clinical assessment and patient self-assessment of acute erythema and induced pigmentation.

The updated 2019 AAD guidelines now recommend that initial NBUVB dosing estimated by skin type starts at 300 mJ/cm^2 for skin types I and II, 500 mJ/cm^2 for skin types III and IV, and 800 mJ/cm^2 for skin types V and VI.[14] Although these guidelines still include recommendations for MED testing for skin types I to IV, for skin types V and VI, they indicate that treatment should be initiated at the aforementioned skin type–based starting dose.

The variation in recommendations emphasizes the importance of metering one's own phototherapy machines, and dosing to clinical effect as a critical component of optimizing therapy for patients. At present, both MED and skin type–based methodologies are acceptable for calculating a starting dose for psoriasis patients undergoing NBUVB. A randomized clinical trial of 210 patients randomized to starting doses of NBUVB via fixed starting dose, 50% of MED, or 70% of MED and subsequent identical protocols found no significant difference in treatment efficacy between groups.[27] Although adequate initial dosing based on MED may contribute to patient safety, it is reasonable to use either protocol for determining starting dose in most populations. In the authors' own practice, they use skin type to initiate therapy; the published equivalence of skin type to MED initiation, the inconvenience to patients returning in 24 hours for reevaluation after MED testing, and the lack of MED testing commonly resulting in significant adjustments all outweigh the potential for initiation by skin type to result in a more prolonged titration to achieve optimal dosing.

DOSE ESCALATION

NBUVB dosage on subsequent visits can be escalated based on percentage, fixed dose, or fixed time. Each method may serve a different need, for example, when considering in-office versus home phototherapy protocols.

Percentage-Based Increase

Dosing decisions are often made based on the patient's extent and duration of erythema as well as their subjective symptoms and tolerance of therapy. As recommended in the new 2019 AAD guidelines, NBUVB dosing should be escalated in subsequent visits using the following protocol[14]:

- Erythema less than 24 hours: increase dose by 20%
- Erythema greater than 24 hours, less than 48 hours: maintain previous dose until erythema duration deceases to less than 24 hours
- Erythema greater than 48 hours: defer next treatment. When erythema subsides, return 1 step down to the last dose that did not produce prolonged erythema and continue dose adjustments as above.

For comparison, the previous 2010 AAD guidelines used an MED-based titration as follows: increasing by 10% of MED for treatments 1 to 20 and increasing as ordered by the treating physician for subsequent treatments, but MED-based

percentage titration was not included in the most recent guidelines.[7,14]

The protocol used at the authors' center is referenced in an earlier article by Matos and colleagues[4] that looked to synthesize 2010 AAD guidelines and 2009 European S3 guidelines[7,8]; this protocol increases the dose by 20% at 48 hours if no erythema was present, increases the dose by 10% if minimal transient erythema or itch was present, maintains the dose if asymptomatic erythema was present but resolved within 48 hours, and holds treatment if there is painful erythema at 48 hours, until resolution.[4] Alternatively, Mehta and Lim[2] suggest a 10% to 15% increase by skin type, as tolerated.

Although these guidelines have slight variations, there has not been recent evidence indicating increased efficacy or minimized side effects with 1 titration protocol over another; rather, clinical judgment should consider a patient's individual symptoms and tolerance. A study of 30 patients with plaque psoriasis receiving NBUVB 3 times per week for 10 weeks on an MED-determined initial dose compared dose increase on a daily versus weekly basis and found no statistically significant difference in treatment efficacy between the groups based on PASI scores, whereas the group with daily dose increases experienced a significantly higher cumulative dose of UVB.[28]

Fixed Dose and Fixed Time Increase

Although percentage titration is used as the standard for in-office phototherapy, fixed dose or fixed time protocols are often safer and more convenient for patients using home phototherapy, where calculation of percentages may be difficult for patients. A fixed dose protocol increases the dosage of phototherapy steadily at a predetermined rate. Published protocols differ slightly in the recommended treatment increase; typically, recommendations are made based on skin type and starting dose. The 2010 AAD guidelines included a skin type–based protocol for fixed dose increases that was not included in the most recent guidelines (**Table 1**).

Fixed timing increases involve escalating patient NBUVB exposure by a time interval rather than by millijoule per square centimeter. This approach has not been as popular nor as well studied in the literature. Although this would theoretically mirror the fixed increases seen in the dosage or percentage protocol, there are inherent potential challenges with this approach because different phototherapy machines have different metering, different numbers of bulbs, and other variations that may interfere with the intended

Table 1
2010 American Academy of Dermatology guidelines for fixed dose narrowband UVB increase based on skin type

Skin Type	UVB Increase After Each Treatment (mJ/cm^2)
I	15
II	25
III	40
IV	45
V	60
VI	65

protocol. This approach may work for individuals going through home phototherapy and consistently using the same machine, as discussed in the section on special considerations for home phototherapy.

Missed Treatments

The 2019 AAD recommendations outline a schedule for managing missed treatments. In summary, if a patient has missed 1 week, the previous dose is held constant. If the patient has missed 1 to 2 weeks, the previous dose is decreased by 25%; if 2 to 4 weeks are missed, it is decreased by 50%, and for a lapse of greater than 4 weeks of therapy, it is recommended to return to the starting dose.[14] This outline is slightly different than the 2010 guidelines, as illustrated in **Table 2**.

As with other treatment parameters, there is variation among missed-dose protocols at different treatment facilities. For example, a protocol from Henry Ford Hospital decreases dosage by 33% for 1 to 2 weeks of missed therapy and by 66% for 3 to 4 weeks of missed therapy.[2] Despite these variations, most published protocols advise returning to the starting dose after more than 1 month of missed therapy.

TREATMENT FREQUENCY

There is general consensus in the literature on the optimal frequency of NBUVB phototherapy treatments. Treatment frequency greater than 3 times per week has been shown to have little value and carries increased risk of UVB-induced erythema. Hallaji and colleagues[29] compared the effects of 3 versus 5 times weekly NBUVB treatment of chronic plaque psoriasis in 65 patients. Although the treatment period was significantly shorter in the 5 times weekly group (mean 14.7 weeks vs 13.7 weeks) to achieve complete clearance, the overall percentage of each group that achieved clearance was not statistically different (78% vs 68%). Whereas the treatment period was shorter, there was no statistically significant difference in the number of treatments, cumulative dose, or rate of side effects. Cameron and colleagues[30] published a study of 113 patients showing that treatment 2 times a week took 1.5 times as long as treatment 3 times per week (88 vs 58 days); treatment groups required an average of 24.4 and 23 treatments, respectively.

Dawe and colleagues[31] similarly showed that clearance was achieved more quickly with 5 times weekly treatment versus 3 times weekly treatment in a study of 21 patients of skin types I to III; however, this study showed increased NBUVB exposures and higher cumulative dose among the group receiving more frequent treatment. Of patients, 93% in the 5 times weekly group also developed at least 1 episode of grade 2 erythema, compared with 19% of patients in the 3 times weekly group. The increased side-effect profile observed in this study may be a reflection of patient selection, with skin types I to III.

A study of 69 Asian patients with psoriasis with skin types III to IV treated with 2 and 4 times weekly NBUVB found no significant difference in PASI or time to clearance (8 weeks); however, patients in the former treatment group required 16 exposures compared with 32 exposures in the treatment group with higher frequency. The twice

Table 2
2010 and 2019 American Academy of Dermatology guidelines regarding missed narrowband UVB phototherapy treatments

2019		2010	
Missed Treatments (wk)	Recommendation	Missed Treatments	Recommendation
1	Hold dose constant	4–7 d	Hold dose constant
1–2	Decrease by 25%	1–2 wk	Decrease by 25%
2–4	Decrease by 50%	2–3 wk	Decrease by 50% or start over
>4	Start over	3–4 wk	Start over

weekly treatment group experienced an average of 12.5 MED multiples compared with 39.7 MEDs in the 4 times weekly group.[32] This study illustrates the same principle in Asian patients of skin types II to IV.

In summary and as concluded in the AAD 2019 guidelines, most patients will receive maximum benefit from treatment 3 times weekly, optimizing for time to clearance, minimization of side effects, and patient convenience. It may be reasonable to increase treatment frequency up to 5 times weekly if the patient's primary goal is reducing time to clearance; however, this could come at the cost of increased inconvenience for patients doing in-office therapy and the risk of erythema in patients with lighter skin types. Similarly, 2 times weekly treatment is a reasonable choice for patients unable to participate in more weekly treatments and should result in the same ultimate clearance rate, albeit potentially over a longer treatment period.

MAXIMUM DOSAGES

Maximum dosage recommendations for patients are based on skin type per the 2019 AAD guidelines; for skin types I and II, a maximum total body dose of 2000 mJ/cm^2 is recommended; for skin types III and IV, a maximum dose of 3000 mJ/cm^2 is recommended; and for skin types V and VI, a maximum dose of 5000 mJ/cm^2 is recommended.[14] This recommendation is unchanged from the 2010 AAD guideline recommendation (**Table 3**), although perhaps slightly more aggressive than some previously published protocols suggesting a maximum total body dose of 1700 to 3500 mJ/cm^2 depending on skin type.[4,7] An NBUVB phototherapy protocol published from Henry Ford Hospital stratifies maximum dosage based on skin area, recommending a maximum dose of 3000 mJ/cm^2 to the body and 1000 mJ/cm^2 to the face, regardless of skin type[2] (see **Table 3**).

It is important to note that there are no explicit data to support the above guidelines regarding maximum dose per treatment. Although the concept of maximum dose protects patients from overtreatment with UV radiation, as discussed above, skin type can be problematic as either an underapproximation or an overapproximation of a patient's MED. It is therefore most important to titrate to clinical effect, which could in certain cases supersede guidelines for a maximum dose per skin type.

It is also important to note that there is no maximum number of lifetime treatments specified by guidelines in the United States. International guidelines, however, have proposed a maximum ceiling for total number of lifetime phototherapy treatments. The British Photodermatology Group Workshop in 2004 recommended a lifetime maximum of 450 treatments, making the assumption that NBUVB has similar carcinogenesis to the sun and that a 50% increased risk for development of nonmelanoma skin cancer would be tolerated by patients.[33] French guidelines state a maximum of 200 lifetime sessions of phototherapy (UVB and PUVA).[34] There is evidently significant variation in international guidelines; in the United States, there is no lifetime maximum nor known evidence to support instituting a maximum. Although most studies to date have not shown an increased risk for skin cancer from NBUVB phototherapy, more studies, which are longer term, larger, and incorporate patient's cumulative dose and lifetime number of treatments, are needed to truly define the risk.[10,35–37] The authors suggest titrating to clinical effect while being careful not to overtreat or maintain patients on a dose or treatment frequency higher than what is necessary, particularly when recommending long-term maintenance programs for patients.

MAINTENANCE DOSE REGIMENS

Maintenance regimens are defined as phototherapy treatment continued after the patient's psoriasis has cleared and may be administered as a taper or indefinitely as needed, depending on the patient's history of recurrence off phototherapy and their preference. For NBUVB phototherapy, an average of 15 to 20 treatments is needed to achieve clearance for psoriasis. Although clearance has been demonstrated in as little as 2 weeks, or 8 to 10 treatments, more treatments are often needed.[7] The last dose before skin clearance is typically used for maintenance therapy (the "clearance dose"), initially twice weekly for 1 month and then tapered to weekly for 1 month, and then discontinued if appropriate. Prolonged maintenance

Table 3	
2019 and 2010 guidelines for maximum narrowband UVB dosages	
Skin Type	Maximum Dosage (mJ/cm^2)
I	2000
II	2000
III	3000
IV	3000
V	5000
VI	5000

therapy, for patients unable to maintain a remission off phototherapy, may be administered at a frequency of 1 treatment every 1 to 2 weeks, as tolerated, at 25% less than the clearance dose.[14]

In contrast, the new 2019 AAD consensus guidelines recommend maintenance therapy at the clearance dose; individual published protocols have increased the dosage by 10% to 15% after the first month of maintenance therapy, as tolerated by the patient and below the maximum acceptable dose, before plateauing and tapering dosage.[2] In the authors' practice, they often lower the dose for maintenance therapy when possible and limit exposure of body parts that likely will not need long-term control.

Phototherapy may induce longer-term remission owing to UV-induced apoptosis of intraepidermal T cells involved in psoriatic pathogenesis.[7] Accordingly, for the patient's first course of phototherapy treatment, the authors strongly recommend a trial off treatment at the end of maintenance taper, before considering a long-term maintenance regimen. A study of 50 patients showed that the group that followed a maintenance protocol of twice weekly NBUVB therapy for 4 weeks and then once weekly therapy for 4 weeks had a remission rate of 55% at 1 year, compared with 33% of patients not receiving maintenance therapy.[7,38] However, another study of 52 patients treated on a 5 times weekly protocol plus topical vitamin D for 1 month found that without maintenance therapy, 27 (56%) were still in remission at 12 months after the end of treatment.[39] The overall cited remission rate for NBUVB according to 2010 AAD guidelines is 38% at 1 year.[7] Previous studies have shown maintenance therapy significantly improves rates of remission.[40]

Although seemingly effective, maintenance protocols are often dependent on the phototherapy center as well as patient preference and availability to return for treatment. Balancing the benefits of disease control with the risks of increased cumulative exposure to UVB should be considered on an individual basis.

Other studies have tried to identify parameters that positively or negatively influence the duration of remission. An analysis of 63 patients who showed marked improvement with NBUVB phototherapy found that age greater than 60, a history of systemic therapy within the last 6 months, and 3 or more total phototherapy cycles were associated with shorter remission periods.[41] Another small study of 17 patients treated with NBUVB found that C-reactive protein levels and PASI score correlated with length of remission.[42] Clinicians should be aware of the possibility of shorter remission periods in these patients and perhaps more strongly consider prolonged maintenance therapy where appropriate.

COMBINATION THERAPY

Newer studies indicate increased efficacy of NBUVB phototherapy when used in combination with other treatments for moderate to severe recalcitrant psoriasis. For example, several studies have shown efficacy and faster time to clearance when etanercept is used in combination with NBUVB[43]; 1 study that used combination therapy in patients who had previously not responded to either phototherapy or etanercept alone cited that all 8 patients achieved a PASI score of 75 and 3 patients had complete remission after 14.6 ± 3.3 NBUVB exposures.[44] A limited number of studies have evaluated monoclonal antibodies adalimumab and ustekinumab; 2 studies found that phototherapy enhances the effect of the monoclonal antibodies in treatment response and time to therapeutic response. Most studies of combination therapy have been well tolerated with no additional adverse effects. More recently, apremilast has been tested in combination with NBUVB for moderate to severe plaque psoriasis; a study that gave patients 30 mg apremilast twice daily along with NBUVB 3 times per week showed 73% (16/22) achieve a PASI 75 response at week 12 without more adverse effects than NBUVB alone.[45]

Combining methotrexate (15 mg/wk, starting 3 weeks before phototherapy treatment) with NBUVB was compared with NBUVB alone in 19 psoriasis patients with skin types III to IV; median time to clearance was 4 weeks in the combination group, significantly shorter than the NBUVB group of which the majority had not cleared at the end of the 24-week study period. The median difference in score reduction between the treatment groups was 5.6 (1.1, 9.7; $P = .013$).[46] Another study of 30 patients compared a treatment group of sequential cyclosporin A (3 mg/kg/d for 4 weeks) followed by NBUVB to NBUVB alone; sequential therapy provided improvement to UV-shielded areas and itch relief, but no significant difference in clearance was found at 9 months of follow-up.[47] In contrast, concomitant use of topical corticosteroids and NBUVB has been reported to have mixed effects in the literature; some trials demonstrated increased rate of clearance, whereas others showed no benefit and even suggested an increase in relapse rate.[7] Topical tazarotene 0.05% added to NBUVB in 10 patients on half of their body resulted in a statistically significant mean PASI reduction of 64% compared with

48% of NBUVB alone.[48] Efficacy of retinoid combined with NBUVB remains unclear, with 1 study demonstrating a 93% success rate with two-thirds of the total irradiation dose, but a high relapse rate of 66% at 6 months.[49]

SPECIAL CONSIDERATIONS FOR HOME PHOTOTHERAPY

In-office phototherapy for psoriasis, which almost always involves treatment multiple times per week, can be burdensome for patients.[50] For certain patients, such as those who live far away from a phototherapy clinic, home phototherapy has emerged as a viable treatment option. NBUVB is particularly well suited for home phototherapy because of its excellent safety profile.[50] Home therapy has been shown to have comparable efficacy to office-based therapy in a randomized controlled trial.[12] Nevertheless, special considerations should be taken into account for home phototherapy patients.

To initiate therapy, patients need a home phototherapy device; there are multiple brands that range in cost and features. Most brands allow for various types of regulation by clinicians to limit misuse and increase the likelihood of patient follow-up.[51] Devices require a prescription and can take up to 2 to 3 weeks to authorize by insurance. Coverage is highly dependent on the patient's insurance. Good documentation of the patient's psoriasis, with objective measures and photographs, can assist in obtaining insurance coverage.[52]

Patients who are candidates for home phototherapy will ideally have already shown good response to in-office treatment. Previous treatment in the dermatology office increases familiarity and subsequent compliance with regular therapy.[51] The most common method for determining starting dose for home phototherapy is based on skin type[52]; MED assessment done in the office before home treatment is also appropriate. The calculations involved in percentage-based dose increases may be difficult for some patients. For these patients, a conservative fixed-time increase may have less potential for error, although with the understanding that the rate of increase will be slower, and therefore, time to clearance will be prolonged. Home phototherapy patients should also receive missed dose and burn protocols, which can be very similar to in-office protocols, although with modified language to ensure patient comprehension.[50] Open communication with the clinician and treatment team is encouraged and vital for patient safety and success.

The authors recommend that the consent process be the same for in-office and home phototherapy patients. The most common adverse effects found in home phototherapy patients are also blistering, erythema, and burning.[12] Clinicians should emphasize to home phototherapy patients the importance of wearing safety goggles and a genital shield and educate them on the dangers of letting others use their phototherapy unit, including safety around small children.[52] Guidelines concerning aforementioned maximum dosages are the same regardless of whether therapy is received at home or in the office. Routine follow-up in clinic is recommended, if possible, once every several months, to assess for therapeutic progress, adverse effects, and any medical changes.[51,52]

SUMMARY

Psoriasis is a significant condition with both skin and systemic manifestations that has great impact on the quality of life of patients. Phototherapy is an effective treatment of psoriasis, and over the last decades, the standard of care in the United States has shifted from PUVA to NBUVB for long-term treatment of psoriasis based on its favorable safety profile, convenience, and cost-effectiveness, with strong evidence favoring its use in the most recent AAD guidelines.[14]

Ultimately, the successful treatment of psoriasis patients with NBUVB requires well-trained staff that sees patients with consistency and is thus able to adapt and tailor treatments based on individual response and tolerability. Although the literature has afforded general consensus concerning the recommended frequency of therapy at 3 times weekly, there are wide variations in published protocols concerning initiation, escalation, and maintenance dosing for NBUVB treatment of psoriasis patients. Recent AAD guidelines, as outlined above, provide a practical standard for the initiation and maintenance of NBUVB phototherapy for psoriasis patients that can be further optimized by experienced clinicians based on individual patient presentations and needs.

REFERENCES

1. Rachakonda TD, Schupp CW, Armstrong AW. Psoriasis prevalence among adults in the United States. J Am Acad Dermatol 2014;70(3):512–6.
2. Mehta D, Lim HW. Ultraviolet B phototherapy for psoriasis: review of practical guidelines. Am J Clin Dermatol 2016;17(2):125–33.
3. Zill JM, Christalle E, Tillenburg N, et al. Effects of psychosocial interventions on patient-reported

outcomes in patients with psoriasis: a systematic review and meta-analysis. Br J Dermatol 2018. [Epub ahead of print].

4. Matos TR, Ling TC, Sheth V. Ultraviolet B radiation therapy for psoriasis: pursuing the optimal regime. Clin Dermatol 2016;34(5):587–93.

5. Chen X, Yang M, Cheng Y, et al. Narrow-band ultraviolet B phototherapy versus broad-band ultraviolet B or psoralen-ultraviolet a photochemotherapy for psoriasis. Cochrane Database Syst Rev 2013;(10): Cd009481.

6. Wan J, Abuabara K, Troxel AB, et al. Dermatologist preferences for first-line therapy of moderate to severe psoriasis in healthy adult patients. J Am Acad Dermatol 2012;66(3):376–86.

7. Menter A, Korman NJ, Elmets CA, et al. Guidelines of care for the management of psoriasis and psoriatic arthritis: section 5. Guidelines of care for the treatment of psoriasis with phototherapy and photochemotherapy. J Am Acad Dermatol 2010;62(1):114–35.

8. Pathirana D, Ormerod AD, Saiag P, et al. European S3-guidelines on the systemic treatment of psoriasis vulgaris. J Eur Acad Dermatol Venereol 2009; 23(Suppl 2):1–70.

9. Archier E, Devaux S, Castela E, et al. Efficacy of psoralen UVa therapy vs. narrowband UVB therapy in chronic plaque psoriasis: a systematic literature review. J Eur Acad Dermatol Venereol 2012; 26(Suppl 3):11–21.

10. Archier E, Devaux S, Castela E, et al. Carcinogenic risks of psoralen UVA therapy and narrowband UVB therapy in chronic plaque psoriasis: a systematic literature review. J Eur Acad Dermatol Venereol 2012;26(Suppl 3):22–31.

11. Lapolla W, Yentzer BA, Bagel J, et al. A review of phototherapy protocols for psoriasis treatment. J Am Acad Dermatol 2011;64(5):936–49.

12. Koek MB, Buskens E, Van Weelden H, et al. Home versus outpatient ultraviolet B phototherapy for mild to severe psoriasis: pragmatic multicentre randomised controlled non-inferiority trial (Pluto Study). BMJ 2009;338:b1542.

13. Almutawa F, Alnomair N, Wang Y, et al. Systematic review of UV-based therapy for psoriasis. Am J Clin Dermatol 2013;14(2):87–109.

14. Elmets CA, Lim HW, Stoff B, et al. Joint American Academy of Dermatology-National Psoriasis Foundation guidelines of care for the management and treatment of psoriasis with phototherapy. J Am Acad Dermatol 2019;81(3):775–804.

15. Stern RS. Genital tumors among men with psoriasis exposed to psoralens and ultraviolet A radiation (PUVA) and ultraviolet B radiation. The photochemotherapy follow-up study. N Engl J Med 1990;322(16): 1093–7.

16. Abdallah MA, El-Khateeb EA, Abdel-Rahman SH. The influence of psoriatic plaques pretreatment with crude coal tar vs. petrolatum on the efficacy of narrow-band ultraviolet B: a half-vs.-half intra-individual double-blinded comparative study. Photodermatol Photoimmunol Photomed 2011;27(5):226–30.

17. Zhang M, Goyert G, Lim HW. Folate and phototherapy: what should we inform our patients? J Am Acad Dermatol 2017;77(5):958–64.

18. Kwon IH, Kwon HH, Na SJ, et al. Could colorimetric method replace the individual minimal erythemal dose (Med) measurements in determining the initial dose of narrow-band UVB treatment for psoriasis patients with skin phototype III-V? J Eur Acad Dermatol Venereol 2013;27(4):494–8.

19. Parlak N, Kundakci N, Parlak A, et al. Narrowband ultraviolet B phototherapy starting and incremental dose in patients with psoriasis: comparison of percentage dose and fixed dose protocols. Photodermatol Photoimmunol Photomed 2015;31(2):90–7.

20. Youn JI, Park JY, Jo SJ, et al. Assessment of the usefulness of skin phototype and skin color as the parameter of cutaneous narrow band UVB sensitivity in psoriasis patients. Photodermatol Photoimmunol Photomed 2003;19(5):261–4.

21. Youn JI, Oh JK, Kim BK, et al. Relationship between skin phototype and med in Korean, brown skin. Photodermatol Photoimmunol Photomed 1997;13(5–6): 208–11.

22. Baron ED, Stern RS, Taylor CR. Correlating skin type and minimum erythema dose. Arch Dermatol 1999; 135(10):1278–9.

23. Haddican MM, Bhutani T, Mcclelland PB, et al. Why are there significant differences in published narrowband ultraviolet B dosimetry recommendations? The need for national standardization of phototherapy treatment. J Am Acad Dermatol 2011;65(2):411–4.

24. Do AN, Koo JY. Initiating narrow-band UVB for the treatment of psoriasis. Journal article in: Psoriasis Forum 2004;10(1):7–11.

25. Zanolli MD, Feldman SR. Phototherapy treatment protocols for psoriasis and other phototherapy-responsive dermatoses. Boca Raton (FL): CRC Press; 2004.

26. Morison WL. Phototherapy and photochemotherapy for skin disease. Boca Raton (FL): CRC Press; 2005.

27. Dawe RS, Cameron HM, Yule S, et al. A randomized comparison of methods of selecting narrowband UVB starting dose to treat chronic psoriasis. Arch Dermatol 2011;147(2):168–74.

28. Altiner DD, Ilknur T, Fetil E, et al. Comparison of weekly and daily incremental protocols of narrowband ultraviolet B phototherapy for psoriasis. J Eur Acad Dermatol Venereol 2006;20(9):1076–80.

29. Hallaji Z, Barzegari M, Balighi K, et al. A comparison of three times vs. five times weekly narrowband ultraviolet B phototherapy for the treatment of chronic plaque psoriasis. Photodermatol Photoimmunol Photomed 2010;26(1):10–5.

30. Cameron H, Dawe RS, Yule S, et al. A randomized, observer-blinded trial of twice vs. three times weekly narrowband ultraviolet B phototherapy for chronic plaque psoriasis. Br J Dermatol 2002;147(5):973–8.

31. Dawe RS, Wainwright NJ, Cameron H, et al. Narrowband (Tl-01) ultraviolet B phototherapy for chronic plaque psoriasis: three times or five times weekly treatment? Br J Dermatol 1998;138(5):833–9.

32. Leenutaphong V, Nimkulrat P, Sudtim S. Comparison of phototherapy two times and four times a week with low doses of narrow-band Ultraviolet B in Asian patients with psoriasis. Photodermatol Photoimmunol Photomed 2000;16(5):202–6.

33. Ibbotson SH, Bilsland D, Cox NH, et al. An update and guidance on narrowband ultraviolet B phototherapy: a British Photodermatology Group Workshop report. Br J Dermatol 2004;151(2):283–97.

34. Amatore F, Villani AP, Tauber M, et al. French guidelines on the use of systemic treatments for moderate-to-severe psoriasis in adults. J Eur Acad Dermatol Venereol 2019;33(3):464–83.

35. Hearn RM, Kerr AC, Rahim KF, et al. Incidence of skin cancers in 3867 patients treated with narrowband ultraviolet B phototherapy. Br J Dermatol 2008;159(4):931–5.

36. Lin TL, Wu CY, Chang YT, et al. Risk of skin cancer in psoriasis patients receiving long-term narrowband ultraviolet phototherapy: results from a Taiwanese population-based cohort study. Photodermatol Photoimmunol Photomed 2019;35(3):164–71.

37. Diffey BL, Farr PM. The challenge of follow-up in narrowband ultraviolet B phototherapy. Br J Dermatol 2007;157(2):344–9.

38. Boztepe G, Karaduman A, Sahin S, et al. The effect of maintenance narrow-band ultraviolet B therapy on the duration of remission for psoriasis: a prospective randomized clinical trial. Int J Dermatol 2006;45(3):245–50.

39. Karakawa M, Komine M, Takekoshi T, et al. Duration of remission period of narrowband ultraviolet B therapy on psoriasis vulgaris. J Dermatol 2011;38(7):655–60.

40. Stern RS, Armstrong RB, Anderson TF, et al. Effect of continued ultraviolet B phototherapy on the duration of remission of psoriasis: a randomized study. J Am Acad Dermatol 1986;15(3):546–52.

41. Ryu HH, Choe YS, Jo S, et al. Remission period in psoriasis after multiple cycles of narrowband ultraviolet B phototherapy. J Dermatol 2014;41(7):622–7.

42. Coimbra S, Oliveira H, Belo L, et al. Principal determinants of the length of remission of psoriasis vulgaris after topical, Nb-UVB, and PUVA therapy: a follow-up study. Am J Clin Dermatol 2013;14(1):49–53.

43. Nakamura M, Farahnik B, Bhutani T. Recent advances in phototherapy for psoriasis. F1000Res 2016;5 [pii:F1000].

44. Calzavara-Pinton PG, Sala R, Arisi M, et al. Synergism between narrowband ultraviolet B phototherapy and etanercept for the treatment of plaque-type psoriasis. Br J Dermatol 2013;169(1):130–6.

45. Bagel J, Nelson E, Keegan BR. Apremilast and narrowband ultraviolet-B combination therapy for treating moderate-to-severe plaque psoriasis. J Drugs Dermatol 2017;16(10):957–62.

46. Asawanonda P, Nateetongrungsak Y. Methotrexate plus narrowband UVB phototherapy versus narrowband UVB phototherapy alone in the treatment of plaque-type psoriasis: a randomized, placebo-controlled study. J Am Acad Dermatol 2006;54(6):1013–8.

47. Calzavara-Pinton P, Leone G, Venturini M, et al. A comparative non randomized study of narrowband (NB) (312 +/- 2 nm) UVB phototherapy versus sequential therapy with oral administration of low-dose Cyclosporin A and Nb-UVB phototherapy in patients with severe psoriasis vulgaris. Eur J Dermatol 2005;15(6):470–3.

48. Behrens S, Grundmann-Kollmann M, Schiener R, et al. Combination phototherapy of psoriasis with narrow-band UVB irradiation and topical tazarotene gel. J Am Acad Dermatol 2000;42(3):493–5.

49. Green C, Lakshmipathi T, Johnson B, et al. A comparison of the efficacy and relapse rates of narrowband UVB (Tl-01) vs. etretinate-PUVA (Re-PUVA) in the treatment of psoriasis patients. Br J Dermatol 1992;127(1):5–9.

50. Hum M, Kalia S, Gniadecki R. Prescribing home narrowband UVB phototherapy: a review of current approaches. J Cutan Med Surg 2019;23(1):91–6.

51. Bhutani T, Liao W. A practical approach to home UVB phototherapy for the treatment of generalized psoriasis. Dermatol Pract 2010;7(2):31–5.

52. Anderson KL, Feldman SR. A guide to prescribing home phototherapy for patients with psoriasis: the appropriate patient, the type of unit, the treatment regimen, and the potential obstacles. J Am Acad Dermatol 2015;72(5):868–78.e1.

The Science and (Lost) Art of Psoralen Plus UVA Phototherapy

Elisabeth G. Richard, MD

KEYWORDS

• PUVA • Psoralen • Photochemotherapy • Psoriasis • Dermatitis • Vitiligo

KEY POINTS

- PUVA phototherapy is the therapeutic use of Psoralen medication and ultraviolet A (UVA) radiation to treat inflammatory skin diseases.
- Psoriasis is the prototype disease treated with PUVA, however numerous other inflammatory dermatoses also respond to PUVA.
- There are risks associated with PUVA, thus the risk-benefit ratio must be considered when making therapeutic choices.
- PUVA remains a valuable tool in dermatology today.

INTRODUCTION

PUVA phototherapy refers to the therapeutic use of *p*soralen medication plus *u*ltraviolet *A* radiation (UVA) (320–400 nm). Introduced in the 1970s and classically used to treat psoriasis, PUVA is effective in 90% of patients. It also may be used in the treatment of more than 30 other skin diseases, primarily inflammatory in nature. Psoralens are a group of phototoxic compounds that, after absorbing photons of light, produce photochemical reactions that alter cellular function[1-3] The inflammatory cells of these dermatoses are sensitive to photons and also the photochemical reactions of PUVA.

At present, innumerable therapeutic options exist for psoriasis, including biologic therapy. This begs the question, is PUVA still valid and important? The answer is yes. Although PUVA may no longer be first line for psoriasis, it still plays a role as an invaluable therapeutic tool for psoriasis and inflammatory dermatoses. Read on for the practical and scientific aspects of PUVA, a lesser used, but not to be forgotten art in dermatology.

CLINICAL USE OF PSORALEN PLUS UVA

The most common indication for PUVA therapy is disabling psoriasis, typically moderate to severe, that is unresponsive to topical therapy.

As PUVA is often a long-term treatment, careful evaluation of the patient is critical. Key elements of the patient history include age, Fitzpatrick skin type, past medical history, including history of skin cancers, immunosuppression, and the patient's current medications.[4]

For psoriasis, the therapeutic ladder is a stepwise progression from topical therapy for mild disease, to phototherapy, which includes both PUVA and ultraviolet B (UVB) therapy for moderate to severe disease, to systemic agents for moderate and severe disease. Systemic agents include oral treatment with methotrexate, retinoids, aprelimast, and cyclosporine, as well as the biologic agents. Efficacy increases stepwise, yet so does the risk associated with these therapeutic choices.

Phototherapy is not effective for the treatment of psoriatic arthritis. For patients with psoriatic arthritis, systemic agents treat both skin and joint

---

Financial Disclosures: Up To Date, author "Psoralen plus ultraviolet A (PUVA) photochemotherapy" for which the author receive an honorarium.

Johns Hopkins University School of Medicine, Johns Hopkins at Green Spring Station, 10753 Falls Road, Suite 355, Lutherville, MD 21093, USA

E-mail address: ericha16@jhmi.edu

Dermatol Clin 38 (2020) 11–23
https://doi.org/10.1016/j.det.2019.08.002

derm.theclinics.com

disease. In some patients, however, the dose of these agents required to control arthritis symptoms does not provide sufficient control of skin disease, and phototherapy can be used as an adjunct treatment.[5,6]

Psoralen Plus UVA Versus UVB

When considering light-based therapy, 4 main differences between UVB and PUVA should be included in the decision-making process, which are discussed in detail in this article:

1. PUVA is more effective than UVB phototherapy in clearing psoriasis in most patients.
2. PUVA is a much more effective maintenance treatment than UVB phototherapy.
3. UVA wavelengths penetrate more deeply into skin than UVB wavelengths.
4. PUVA has a greater risk of long-term adverse events compared with UVB.

Of note, with the advent of narrowband UVB phototherapy (NBUVB) in the 1980s, treatment with NBUVB (311–313 nm) is presently preferred over broad-band UVB phototherapy (BB-UVB) (290–320 nm).[7–10] Regarding UVB phototherapy in the previous comparison with PUVA, the same conclusions may be applied to both forms of UVB phototherapy, NBUVB and BB-UVB, hence the general use of the term UVB phototherapy.

Factors that favor the use of PUVA phototherapy include Fitzpatrick skin types III-VI, as there is a lower inherent risk of skin cancer in these patients, age older than 50 years, long history of psoriasis, extensive disease with thick and/or inflamed plaques, no arthritis or arthritis controlled at doses of disease-modifying antirheumatic drugs not clearing psoriasis, incomplete response to UVB phototherapy and/or sunlight, palm and/or sole disease, and erythrodermic or pustular psoriasis.

Factors that favor the use of UVB phototherapy include Fitzpatrick skin types I-II with inherently higher risk of skin cancer, age younger than 50 years, psoriasis of recent onset, thin psoriasis plaques (macular), history of rapid clearance with sunlight, pregnancy, young age, and high risk for noncompliance with patient protective measures required by PUVA.[2,11]

In plaque psoriasis, NBUVB is almost as effective as PUVA. However, direct comparison of PUVA with NBUVB in a double-blind, randomized, single-center study with 93 patients demonstrated that PUVA achieves clearance in more patients and fewer treatment sessions than NBUVB. PUVA also results in longer remission times than NBUVB and maintenance therapy is more viable

option with PUVA then NBUVB. Using a tapering schedule of PUVA, it is possible to extend the time interval between maintenance treatments to as far apart as 4 weeks in many patients. Last, BB-UVB is much less effective than PUVA therapy for plaque psoriasis[2,12–15]

Special Sites Requiring Psoralen Plus UVA

When psoriasis involves the palms and soles, significant morbidity occurs. Pain, discomfort, and interference with activities of daily living accompany palm and sole disease. There are 3 main variants of psoriasis at these sites: (1) pustular psoriasis, (2) hyperkeratotic psoriasis, and (3) psoriasis vulgaris (classic plaques extending onto palms and soles).

The thickened epidermis on the palms and soles decreases transmission of UVB wavelengths. The longer wavelength of UVA light is better able to penetrate the thick stratum corneum and reach the dermis where it can induce its therapeutic effect. For this reason, PUVA may be required to clear most palm and sole disease.[16–19]

Dermatoses Other than Psoriasis Treatable with Psoralen Plus UVA

Based on the scientific understanding of PUVA's mechanism of action, namely its immunosuppressive and antiproliferative effects, PUVA is used to treat many inflammatory dermatoses. Currently, PUVA is approved by the Food and Drug Administration (FDA) for the treatment of psoriasis and vitiligo. Other common uses of PUVA include mycosis fungoides, eczematous dermatitis such as atopic dermatitis, and chronic graft versus host disease.

PSORALENS

Psoralens are naturally occurring compounds occurring in plants, where they function as natural insecticides. They are phototoxic compounds that belong to the furocoumarin group of compounds. When humans come in contact with psoralen-containing plants (eg, limes, figs, parsnips) followed by exposure to sunlight, a phytophotodermatitis can occur manifesting as an acute phototoxic reaction with erythema, blistering, and pigmentation. The medicinal properties of psoralens have been known for centuries, and their use in treating vitiligo was recorded as long ago as 1550 BC.[20]

Four psoralens are used in PUVA therapy; however, only one, methoxsalen or 8-methoxypsoralen, is approved for use in the United States (**Table 1**). Methoxsalen is marketed in the

Table 1
Methoxsalen (also known as 8-methoxypsoralen or 8-MOP)

Drug	Brand vs Generic	Trade Name	Manufacturer	Preparation
Methoxsalen	Brand	Oxsoralen Ultra	Valeant	10-mg soft gelatin capsules (green)
	Generic	Not applicable	Oceanside, a division of Valeant	10-mg soft gelatin capsules (green)
	Generic	Not applicable	Strides	10-mg soft gelatin capsules (green)
	Brand[a]	8-MOP	Valeant	10-mg hard gelatin caps (pink)

[a] Older formulation with lower bioavailability and longer time to onset.

United States as 10-mg soft gelatin capsules under the name Oxsoralen Ultra by Bausch Health Pharmaceuticals (US headquarters in Bridgewater, NJ). Generic methoxsalen soft gelatin capsules are also available, produced by several generic drug manufacturers[21-24] (see **Table 1**).

Mechanism of Action

Psoralens rapidly penetrate into the cell and intercalate between DNA base pairs and, on exposure to UVA radiation, cause a linkage of the psoralen to pyrimidine bases forming C_4 cycloadducts. As a result of these cycloadducts, DNA synthesis and epidermal proliferation are inhibited. Inhibition of epidermal growth factor binding occurs with PUVA therapy and acts to downregulate the hyperproliferative state that is the hallmark of psoriasis. Additional therapeutic effects of PUVA include mitochondrial dysfunction, creation of reactive oxygen species, toxicity to Langerhans cells, and apoptosis of both keratinocytes and lymphocytes.[11,25-28]

PHOTOBIOLOGY OF PSORALEN PLUS UVA

In vivo, the action spectrum for activating psoralens peaks in the UVA-2 spectrum, 320 to 340 nm. Psoralen activation occurs as well by radiation from the UVB spectrum. Ground state psoralen molecules are activated to a singlet state by absorption of photons. The singlet state undergoes decay to the triplet state, which is a long-lived state and is responsible for most of the photochemical effects. Type I (direct) photochemical reactions result in cross-linking of adjacent strands of DNA and formation of cycloadducts via the photoaddition of the psoralen to pyrimidine bases. Type II (indirect) photochemical reactions produce the reactive oxygen species that damage cell membranes and cytoplasmic elements.[2,29,30]

The most common source of UVA radiation is fluorescent light bulbs having a maximum emission at 352 nm, as well as some emission in the UVB and visible light ends of the spectrum. Current understanding is that psoralen activation peaks between 320 and 330 nm; however, early psoralen research indicated maximum psoralen activation to be in the 340 to 380 nm range.[31] Treatment protocols were developed based on the initial research using PUVA bulbs with maximum emission at 352 nm. With current understanding, it is apparent that the 352-nm bulbs are not optimal for activating psoralens; however, treatment protocols with these bulbs are well established. Changing the emission spectrum of PUVA bulbs would require new parameters and protocols to be written.

Although sunlight is a convenient source of UVA radiation, it is not a safe source of UVA, as the therapeutic dose is close to the phototoxic dose, hence severe erythema can occur.[32] Likewise the use of tanning beds, which have a peak emission spectrum between 320 and 340 nm, will unpredictably activate psoralens and carry a tremendous risk of severe erythema.

Overview of Ultraviolet Radiation

Electromagnetic radiation is a form of energy derived from the sun or produced artificially (**Fig. 1**). Biological responses observed in photomedicine are the result of absorption of the energy from the UV and visible portion of the electromagnetic spectrum by cells. Energy of photons is inversely proportional to wavelength, thus as wavelength increases, the energy of the photon decreases. UV radiation (UVR) comprises only 5% of the solar radiation on the earth's surface and cumulative exposure to UVR leads to photoaging.

UVA radiation (320–400 nm) has the longest UV waves, and represents the greatest fraction of

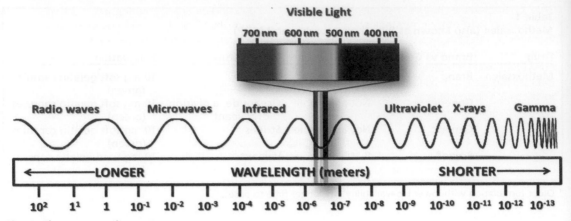

Fig. 1. Electromagnetic spectrum.

solar UVR present on the earth's surface. The UVA waveband is subdivided into UVA-2 (320–340 nm) and UVA-1 (340–400 nm). UVA-1 induces mainly oxygen-dependent photochemistry, whereas UVA-2 induces UVB-type photochemistry with direct absorption by DNA molecules. UVA is not blocked by glass, and the intensity varies little with season or time of day. Although of lower energy than UVB, it is the longer wavelength of UVA that penetrates deeper into the skin to reach deeper dermal layers and structures.

UVB radiation (290–320 nm) has the most biologically active wavelengths of UVR in sunlight. Clinically, sun-induced erythema (or "sunburn") is primarily the result of UVB waves. UVB primarily affects the epidermis and is absorbed by cellular DNA. Despite DNA repair mechanisms, the UVB-induced DNA damage is incompletely repaired, ultimately leading to apoptosis, mediated mostly by tumor suppressor protein p53. UV-induced mutations that inactivate p53 are found in most nonmelanoma skin cancers.

UVC radiation (200–290 nm) is filtered out by ozone and water vapor in the atmosphere and does not reach the surface of the earth. UVC is of high energy, the effect of which provides for the germicidal properties of UVC. UVC (artificially produced) is used for sterilization, but otherwise does not have applications in photomedicine.[2,33–35]

Nontherapeutic Cutaneous Responses to Psoralen Plus UVA

In addition to the therapeutic effects of PUVA on psoriasis and other dermatoses, the skin can respond to PUVA phototherapy in additional ways: erythema, pruritus, and pigment production. The occurrence of these responses is influenced greatly by several factors, including dose of psoralen, dose of UVA radiation, prior exposure to UV radiation, individual susceptibility (eg, Fitzpatrick skin type), and body site.

Erythema induced by PUVA usually appears 36 to 48 hours after exposure to UVA radiation; however, can be as late as 72 hours after treatment. PUVA erythema appears later and lasts longer than sunlight-induced erythema (ie, a sunburn). When erythema develops, the peak is also delayed, often not reached until 96 to 120 hours after UVA exposure. At the extreme, this erythema can persist for up to 2 to 3 weeks. Erythema is the most common phototoxic reaction and occurs in 10% of patients.

When PUVA-induced erythema occurs, pruritus is a characteristic feature, which can be described as a deep, burning itch akin to insects crawling on or under the skin. Direct phototoxic injury of cutaneous nerves is the proposed cause of this adverse effect. PUVA-induced pruritus also can occur in the absence of erythema, and generally begins on the outer arms, thighs, and buttocks, and in women, on the breasts. Treatment of this pruritus is primarily with supportive measures. Gabapentin has been reported to be beneficial as well.[36]

Functional melanocytes respond to PUVA by producing pigment. This pigmentation is darker and longer-lasting than that produced by sunlight. It is important to keep in mind that if pigmentation induced by the PUVA treatments becomes too great, the efficacy of PUVA in clearing psoriasis can decrease.[36–40]

PSORALEN PHARMACOLOGY

With psoralens, the drug itself has no therapeutic effect unless there is exposure to UV radiation and consequent absorption of photons by the psoralen to activate and excite the molecule.

This characteristic makes psoralens unique in comparison with other oral medications in which therapeutic effect is not UV dependent. Furthermore, the pharmacologic goal is to produce a consistent and high level of psoralen delivered to the target organ, the skin, at the time of exposure to UV radiation to achieve therapeutic effect.

As psoralens are lipophilic and poorly soluble in water, the absorption from the gastrointestinal tract is limited. Dissolved formulation of the drug helps to overcome the absorption problem, as compared with the crystalline form. Soft gelatin capsules containing dissolved methoxsalen (Oxsoralen Ultra) are more completely and rapidly absorbed.

Psoralens are best taken on an empty stomach, as food, especially foods high in fat, delay absorption and reduce peak blood levels. There is tremendous variation among individuals regarding both the amount of drug absorbed as well as the rate of absorption. Consequently, peak blood levels vary widely among patients, and it is thus critical to administer the UVA treatment at a consistent time after ingestion of the psoralen. When high blood levels of psoralen drug occur, nausea can develop as a result of central mechanisms triggered by high serum levels. This can be alleviated by taking methoxsalen with a small amount of food with a high fat content to slow down the rate of absorption. If nausea persists, the dose of methoxsalen can be reduced by 10 mg.[24,41–43]

Psoralen binding to protein, serum albumin, is relatively high. Oral administration yields 75% to 80% of methoxsalen, which is reversibly bound to protein. Distribution of psoralen is to all organs, but without exposure to UVA radiation, binding is short lived and excretion is rapid. Methoxsalen is metabolized in the liver rapidly and completely with only a small amount of parent compound detectable in urine and bile. The metabolites do not accumulate nor are they biologically active. Drugs that induce cytochrome P-450 enzymes accelerate the metabolism of methoxsalen and theoretically decrease the biologic effect of PUVA.[43–46]

Drug Interactions

Phototoxic drugs, such as tetracyclines, fluoroquinolones, phenothiazines, sulfonamides, and voriconazole, may augment the action of PUVA and increase the risk of acute phototoxic erythema.[47]

Pregnancy

Methoxsalen is pregnancy category C, and, consequently, PUVA phototherapy is contraindicated in pregnancy. Likewise, PUVA during lactation is contraindicated, as psoralens are likely excreted in breast milk.

PSORALEN PLUS UVA TREATMENT PROTOCOL

Methoxsalen capsules are taken orally at a dose of 0.4 to 0.6 mg/kg actual body weight, 1 to 2 hours before exposure to UVA radiation. As the soft gelatin capsule formulation of methoxsalen has better and more predictable absorption, a dose of 0.4 mg/kg is recommended in practice. Adverse reactions are reduced (less nausea) and cost savings over time can be realized with a lower dose of the methoxsalen required for each treatment. If nausea develops associated with drug administration, it is the result of high blood level of the drug, thus taking the drug with a small amount of food with high fat content (eg, cheese) alleviates this problem. UVA radiation is delivered 1 hour after medication administration.

Psoralen Plus UVA Schedule for Disease Clearance

The dose of UVA radiation is determined by Fitzpatrick skin type (**Table 2**). Treatments are delivered twice or 3 times weekly, at least 48 hours apart. If no erythema is noted, the dose of UVA is increased each treatment until satisfactory control of the disease has been obtained, then dose is held. If faint erythema is present, the dose of radiation is held constant. If skin tenderness and/or definite erythema is present, treatment is stopped until erythema has faded, then treatments are resumed at a lower dose than the last treatment. If localized erythema develops, such as on the breast or buttocks, clothing or sunscreens may be used as shielding, and treatment may be continued. Improvement is noted initially between treatments 8 through 10, and the average number of

Table 2
Psoralen plus UVA treatment schedule

Fitzpatrick Skin Type	UVA Radiation in J/cm²		
	Initial	Increments	Max UVA Dose
I	1.5	0.5	5
II	2.5	0.5	8
III	3.5	0.5	12
IV	4.5	0.5–1.0	14
V	5.5	1.0	16

Data from Morison WL. Phototherapy and photochemotherapy for skin disease. Vol 34. Baton Rouge: CRC Press; 2005. http://www.crcnetbase.com/isbn/9780849360183.

treatments to "clear" psoriasis (or other inflamma-tory skin diseases) is 25 to 30.[2,48–50]

For patients who have extensive disease on the arms and legs, these areas are generally slower to clear than the trunk. Additional exposure to UVA radiation to the extremities is given after the whole-body dose. After the whole-body dose, the patient puts on a gown (tied in the back) or shorts and t-shirt, and covers the head with a pillowcase. For patients with type I or II skin, an additional 1 J/cm^2 is given to the limbs and increased by 0.5 J/cm^2 each treatment. Patients with type III or higher skin type, are started with an additional 2 to 4 J/cm^2 to the limbs and increased by 1 J/cm^2 each treatment. These additional treatments can be discontinued once disease has been controlled and clearance obtained.

It is important for the patients to understand that compliance with treatment schedule is critical for success. PUVA delivered twice or 3 times weekly is considered a clearance schedule. In comparison, once-weekly PUVA will maintain the current disease burden, but will not clear a significant portion more.

Of note, in Europe, the starting dose of PUVA is frequently determined by an alternative approach. The minimum phototoxic dose (MPD) is determined, and then treatments are begun at 70% of the MPD.[51,52]

Although the obvious goal of PUVA is to clear psoriasis (or other skin disease), 2 key considerations regarding the treatment protocol must be recalled. There is a risk of PUVA erythema from being too aggressive and the symptoms (pruritus) of this erythema are unpleasant and may last for weeks. Furthermore, too much pigment may develop with PUVA treatment if too conservative a protocol is used (especially in skin types III to VI) and the pigmentation ultimately decreases the efficacy of the treatment.

Use of Psoralen Plus UVA as Maintenance Treatment

Once 90% of original disease is cleared, a patient may be transitioned to a maintenance schedule. In most studies, 90% of patients are clear by 30 treatments and transition to maintenance is appropriate for long-term disease management.[14,15,53]

As opposed to UVB, one of the main advantages of PUVA is that patients can be maintained in an improved state from baseline, relatively clear, using infrequent treatments once control is obtained. Furthermore, even if maintenance with PUVA is not used, the duration of remission after clearance with PUVA is longer than with UVB phototherapy.

For maintenance treatment, the final dose of UVA radiation is held constant and the frequency of treatments is gradually reduced. At first, treatment is weekly for 4 treatments, then every 2 weeks for 4 treatments, then every 3 weeks for 4 treatments, and then every 4 weeks for 4 treatments. The greatest interval between treatments without needing to decrease the dose of UVA radiation is 4 weeks.

Each patient's response to the maintenance phase is unique, and the interval between maintenance treatments that can be tolerated and still suppress disease is determined on a patient-by-patient basis. Once the interval between maintenance treatments (up to every 4 weeks) is ascertained for a given patient, treatment can typically continue at this interval to maintain the patient in his or her improved state of disease control.

During the maintenance phase, physician involvement is essential. The goal is to use the minimal number of treatments to control disease, thus minimizing long-term adverse effects. Office visits with the physician every 3 months, at a minimum, are of vital importance to assess the effectiveness of treatment and long-term sequelae of treatment. If the patient still has some level of active disease, albeit decreased 80% to 90% from baseline, on maintenance PUVA, then continued maintenance therapy is appropriate. When recurrence does develop, a rebound phenomenon is not seen as can occur with other therapeutic modalities.

Treatment of Disease Relapses

If a significant relapse of the disease occurs during the maintenance phase, stop the sequential reduction in frequency of PUVA treatments. If the disease recurs rapidly and in a widespread fashion, resume clearance schedule including resuming increases in UVA dose (as tolerated). Once disease is clear again, transition again into the maintenance phase of PUVA therapy. In contrast, if disease recurrence is insidious and/or minor, increasing the frequency of treatments, without an increase in UVA radiation, back to twice weekly until controlled, is the optimal course. Once the disease breakthrough is cleared, maintenance phase and sequential decrease in frequency of treatment can be resumed.

Topical Psoralen Plus UVA

Direct application of psoralen to the skin followed by exposure to UVA radiation can been used as treatment for several skin conditions, most commonly psoriasis and vitiligo.

Topical PUVA using methoxsalen lotion is an FDA-approved treatment for vitiligo. Methoxsalen lotion (10 mg/mL) is diluted 1:10 with ethanol to yield a 0.1% solution, which is then applied to affected skin 15 minutes before exposure to UVA radiation. Initial exposure is 0.5 J/cm^2 and increased in increments of 0.25 J/cm^2 until a light pink erythema is achieved in the vitiliginous skin. UVA dose is either held at this level or adjusted with the goal of maintaining a faint erythema in affected skin, as repigmentation occurs. Treatment is 2 or 3 times per week. Appropriate patients for topical PUVA have small areas of localized vitiligo. Unfortunately, a frequent complication of topical PUVA is an unexpected phototoxic reaction, usually bullous in nature. Phototoxicity occurring with topical PUVA is generally caused by inadvertent and unexpected exposure to natural sunlight after treatment.[54]

Bath PUVA uses a dilute solution of methoxsalen in which the affected area is soaked for 20 to 30 minutes followed by exposure to UVA radiation; 50 mg of methoxsalen is added to 100 L of bathwater for a 0.5 mg/L final concentration. Caution must be exercised by all parties (patient and provider) involved in bath PUVA treatment to avoid unintentional exposure of previously nonexposed skin to the topical psoralen. For whole-body exposure, a bathtub is used for soaking, whereas a basin is used for localized soaking, such as for the hands and/or feet. At present, bath PUVA is not FDA-approved.

Topical route of administration has the advantage of avoiding the systemic side effects, namely nausea, from oral administration of psoralens. Topical administration also has a shorter duration of photosensitivity, lasting approximately 2 hours after application of psoralen. Eye protection is still required, however, as serum levels are detectable after topical application of methoxsalen.[55]

The disadvantages of topical PUVA are generally considered greater than the advantages, hence its infrequent use as a treatment modality. Disadvantages include frequent and unpredictable bullous phototoxicity in addition the medicolegal implications of using a non–FDA-approved treatment (ie, bath PUVA).

OTHER PRACTICAL CONSIDERATIONS IN PSORALEN PLUS UVA THERAPY

Remembering the principles and mechanism of action of PUVA therapy is paramount in patient safety and patient education. Psoralens enter all cells of the body after oral administration of methoxsalen. UVA radiation is present in great amounts in sunlight, with little temporal or seasonal variation, and can activate psoralens until the drug is metabolized and excreted. Consequently, protective measures must be used for patient safety and to minimize adverse effects.

Protective Safety Measures

Once exposure occurs to methoxsalen, patients must use several safety measures to prevent inadvertent exposure to UVA light. The eyes must be protected with the use of wraparound UV-blocking glasses while exposed to sunlight (ie, in transit to and from treatment) from the time methoxsalen is ingested until sunset that same day. Likewise, skin should be protected from natural sunlight through appropriate clothing and avoidance.

The amount of UVA emitted by fluorescent lights is not adequate to activate psoralens, thus photoprotection is not required while in a home or office setting. Metabolism of methoxsalen is rapid and metabolites are not biologically active, thus by the following morning, no active psoralens remain.

While in the PUVA unit, small UV-blocking goggles are used to protect the eye. The face, if unaffected, is protected through the use of sunscreen and/or a pillowcase so as to prevent unnecessary exposure to UVA and prevent photodamage. Men are instructed to protect the genitals with the use of underwear or a jock strap.

On nontreatment days, sun avoidance is advised to minimize pigmentation from natural sunlight. This pigmentation may ultimately limit the effectiveness of PUVA therapy.

Combination with Systemic Treatments

For patients on systemic therapies, such as biologic therapy, lessening of response is a not infrequent occurrence. Often combination therapies are used, including combination with phototherapy to enhance efficacy and maintain therapeutic response.[56,57] Combination of systemic therapy and PUVA phototherapy has the advantage of increasing the success rate of both therapies, as well as potentially decreasing the overall exposure to UVA radiation. Common indications for combination therapy are erythrodermic psoriasis, generalized pustular psoriasis, thick asbestoslike plaques, and very active, recalcitrant, and/or inflammatory psoriasis.[58]

Oral retinoids (acitretin) in combination with PUVA, is more effective than monotherapy with either PUVA or acitretin alone.[59] Acitretin therapy is best initiated first and used for 2 weeks before initiating PUVA therapy. Both therapies are continued until the patient is clear, then acitretin is discontinued and PUVA used to maintain clearance. When retinoids are combined with PUVA phototherapy, there is an associated decreased incidence of cutaneous squamous cell carcinoma.[60] Retinoids are teratogens, hence contraindicated in women of childbearing potential.

Methotrexate also may be used in combination with PUVA phototherapy. Some studies suggest that the combination is more effective than either therapy alone; however, the safety of this combination has also been raised.[6,61] Two to 3 weeks before beginning PUVA, methotrexate can be initiated. PUVA is then added and used together with methotrexate until the patient is clear. Once clear, tapering of both methotrexate dose and PUVA frequency can occur.

Cyclosporine is contraindicated for use with PUVA. Patients who have received PUVA therapy have an increased risk of developing squamous cell carcinoma when later treated with cyclosporine. This combination should be avoided in all but the most extreme situations.[62,63]

Combination with UVB

A regimen of PUVA with BB-UVB radiation results in marked reduction in cumulative exposure to both UVA and UVB, with more rapid clearance of psoriasis than with PUVA alone. The combination is especially effective in Fitzpatrick skin types IV to VI, as the pigmentation induced by PUVA can limit the effectiveness of PUVA in these patients. Expediting clearance with PUVA plus BB-UVB helps prevent the limitations on treatment success that occur as a result of PUVA-induced skin darkening.

Of critical importance, however, is that only BB-UVB can be used in combination therapy. NBUVB activates psoralen to a similar degree as UVA radiation, whereas BB-UVB does not have such activating properties for psoralen. If NBUVB is used in combination with PUVA, then the patient is receiving 3 treatments: (1) PUVA, (2) NBUVB, and (3) psoralen plus NBUVB. There is to date no defined treatment protocol or appropriate dosing determined for this combination.

ADVERSE EFFECTS

As in any therapy, with PUVA phototherapy, there are potential adverse effects both short-term and long-term.

Short-Term Adverse Effects of Psoralen Plus UVA

Nausea is the most common adverse reaction induced by PUVA. As described previously, nausea correlates with the serum level of drug. Absorption can be slowed down by taking methoxsalen with a small amount of food with high fat content. If gastrointestinal disturbance continues, the dose of methoxsalen can be decreased by 10 mg (1 capsule). Rarely, antiemetics are needed, but could be used.

Symptomatic erythema is the most common phototoxic reaction seen in PUVA therapy and occurs in 10% of patients during the clearance phase. Erythema from PUVA peaks at 48 to 96 hours after exposure to UVA. Treatment is to withhold treatment until erythema resolves and treat symptoms with supportive measures such as cool baths, liberal use of emollients, and antipruritics. Symptoms are likely to persist for 7 to 10 days, and may last 2 weeks depending on the severity of the erythema. When treatment is resumed, decrease UVA dose by 10% to 20%.

Mild pruritus is common, and is usually the result of skin dryness. Emollients are usually sufficient to relieve this symptom. If intense pruritus ("PUVA-itch") and/or subacute phototoxicity develop, PUVA therapy should be discontinued until the symptoms resolve, then PUVA resumed at a UVA dose reduced by 10% to 20%.

Other short-term adverse effects include reactivation of herpes simplex, bronchoconstriction, drug fever, cardiovascular stress, photo-onycholysis and melanonychia, friction blisters, and ankle edema. Potential short-term central nervous system disturbances reported with PUVA therapy include headache, dizziness, depression, insomnia, hyperactivity, and a feeling of detachment from the environment.

Long-Term Adverse Effects of Psoralen Plus UVA

Photoaging

Photoaging occurs in all patients with Fitzpatrick skin types I through IV who have long-term exposure to PUVA therapy. These changes are partially reversible on discontinuation of therapy, with more reversibility if discontinued earlier in the course of treatment. Likewise, type I and II skin have more marked changes than types III and IV. UVA dose is an important factor as well, as more marked changes occur with higher exposure.

The photoaging changes produced are similar to those produced by natural sunlight: hyperpigmentation and hypopigmentation, telangiectasia, formation of wrinkles, and actinic keratosis. Hypertrichosis also has been reported to occur with long-term PUVA. The lentigines seen with long-term PUVA therapy are composed of melanocytes of larger size and with some cellular atypia compared with melanocytes in untreated skin. Despite the histologic changes, there is no evidence that "PUVA lentigos" are precursors of melanoma.[64–66]

Skin cancer

Long-term studies have demonstrated a dose-related increase in nonmelanoma skin cancers, particularly cutaneous squamous cell carcinoma, with high cumulative exposure to oral PUVA.

The risk of squamous cell carcinoma is dose dependent, with increased incidence in patients who have received more than 200 treatments. These findings have been found in multiple studies. The risk for squamous cell of the male genitalia is particularly elevated, hence the standard recommendation for shielding this area. Patients treated with PUVA who then receive subsequent treatment with cyclosporine are also at a tremendously increased risk for developing squamous cell carcinoma. This increased risk is not seen with bath PUVA or in non-white populations.[62,63,66–78]

Controversy surrounds the issue of long-term PUVA and melanoma. In a long-term multicenter study, melanoma incidence increased in patients treated with more than 200 PUVA treatments following a 15-year latency. In contrast, other data primarily from Europe do not show the increased risk.[68,79]

Regardless, squamous cell carcinoma is the primary cause of cancer morbidity and mortality in patients with psoriasis treated with long-term PUVA phototherapy. Routine skin cancer screenings are important for PUVA patients.

Cataracts

Long-term PUVA carries with it the potential risk of cataract formation. Methoxsalen does enter the lens, and UVA exposure induces formation of photoproducts. Eye protection throughout the day of treatment, following methoxsalen ingestion, is important to protect the eye from natural UVA. Long-term studies have failed to show an increased risk of visual impairment or cataract formation in PUVA-treated patients.[80]

Subacute phototoxicity

When pruritus is accompanied by a widespread eruption on the skin, subacute phototoxicity has occurred. Subacute phototoxicity can occur at any point during treatment, even if the UVA dose has been stable for some time. Often the patient feels there has been a flare in his or her baseline disease; however, a key difference is the presence of intense pruritus. Furthermore, the skin eruption spares areas that are not exposed to UVA during PUVA treatment, namely the axillae and inner thighs.[38]

Management includes cessation of PUVA therapy, emollients and cool baths, and antipruritics until the eruption has cleared. PUVA can then be resumed at a dose of UVA decreased by 30% to 40%, with gradual increases as tolerated to continue clearance of the skin.

MONITORING

As with any treatment, the potential benefits of PUVA phototherapy must be considered on a patient-by-patient basis, weighing benefits against the dose-related risks of long-term therapy.

Both baseline and annual monitoring for skin cancer is appropriate in patients receiving PUVA.[4] Furthermore, regular appointments, every 3 to 4 months, with the treating physician is important for monitoring disease activity and treatment efficacy. Skin cancer is the most important

---

Box 1
Other dermatologic uses of psoralen plus UVA

Dermatitis & Papulosquamous Disorders
  Atopic dermatitis
  Chronic hand dermatitis
  Lichen planus
  Lymphomatoid papulosis
  Palmoplantar pustulosis
  Parapsoriasis
  Pityriasis lichenoides

Photosensitive Disorders
  Chronic actinic dermatitis
  Polymorphous light eruption (PMLE)
  Solar Urticaria

Autoimmune Disorders
  Alopecia areata
  Graft vs host disease
  Morphea and scleroderma

Other Pruritic Disorders
  Chronic urticaria
  Idiopathic pruritus
  Prurigo nodularis
  Urticaria pigmentosa

Miscellaneous
  Granuloma annulare
  Grover's disease

Data from Morison WL, Richard EG. PUVA photochemotherapy and other phototherapeutic modalities. In: Wolverton SE editor. *Comprehensive dermatologic drug therapy.* 3. ed. Edinburgh [u.a.]: Saunders; 2013. http://www.gbv.de/dms/bs/toc/720747023.pdf.

adverse effect of long-term PUVA treatment, and patient education is critical in addition to routine skin examination by both physician and patient.

CLINICAL USE BEYOND PSORIASIS

A myriad of other disease beyond psoriasis may be treated with phototherapy (**Box 1**). Based on the scientific understanding of the mechanism of action of PUVA, namely its immunosuppressive and antiproliferative effects, PUVA is used to treat many inflammatory dermatoses. At present, the FDA has approved PUVA only for use in the treatment of psoriasis (oral PUVA), vitiligo (topical PUVA using methoxsalen lotion), and increasing tolerance to sunlight (oral PUVA).

When using oral PUVA phototherapy to treat nonpsoriatic disorders, the same general protocol and guidelines as outlined previously for psoriasis in the clearance phase may be used. Likewise, once the patient is adequately responding to PUVA and disease control is obtained, transition into maintenance therapy can be effective and appropriate for long-term management of certain more chronic processes, such as atopic dermatitis. As with psoriasis treatment, once control is obtained, the risk of long-term PUVA treatment for maintenance should be balanced against the alternative therapies available for that disease process.

SUMMARY AND RECOMMENDATIONS

Psoriasis and other inflammatory dermatoses can be challenging to manage for the clinician, despite the ever-enlarging armamentarium of systemic and biologic therapies in dermatology. PUVA therapy allows for control of moderate to severe disease with the option of transitioning into maintenance for long-term control. Although the risk-benefit ratio must be considered, PUVA remains a powerful tool for the dermatologist, and continues to play an important role in the stepwise treatment algorithm for many cases of psoriasis and other inflammatory dermatoses.

REFERENCES

1. Abel EA. Photochemotherapy in dermatology. New York: Igaku-Shoin; 1993.
2. Morison WL. Phototherapy and photochemotherapy for skin disease, vol. 34. Baton Rouge (LA): CRC Press; 2005. Available at: http://www.crcnetbase.com/isbn/9780849360183.
3. Parrish JA, Fitzpatrick TB, Tanenbaum L, et al. Photochemotherapy of psoriasis with oral methoxsalen and longwave ultraviolet light. N Engl J Med 1974; 291(23):1207–11.
4. Menter A, Korman NJ, Elmets CA, et al. Guidelines of care for the management of psoriasis and psoriatic arthritis: Section 5. Guidelines of care for the treatment of psoriasis with phototherapy and photochemotherapy. J Am Acad Dermatol 2010;62(1): 114. Available at: https://www.ncbi.nlm.nih.gov/pubmed/19811850.
5. Leonardi CL, Powers JL, Matheson RT, et al. Etanercept as monotherapy in patients with psoriasis. N Engl J Med 2003;349(21):2014–22. Available at: http://content.nejm.org/cgi/content/abstract/349/21/2014.
6. Morison WL, Momtaz K, Parrish JA, et al. Combined methotrexate-PUVA therapy in the treatment of psoriasis. J Am Acad Dermatol 1982;6(1):46–51. Available at: https://www.sciencedirect.com/science/article/pii/S0190962282700052.
7. Walters IB, Burack LH, Coven TR, et al. Suberythemogenic narrow-band UVB is markedly more effective than conventional UVB in treatment of psoriasis vulgaris. J Am Acad Dermatol 1999;40(6): 893–900. Available at: https://www.sciencedirect.com/science/article/pii/S0190962299700769.
8. Karvonen J, Kokkonen EL, Ruotsalainen E. 311 nm UVB lamps in the treatment of psoriasis with the ingram regimen. Acta Derm Venereol 1989;69(1):82. Available at: https://www.ncbi.nlm.nih.gov/pubmed/2563617.
9. Larkö O. Treatment of psoriasis with a new UVB-lamp. Acta Derm Venereol 1989;69(4):357. Available at: https://www.ncbi.nlm.nih.gov/pubmed/2568064.
10. Coven TR. Narrowband UV-B produces superior clinical and histopathological resolution of moderate-to-severe psoriasis in patients compared with broadband UV-B (Archives of Dermatology 1997;133:1514-1522. JAMA J Am Med Assoc 1998;279(17):1330E.
11. Stern RS. Psoralen and ultraviolet A light therapy for psoriasis. N Engl J Med 2007;357(7):682–90. Available at: http://content.nejm.org/cgi/content/extract/357/7/682.
12. Yones SS, Palmer RA, Garibaldinos TT, et al. Randomized double-blind trial of the treatment of chronic plaque psoriasis: efficacy of Psoralen–UV-A therapy vs narrowband UV-B therapy. Arch Dermatol 2006;142(7):836–42.
13. Tanew A. Narrowband UV-B phototherapy vs photochemotherapy in the treatment of chronic plaque-type psoriasis: paired comparison study. J Am Med Assoc 1999;282(4):312.
14. Melski JW. Annual rate of psoralen and ultraviolet-A treatment of psoriasis after initial clearing. Arch Dermatol 1982;118(6):404–8.
15. Stern RS, Melski JW. Long-term continuation of psoralen and ultraviolet-A treatment of psoriasis. Arch Dermatol 1982;118(6):400–3.

16. Morison WL, Parrish JA, Fitzpatrick TB. Oral methoxsalen photochemotherapy of recalcitrant dermatoses of the palms and soles. Br J Dermatol 1978; 99(3):293. Available at: https://www.ncbi.nlm.nih. gov/pubmed/708596.

17. Hönigsmann H, Gschnait F, Konrad K, et al. Photochemotherapy for pustular psoriasis (von Zumbusch). Br J Dermatol 1977;97(2): 119–26. Available at: https://www.ncbi.nlm.nih. gov/pubmed/911672.

18. Hawk JL, Grice PL. The efficacy of localized PUVA therapy for chronic hand and foot dermatoses. Clin Exp Dermatol 1994;19(6):479–82. Available at: https://www.ncbi.nlm.nih.gov/pubmed/7889668.

19. Agren-Jonsson S, Tegner E. PUVA therapy for palmoplantar pustulosis. Acta Derm Venereol 1985;65(6):531. Available at: https://www.ncbi.nlm. nih.gov/pubmed/2420119.

20. Pathak MA, Fitzpatrick TB. The evolution of photochemotherapy with psoralens and UVA (PUVA): 2000 BC to 1992 AD. J Photochem Photobiol B 1992;14(1):3–22.

21. Morison WL, Richard EG. PUVA photochemotherapy and other phototherapeutic modalities. In: Wolverton SE, editor. Comprehensive dermatologic drug therapy. 3rd edition. Edinburgh (Scotland): Saunders; 2013. p 279–90. Available at: http://www. gbv.de/dms/bs/toc/720747023.pdf.

22. Sullivan TJ. Bioavailability of a new oral methoxsalen formulation. A serum concentration and photosensitivity response study. Arch Dermatol 1986;122(7):768–71.

23. Levins PC, William Gange R, Momtaz-T K, et al. A new liquid formulation of 8-methoxypsoralen: bioactivity and effect of diet. J Invest Dermatol 1984; 82(2):185–7. Available at: https://www.science direct.com/science/article/pii/S0022202X15433172.

24. Hönigsmann H, Jaschke E, Nitsche V, et al. Serum levels of 8-methoxypsoralen in two different drug preparations: correlation with photosensitivity and UV-A dose requirements for photochemotherapy. J Invest Dermatol 1982;79(4):233–6. Available at: https://www.sciencedirect.com/science/article/pii/ S0022202X15464693.

25. McEvoy MT, Stern RS. Psoralens and related compounds in the treatment of psoriasis. Pharmacol Ther 1987;34(1):75–97. Available at: https://www. sciencedirect.com/science/article/pii/01637258879 00933.

26. Zanolli M. Phototherapy treatment of psoriasis today. J Am Acad Dermatol 2003;49(2):78–86. Available at: https://www.sciencedirect.com/science/article/pii/ S0190962203011393.

27. Erkin G, Uğur Y, Gürer CK, et al. Effect of PUVA, narrow-band UVB and cyclosporin on inflammatory cells of the psoriatic plaque. J Cutan Pathol 2007; 34(3):213–9. Available at: https://www.ncbi.nlm.nih. gov/pubmed/17302604.

28. Laskin JD, Lee E, Laskin DL, et al. Psoralens potentiate ultraviolet light-induced inhibition of epidermal growth factor binding. Proc Natl Acad Sci U S A 1986;83(21):8211–5.

29. Morison WL. In vivo effects of psoralens plus long-wave ultraviolet radiation on immunity. Natl Cancer Inst Monogr 1984;66:243. Available at: https://www. ncbi.nlm.nih.gov/pubmed/6335739.

30. Farr PM, Diffey BL, Higgins EM, et al. The action spectrum between 320 and 400 nm for clearance of psoriasis by psoralen photochemotherapy. Br J Dermatol 1991;124(5):443–8. Available at: https:// www.ncbi.nlm.nih.gov/pubmed/2039720.

31. Cripps DJ, Lowe NJ, Lerner AB. Action spectra of topical psoralens: a re-evaluation. Br J Dermatol 1982;107(1):77–82. Available at: https://www.ncbi. nlm.nih.gov/pubmed/7104210.

32. Parrish JA, White HAD, Kingsbury T, et al. Photochemotherapy of psoriasis using methoxsalen and sunlight: a controlled study. Arch Dermatol 1977; 113(11):1529–32.

33. Midelfart K, Moseng D, Kavli G, et al. One-year measurements of solar UVB and UVA radiation at latitude 70 degrees north. Photodermatol 1984;1(5): 252. Available at: https://www.ncbi.nlm.nih.gov/ pubmed/6543391.

34. de Gruijl FR. Photocarcinogenesis: UVA vs. UVB radiation. Skin Pharmacol Physiol 2002;15(5): 316–20. Available at: https://www.karger.com/ Article/Abstract/64535.

35. Brash DE, Ziegler A, Jonason AS, et al. Sunlight and sunburn in human skin cancer: p53, apoptosis, and tumor promotion. J Investig Dermatol Symp Proc 1996;1(2):136–42.

36. Zamiri M, Bilsland D. Treatment of bath PUVA-induced skin pain with gabapentin. Br J Dermatol 2004;151(2):516–7. Available at: https://online library.wiley.com/doi/abs/10.1111/j.1365-2133.2004. 06090.x.

37. Kumakiri M, Hashimoto K, Willis I. Biological changes of human cutaneous nerves caused by ultraviolet irradiation: an ultrastructural study. Br J Dermatol 1978;99(1):65–75. Available at: https:// www.ncbi.nlm.nih.gov/pubmed/678467.

38. Morison WL, Marwaha S, Beck L. PUVA-induced phototoxicity: incidence and causes. J Am Acad Dermatol 1997;36(2):183–6. Available at: https:// www.sciencedirect.com/science/article/pii/S01909 62297702779.

39. Norris PG, Maurice PD, Schott GD, et al. Persistent skin pain after PUVA. Clin Exp Dermatol 1987;12(6): 403–5. Available at: https://www.ncbi.nlm.nih.gov/ pubmed/3504747.

40. Ibbotson SH, Farr PM. The time-course of psoralen ultraviolet A (PUVA) erythema. J Invest Dermatol 1999;113(3):346–9. Available at: https://www.

sciencedirect.com/science/article/pii/S0022202X15
405925.

41. Brickl R, Schmid J, Koss FW. Clinical pharmacology of oral psoralen drugs. Photodermatol 1984;1(4): 174–86.

42. Roelandts R, Van Boven M, Deheyn T, et al. Dietary influences on 8-MOP plasma levels in PUVA patients with psoriasis. Br J Dermatol 1981;105(5):569–72. Available at: https://www.ncbi.nlm.nih.gov/pubmed/7295571.

43. Herfst MJ, Wolff FAD. Intraindividual and interindividual variability in 8-methoxypsoralen kinetics and effect in psoriatic patients. Clin Pharmacol Ther 1983;34(1):117–24.

44. Artuc M, Stuettgen G, Schalla W, et al. Reversible binding of 5- and 8-methoxypsoralen to human serum proteins (albumin) and to epidermis in vitro. Br J Dermatol 1979;101(6):669–77. Available at: https://www.ncbi.nlm.nih.gov/pubmed/534612.

45. Wulf HC, Andreasen MP. Distribution of 3H-8-MOP and its metabolites in rat organs after a single oral administration. J Invest Dermatol 1981;76(4):252–8. Available at: https://www.sciencedirect.com/science/article/pii/S0022202X15460580.

46. Schmid J, Prox A, Reuter A, et al. The metabolism of 8-methoxypsoralen in man. Eur J Drug Metab Pharmacokinet 1980;5(2):81–92. Available at: https://www.ncbi.nlm.nih.gov/pubmed/7398681.

47. Stern RS, Kleinerman RA, Parrish JA, et al. Phototoxic reactions to photoactive drugs in patients treated with PUVA. Arch Dermatol 1980;116(11): 1269–71.

48. Wolff K, Fitzpatrick TB, Parrish JA, et al. Photochemotherapy for psoriasis with orally administered methoxsalen. Arch Dermatol 1976;112(7):943–50.

49. Melski JW, Tanenbaum L, Parrish JA, et al. Oral methoxsalen photochemotherapy for the treatment of psoriasis: a cooperative clinical trial. J Invest Dermatol 1977;68(6):328–35. Available at: https://www.sciencedirect.com/science/article/pii/S0022202X15450407.

50. Henseler T, Hönigsmann H, Wolff K, et al. Oral 8-methoxypsoralen photochemotherapy of psoriasis: the European PUVA study: a cooperative study among 18 European centres. Lancet 1981;317(8225):853–7. Available at: https://www.sciencedirect.com/science/article/pii/S0140673681921371.

51. Buckley DA, Phillips WG. 8-methoxypsoralen PUVA for psoriasis: a comparison of a minimal phototoxic dose-based regimen with a skin-type approach. Br J Dermatol 1997;136(5):800–1. Available at: https://www.ncbi.nlm.nih.gov/pubmed/9205529.

52. Collins P, Wainwright NJ, Amorim I, et al. 8-MOP PUVA for psoriasis: a comparison of a minimal phototoxic dose-based regimen with a skin-type approach. Br J Dermatol 1996;135(2):248–54. Available at: https://www.ncbi.nlm.nih.gov/pubmed/8881668.

53. Stern RS. Long-term use of psoralens and ultraviolet A for psoriasis: evidence for efficacy and cost savings. J Am Acad Dermatol 1986;14(3):520–6. Available at: https://www.sciencedirect.com/science/article/pii/S0190962286700662.

54. Gange RW, Levins P, Murray J, et al. Prolonged skin photosensitization induced by methoxsalen and subphototoxic UVA irradiation. J Invest Dermatol 1984;82(3):219–22. Available at: https://www.sciencedirect.com/science/article/pii/S0022202X15433263.

55. Lowe NJ, Weingarten D, Bourget T, et al. PUVA therapy for psoriasis: comparison of oral and bathwater delivery of 8-methoxypsoralen. J Am Acad Dermatol 1986;14(5):754–60. Available at: https://www.sciencedirect.com/science/article/pii/S0190962286700893.

56. Busard CI, Cohen AD, Wolf P, et al. Biologics combined with conventional systemic agents or phototherapy for the treatment of psoriasis: real-life data from PSONET registries. J Eur Acad Dermatol Venereol 2018;32(2):245–53.

57. Cather JC, Crowley JJ. Use of biologic agents in combination with other therapies for the treatment of psoriasis. Am J Clin Dermatol 2014;15(6):467–78.

58. Menter MA, See J, Amend WJC, et al. Proceedings of the psoriasis combination and rotation therapy conference. J Am Acad Dermatol 1996;34(2):315–21.

59. Tanew A, Guggenbichler A, Hönigsmann H, et al. Photochemotherapy for severe psoriasis without or in combination with acitretin: a randomized, double-blind comparison study. J Am Acad Dermatol 1991; 25(4):682–4. Available at: https://www.sciencedirect.com/science/article/pii/019096229170253X.

60. Nijsten TEC, Stern RS. Oral retinoid use reduces cutaneous squamous cell carcinoma risk in patients with psoriasis treated with psoralen-UVA: a nested cohort study. J Am Acad Dermatol 2003;49(4): 644–50. Available at: https://www.sciencedirect.com/science/article/pii/S0190962203015871.

61. Shehzad T, Dar NR, Zakria M. Efficacy of concomitant use of PUVA and methotrexate in disease clearance time in plaque type psoriasis. J Pak Med Assoc 2004;54(9):453. Available at: https://www.ncbi.nlm.nih.gov/pubmed/15518366.

62. Marcil I, Stern RS. Squamous-cell cancer of the skin in patients given PUVA and ciclosporin: nested cohort crossover study. Lancet 2001;358(9287): 1042–5. Available at: https://www.sciencedirect.com/science/article/pii/S0140673601061797.

63. Paul CF, Ho VC, McGeown C, et al. Risk of malignancies in psoriasis patients treated with cyclosporine: a 5 y cohort study. J Invest Dermatol 2003;120(2):211–6. Available at: https://www.sciencedirect.com/science/article/pii/S0022202X15301731.

64. Gschnait F, Wolff K, Hönigsmann H, et al. Long-term photochemotherapy: histopathological and

immunofluorescence observations in 243 patients. Br J Dermatol 1980;103(1):11–22. Available at: https://www.ncbi.nlm.nih.gov/pubmed/7000141.

65. Rhodes AR, Harrist TJ, Momtaz-T K. The PUVA-induced pigmented macule: a lentiginous proliferation of large, sometimes cytologically atypical, melanocytes. J Am Acad Dermatol 1983;9(1):47–58. Available at: https://www.sciencedirect.com/science/article/pii/S0190962283701064.

66. Stern RS. Actinic degeneration and pigmentary change in association with psoralen and UVA treatment: a 20-year prospective study. J Am Acad Dermatol 2003;48(1):61–7. Available at: https://www.sciencedirect.com/science/article/pii/S0190962203500123.

67. Stern RS, Laird N, Melski J, et al. Cutaneous squamous-cell carcinoma in patients treated with PUVA. N Engl J Med 1984;310(18):1156–61.

68. Morison WL, Baughman RD, Day RM, et al. Consensus workshop on the toxic effects of long-term PUVA therapy. Arch Dermatol 1998;134(5):595–8.

69. Nijsten TEC, Stern RS. The increased risk of skin cancer is persistent after discontinuation of Psoralen+Ultraviolet A: a cohort study. J Invest Dermatol 2003;121(2):252–8. Available at: https://www.sciencedirect.com/science/article/pii/S0022202X15303638.

70. Stern RS, Lange R. Non-melanoma skin cancer occurring in patients treated with PUVA five to ten years after first treatment. J Invest Dermatol 1988;91(2):120–4. Available at: https://www.sciencedirect.com/science/article/pii/S0022202X88900358.

71. Stern RS, Laird N. The carcinogenic risk of treatments for severe psoriasis. Cancer 1994;73(11):2759–64.

72. Reshad H, Challoner F, Pollock DJ, et al. Cutaneous carcinoma in psoriatic patients treated with PUVA. Br J Dermatol 1984;110(3):299–305. Available at: https://www.ncbi.nlm.nih.gov/pubmed/6696845.

73. Forman AB, Roenigk HH, Caro WA, et al. Long-term follow-up of skin cancer in the PUVA-48 cooperative study. Arch Dermatol 1989;125(4):515–9.

74. Lindelöf B, Sigurgeirsson B, Tegner E, et al. PUVA and cancer: a large-scale epidemiological study. Lancet 1991;338(8759):91–3. Available at: https://www.sciencedirect.com/science/article/pii/0140673691900832.

75. Stern RS, Lunder EJ. Risk of squamous cell carcinoma and methoxsalen (psoralen) and UV-A radiation (PUVA): a meta-analysis. Arch Dermatol 1998;134(12):1582–5.

76. Stern RS. Genital tumors among men with psoriasis exposed to psoralens and ultraviolet A radiation (PUVA) and ultraviolet B radiation. N Engl J Med 1990;322(16):1093–7.

77. Murase JE, Lee EE, Koo J. Effect of ethnicity on the risk of developing nonmelanoma skin cancer following long-term PUVA therapy. Int J Dermatol 2005;44(12):1016–21. Available at: https://onlinelibrary.wiley.com/doi/abs/10.1111/j.1365-4632.2004.02322.x.

78. Lim JL, Stern RS. High levels of ultraviolet B exposure increase the risk of non-melanoma skin cancer in psoralen and ultraviolet A-treated patients. J Invest Dermatol 2005;124(3):505–13. Available at: https://www.sciencedirect.com/science/article/pii/S0022202X15321837.

79. Stern RS, Nichols KT, Vakeva LH. The PUVA follow-up study. Malignant melanoma in patients treated for psoriasis with methoxsalen (psoralen) and ultraviolet A radiation (PUVA). N Engl J Med 1997;336(15):1041–5. Available at: http://content.nejm.org/cgi/content/abstract/336/15/1041.

80. Malanos D, Stern RS. Psoralen plus UVA does not increase the risk of cataracts: a 25-year prospective study. J Am Acad Dermatol 2007;57(2):231–7.

Distinguishing Myth from Fact
Photocarcinogenesis and Phototherapy

Katherine G. Thompson, BS, Noori Kim, MD*

KEYWORDS

- Photocarcinogenesis • Skin cancer • PUVA • Narrowband UVB • Broadband UVB • UVA1
- Phototherapy

KEY POINTS

- There is a dose-dependent increase in the risk of squamous cell carcinoma in patients treated with psoralen and UVA (PUVA), which begins to manifest after 150 treatments.
- There is minimal increased risk of basal cell carcinoma following PUVA; the risk of melanoma has a delayed onset, appearing approximately 15 years following initiation of PUVA treatment.
- Current evidence suggests minimal risk of photocarcinogenesis following broadband or narrowband UVB treatment.
- There is insufficient evidence for the risk of photocarcinogenesis following UVA1 treatment.

INTRODUCTION

The risk of cutaneous carcinogenesis following repeated ultraviolet (UV) light exposures is well established.[1] UVB radiation directly damages DNA in an oxygen-independent manner, promoting the formation of characteristic pyrimidine photoproducts: cyclobutane dimers and 6,4-photoproducts.[2] These mutations may lead to errors in DNA replication, initiating the development of skin cancer if not repaired.[3] UV radiation also indirectly damages DNA through the absorption of photons by other chromophores, including cytochromes, flavin, heme, nicotinamide adenine dinucleotide plus hydrogen, and porphyrins.[4] The energy of the absorbed photons can be either transferred to DNA in a type I photosensitized reaction or to molecular oxygen in a type II photosensitized reaction. UVA radiation may contribute to the formation of pyrimidine dimers through a type I photosensitized reaction in addition to producing reactive oxygen species capable of damaging DNA.[5] Reactive oxygen species act on guanosine to produce 7,8-dihydro-8-oxoguanosine (8-oxoG), a mutagenic lesion that may be involved in promoting inflammation.[6]

Antigen-specific immunosuppression induced by UV radiation, in part responsible for the efficacy of phototherapy,[7] also contributes to photocarcinogenesis.[8] Biopsies of basal and squamous cell carcinomas have demonstrated regulatory T cells (Tregs), which may be induced by UV exposure, infiltrating the tumors.[9] Tregs in cutaneous squamous cell carcinomas have been shown to suppress proliferation of effector T cells, promoting tumor growth and subsequent metastasis.[10] These mechanisms may in part explain the exceptionally increased risk of skin cancer, particularly squamous cell carcinoma, in chronically immunosuppressed organ transplant recipients.[11]

The induction of DNA damage and immunosuppression by UV radiation raises a concern for the potential risk of carcinogenesis in phototherapy.

Disclosure Statement: The authors have nothing to disclose.
Department of Dermatology, Johns Hopkins University School of Medicine, 601 North Caroline Street, Suite 8033, Baltimore, MD 21287, USA
* Corresponding author.
E-mail address: nkim34@jhmi.edu

Dermatol Clin 38 (2020) 25–35
https://doi.org/10.1016/j.det.2019.08.003
0733-8635/20/© 2019 Elsevier Inc. All rights reserved.

derm.theclinics.com

Specific wavelength ranges are selected in phototherapy to provide targeted treatment and ameliorate the risk of skin cancer.

PSORALEN PLUS UVA

Approximately 3500 years ago, ancient Egyptians administered *Ammi majus* extract, a natural source of psoralen derivatives, in addition to sunbathing for the treatment of vitiligo.[12] In the 1970s, oral 8-methoxypsoralen (8-MOP) in combination with high-intensity UVA irradiation was demonstrated to be highly successful in the treatment of psoriasis, giving rise to modern psoralen-UVA (PUVA) phototherapy.[13] Psoralens intercalate into DNA, and UVA radiation promotes their linkage with pyrimidine bases to form C_4 cycloadducts, which can inhibit DNA synthesis and epidermal proliferation.[14] The role of UV radiation in DNA damage as well as the direct action of psoralens themselves on DNA gave rise to concern for the carcinogenic potential of PUVA.

Numerous studies have examined the long-term risk of developing melanoma and nonmelanoma skin cancer (NMSC) following treatment with PUVA (**Table 1**). The PUVA Follow-Up Study prospectively followed 1380 patients with psoriasis at 16 collaborating university centers who were first treated in 1975 to 1976 with PUVA. At a mean follow-up of 20.2 years, the incidence of melanoma (invasive or in situ) in this cohort was evaluated.[15] Incidence of melanoma in the patient cohort was compared over 2 time periods: 1975 to 1990 and 1991 to 1998. The risk of melanoma was not detectable until approximately 15 years after the first PUVA treatment. After adjusting for age, sex, and the expected increase in melanoma risk over time, the incidence of melanoma was found to be 6.9 times higher in the cohort from 1991 to 1998 than it was in the same cohort between 1975 to 1990. Although the risk of melanoma was greatest in patients treated with high-dose PUVA (>200 treatments), approximately 15 years after the first treatment, even patients treated with lower doses of PUVA demonstrated a fivefold increase in melanoma risk compared with the general white US population.

At a mean 28 years of follow-up, the risk of squamous cell (SCC) and basal cell carcinoma (BCC) following PUVA was evaluated.[16] A clear dose-dependent increase in SCC risk compared with the general population was observed in patients treated with PUVA. Although no meaningful increase in SCC risk was observed in patients who had received fewer than 150 treatments, the SCC incidence rate ratio (IRR) was shown to increase with increasing PUVA exposure: IRR 3.10

(95% confidence interval [CI] 2.32–4.14) for 151 to 250 treatments, IRR 3.82 (95% CI 2.83–5.14) for 251 to 350 treatments, IRR 6.16 (95% CI 4.55–8.35) for 351 to 450 treatments, and IRR 8.71 (95% CI 6.55–11.59) for more than 450 treatments. Although the risk of SCC in the PUVA cohort was approximately 30 times higher than that of the general population, the risk of BCC was only approximately 5 times higher, suggesting that PUVA has a smaller effect on the risk of the development of BCC compared with SCC. Of note, no increased risk of NMSC has been observed in non-Caucasian populations receiving long-term PUVA.[17]

BROADBAND AND NARROWBAND UVB

The action spectrum of UVB in the treatment of psoriasis has been identified at the wavelengths of 304 and 313 nm, at which patients experience optimal treatment efficacy with minimal erythema.[18] The minimal erythema dose elicited by narrowband UVB (NBUVB) (311–313 nm) is significantly higher than that of broadband (BB-) UVB, suggesting that NBUVB is a safer alternative to BB-UVB.[19] To date, no prospective cohort studies following skin cancer risk due to BB-UVB or NBUVB alone have been completed (**Table 2**). A study evaluating incidence of skin cancers in patients treated with BB-UVB or NBUVB over 7.8 years of follow-up found 0 occurrences of skin cancer with BB-UVB and 1 melanoma-in-situ with NBUVB, which is not significantly different from the general population's risk.[20] The PUVA Follow-Up Study also examined incidence of NMSC in patients who additionally received UVB phototherapy.[21] Although the study did not distinguish patients treated with NBUVB or BB-UVB, the cohort was predominantly exposed to BB-UVB. In patients receiving fewer than 100 PUVA treatments, high UVB exposure, defined as ≥300 UVB treatments, was modestly associated with future development of SCC compared with lower-dose UVB exposure (IRR 1.37) and BCC (IRR 1.45). The largest retrospective review examined 3867 patients treated with NBUVB over a median 5.5-year follow-up period.[22] No significant association was discovered between NBUVB therapy and the future development of SCC, BCC, or melanoma compared with the general population of the country.

UVA1

High-dose UVA1 (340–400 nm) therapy, first used successfully in the treatment of atopic dermatitis, is ideally suited for diseases affecting the dermis

Table 1
Clinical studies on the photocarcinogenic risk of psoralen plus UVA

Authors, publication year	PubMed ID	Sample Size	Study Design and Setting	Dose	Outcome Measures	Outcome
Roenigk HH & Caro WA,[29] 1981	7217399	631	Prospective. United States; 12 sites. Follow-up of 4 y.	Mean number of treatments to clear by site ranged from 22–38. Mean cumulative dose ranged from 557–2032 J by site.	Incidence of BCC, SCC in patients with psoriasis treated with PUVA.	10 BCCs and 3 SCCs developed in 10 patients during the 4-y follow-up period. No comparison against incidence in control/ general population was reported.
Stern et al,[30] 1984	6709010	1380	Prospective cohort study. United States. Mean follow-up of 5.7 y.	Median cumulative dose was nearly 1500 J/cm². More than 60% of cohort received >1000 J/cm².	Dose-dependent risk of SCC in patients with psoriasis treated with PUVA.	50-fold increase in incidence of SCC in high-dose PUVA group compared with that of general population. Risk of developing SCC at least 22 mo after first exposure to PUVA was 12.8 times higher in patients treated with high-dose compared with low-dose PUVA.
Forman et al,[31] 1989	2649011	551	Retrospective. United States. Mean follow-up of 57.2 mo.	Mean cumulative dose of 1861 J/cm². 37.6% of cohort received >1500 J/cm².	Incidence of BCC and SCC in patients with psoriasis receiving PUVA.	Statistically significant increase in incidence of SCCs compared with general population.
Lindelof et al,[32] 1991	1676477	4799	Retrospective chart review. Swedish. Mean follow-up of 6.9 y (men) and 7.2 y (women).	9.6% of cohort received cumulative dose of >1200 J/cm². 7.7% received >200 txs.	Relative risk of SCC and melanoma in patients receiving PUVA.	No significant increase in risk of melanoma in PUVA patients compared with general Swedish population. Risk of SCC increased six-fold in men and 5-fold in women. Men receiving >200 txs (corresponding to approximately 1200 J/cm²) had 30-fold increase in SCC incidence.

(continued on next page)

Table 1
(continued)

Authors, publication year	PubMed ID	Sample Size	Study Design and Setting	Dose	Outcome Measures	Outcome
Chuang et al,[33] 1992	1552048	492	Historical cohort study. United States. Mean follow-up of 5.4 y (8.9 y for high-dose group; 4.5 y for low-dose group).	20.9% received total dose of >1000 J/cm^2; 79.1% received total dose of <200 J/cm^2.	Incidence of skin cancer in patients with psoriasis receiving high-dose (>200 J/cm^2 cumulative) or low-dose PUVA compared with general population.	Incidence of SCC in high-dose group was significantly higher than expected (P<.0005). No observed increase in BCC, genital tumors, or melanoma.
McKenna et al,[34] 1996	8733363	245	Retrospective chart review. United Kingdom. Median follow-up of 9.5 y.	Median number of exposures of 59, and median total dose of 133 J/cm^2 in entire cohort. Median of 225 txs and dose of 654 J/cm^2 in group developing NMSC.	Incidence of skin cancer in patients with psoriasis receiving PUVA compared with general population.	NMSCs in 2.4%, melanoma in 0%; 1.4 times increased risk of NMSC compared with control population of Wales. Significantly increased risk of NMSC in patients receiving >100 exposures (>250 J/cm^2). Minimal increase in NMSC risk with dose <250 J/cm^2 or <100 txs.
Stern et al,[35] 1997	9091799	1380	Prospective cohort study. United States. Median interval from 1st tx to most recent follow-up was 19 y.	29% of cohort received >250 txs (high-dose group).	Occurrence of melanoma in patients treated with PUVA within first few years of tx and after 15 y of tx.	Significantly higher overall risk of melanoma (RR 2.3) in PUVA patients compared with general population. After 15+ y since 1st tx, risk of melanoma significantly higher (RR 5.4). Greatest increase in melanoma risk in patients receiving >250 tx.
Stern & Vakeva,[36] 1997	9182818	1380	Prospective cohort study. United States. Mean follow-up 19.2 y.	Not reported.	Occurrence of noncutaneous cancers among patients with psoriasis treated with PUVA compared with general population.	Overall risk of noncutaneous cancer was not different from that expected in the general population. No association between higher PUVA dose and risk of any noncutaneous cancer.

Reference						
Cockayne & August,[37] 1997	9604461	178	Retrospective chart review. United Kingdom. Mean follow-up period of 10 y (range 5–17).	24% of cohort received cumulative dose >1000 J/cm² (mean 2250 J/cm²) with mean 409 txs.	Incidence of cutaneous carcinomas in patients with psoriasis undergoing PUVA.	NMSC incidence was 169.5 times higher in PUVA group compared with Mersey Cancer Registry. All patients developing SCC had received a cumulative dose of more than 1500 J/cm² or 200 treatment sessions.
Lunder & Stern,[38] 1998	9786759	1380	Prospective cohort study. United States.	Two-thirds of the patients received >300 txs.	Incidence of Merkel cell carcinoma.	Merkel cell carcinomas have developed in 3 (0.2%) of the cohort, which is 100 times higher than expected in the general population.
Stern & Lunder,[39] 1998	9875197		Meta-analysis. Included PUVA Follow-Up Study and 8 others.	Not reported.	Risk of SCC and relation to dose of PUVA in patients with psoriasis.	Long-term, high-dose PUVA (>200 txs or 2000 J/cm²) significantly increased risk of SCC.
Hannuksela-Svahn et al,[40] 1999	10583054	944	Retrospective. Sweden/Finland. Mean follow-up period of 14.7 y.	Sweden: 4.3% received >200 txs; mean cumulative dose of 33 J/cm², mean 55 txs. Finland: 12.3% received >200 txs; mean cumulative dose of 65 J/cm², mean 112 txs.	Incidence of cancers in patients who underwent bath PUVA compared with national cancer incidence rates.	No significant increase in incidence rates of SCC, melanoma, or all noncutaneous cancers in bath PUVA group compared with national registry rates. BCC was not studied. Significant increase in standardized incidence ratio for kidney cancer and non-Hodgkin lymphoma in bath PUVA group.
Stern,[15] 2001	11312420	822	Prospective cohort study. United States. Mean follow-up period of 20.2 y.	44% received >200 txs and 35% received >250 txs.	Incidence of melanoma in patients with psoriasis treated with PUVA.	Incidence of melanoma was 6.9 times higher in the cohort studied from 1991–1998 than it was among the same cohort from 1975–1990.

(continued on next page)

Table 1
(continued)

Authors, publication year	PubMed ID	Sample Size	Study Design and Setting	Dose	Outcome Measures	Outcome
Stern et al,[41] 2002	12077578	892	Prospective cohort study. United States.	Not reported.	Incidence of genital neoplasms in men with psoriasis treated with PUVA.	52.6-fold increase in incidence of invasive penile and scrotal SCCs in PUVA patients compared with general population; 90-fold increased risk among high-dose PUVA patients compared with general population.
Nijsten & Stern,[42] 2003	12880415	1380	Prospective cohort study. United States. Mean follow-up of 20 y.	36.0% of cohort received <100 txs; 37.1% of cohort received >200 txs.	Incidence of NMSC in patients with psoriasis who have discontinued PUVA.	Risk of SCC associated with PUVA persists for at least 15 y after discontinuing PUVA. Risk of BCC continues to increase after stopping PUVA.
Murase et al,[17] 2005	16409267	4294	Retrospective review. Asia, Africa, and South America. Minimum follow-up of 5 y.	Mean number of treatments ranged by site from 12-125.5. Mean cumulative dose reported in only 2 studies: 459 and 785.2 J/cm².	Incidence of NMSC in PUVA patients in Japan, Korea, Thailand, Egypt, and Tunisia compared with country-specific incidence rates.	Relative risk of NMSC in PUVA patients compared with general population was nonsignificant in Japanese/Korean patients (RR = 0.73; CI = 0.22–1.25) and Thai/Egyptian/Tunisian patients (RR = 1.29; CI = 0–2.58).
Stern,[16] 2012	22264671	1380	Prospective cohort study. United States. Mean interval from 1st tx to most recent follow-up was 28 y.	Not reported.	Incidence of SCC and BCC in patients with psoriasis treated with PUVA.	Significant increase in risk of SCC after exposure to >350 PUVA txs. High-dose PUVA does not greatly increase BCC risk.

Abbreviations: BB-UVB, broadband ultraviolet B; BCC, basal cell carcinoma; CI, confidence interval; IRR, incidence rate ratio; NBUVB, narrowband ultraviolet B; NMSC, nonmelanoma skin cancer; PUVA, psoralen and UVA; RR, relative risk; SCC, squamous cell carcinoma; txs, treatments.

Table 2
Clinical studies on the photocarcinogenic risk of broadband (BB-) and narrowband (NB-) UVB

Authors, publication year	PubMed ID	Sample Size	Study Design & Setting	Dose	Outcome Measures	Outcome
Weischer et al,[20] 2004	15370703	BB: 69 NB: 126	Retrospective chart review. Germany. Mean follow-up of 7.8 y (range 2.4–9.3).	BB: mean 17.8 txs and 2.34 J/cm² cumulative dose. NB: mean 44.2 txs and 35.75 J/cm² cumulative dose.	Incidence of skin tumors in patients with psoriasis treated with BB-UVB or NBUVB.	BB: no skin cancers developed. NB: 1 MIS developed within 1 y of treatment. Compared with incidence of skin tumors in general German population, there is no significant increase in risk.
Man et al,[43] 2005	15840109	1908	Retrospective chart review. Scotland. Median follow-up time of 4 y (range 0.04–13).	Median 23 treatments and cumulative 13.337 J/cm² dose.	Incidence of melanoma, SCC, and BCC in patients treated with NB TL-01 UVB.	No increased incidence of melanoma or SCC. Small increase in incidence of BCC compared with general Scottish population ($P<.05$).
Lim & Stern,[21] 2005	15737190	1380	Prospective cohort study. United States.	Mean 403 UVB treatments (median 200).	Association between UVB and development of NMSC among patients with <100 PUVA txs.	Significant association between high UVB exposure (≥300 txs) and development of SCC (IRR 1.37) and BCC (IRR 1.45) compared with low UVB exposure (<300 txs) in patients with <100 PUVA txs.
Black & Gavin,[44] 2006	16445801	484	Retrospective chart review. Northern Ireland.	Not reported.	Incidence of melanoma and NMSC in patients treated with NB TL-01 UVB.	No significant increase in melanoma or NMSC in NBUVB treated group compared with general Northern Irish population.

(continued on next page)

Table 2
(continued)

Authors, publication year	PubMed ID	Sample Size	Study Design & Setting	Dose	Outcome Measures	Outcome
Hearn et al,[22] 2008	18834483	3867	Retrospective chart review. Scotland. Median follow-up 5.5 y (range 0–18 y).	Median 29 treatments. 9.1% of patients received ≥100 txs.	Incidence of melanoma, SCC, and BCC in patients treated with NB TL-01 UVB.	No significant association between NBUVB and BCC, SCC, or melanoma compared with general Scottish population.
Maiorino et al,[45] 2016	26822468	NB: 50 PUVA: 42	Retrospective. Italy. Median follow-up time of 7.1 y for PUVA and 7.9 y for NB.	NB: 34% of patients underwent ≤200 txs (mean cumulative dose 140 J/cm², 66% of patients underwent >200 txs (mean cumulative dose 2007 J/cm²).	Occurrence of melanoma and NMSC in patients with psoriasis treated with NBUVB or PUVA.	NB: 14 skin cancers identified (2 melanoma, 4 BCC, 8 SCC) in 6 patients (12%). PUVA: 9 skin cancers identified (1 melanoma, 7 BCC, 1 SCC) in 2 patients (4.7%). No comparison against incidence in general population was conducted.
Ortiz-Salvador et al,[46] 2018	29463381	474	Retrospective chart review. Spain. Mean (SD) follow-up period of 5.8 (3) y.	Mean cumulative dose of 36.6 J/cm² in patients not developing tumors and 38.2 J/cm² in patients developing tumors.	Incidence of NMSC in patients treated with whole-body NBUVB (data from at least 1 y of follow-up).	Standard incidence rate of NMSC was not significantly different from that of the general population in that geographic area. Number needed to treat with NBUVB to cause 1 case of NMSC is 1900.

Abbreviations: BB-UVB, broadband ultraviolet B; BCC, basal cell carcinoma; IRR, incidence rate ratio; NBUVB, narrowband ultraviolet B; NMSC, nonmelanoma skin cancer; PUVA, psoralen and UVA; SCC, squamous cell carcinoma; txs, treatments.

as it penetrates more deeply into the skin.[23] The mechanisms of action of UVA1 phototherapy may differ depending on the disease that is being treated. Apoptosis of skin-infiltrating CD4+ T cells induced by UVA1 likely contributes to the efficacy of UVA1 in diseases including atopic dermatitis and mycosis fungoides.[24] UVA1 induction of interstitial collagenases may promote skin softening with UVA1 phototherapy for morphea and other sclerosing conditions.[25]

UVA is the predominant wavelength in indoor tanning beds, frequent use of which is known to contribute to skin cancer risk.[26] There are no large-scale studies that have been conducted to date concerning the risk of skin cancer following UVA1 phototherapy (**Table 3**). Two case reports exist describing the development of skin cancer in patients treated with UVA1. In the first case, a patient receiving 18 months of UVA1 and bath PUVA developed a melanoma.[27] In the second, 2 immunosuppressed patients each developed a Merkel cell carcinoma soon after treatment with high-dose UVA1.[28] The simultaneous treatment with bath PUVA in the first report and the immunosuppressive comorbidities in the second report limit the interpretation of these findings.

DISCUSSION

In this study, we reviewed the available evidence concerning the risk of photocarcinogenesis following phototherapy. Although there is abundant evidence for the dose-related risk of skin cancer in PUVA, studies investigating the risk of photocarcinogenesis in UVB and UVA1 are limited to retrospective chart reviews and case reports. In addition, the patient populations studied may not be representative of the general population receiving phototherapy. These patients may already be at an inherently increased risk of developing skin cancer because of other comorbidities. Our analysis was furthermore limited by the lack of standardized outcome measures, such as follow-up period and dosing, which could be used to compare outcomes across all studies.

In patients treated with PUVA, there is a dose-dependent increase in the risk of SCC, which becomes apparent after approximately 150 treatments. The risk of BCC even in patients who received high PUVA doses is smaller than that of SCC. The increased risk of melanoma following even low doses of PUVA does not manifest until

Table 3
Clinical studies on the photocarcinogenic risk of UVA1

Authors, publication year	PubMed ID	Sample Size	Study Design & Setting	Dose	Outcome Measures	Outcome
Wallenfang & Stadler,[27] 2018	11544941	1	Case Report. Germany. [Article in German].	UVA1: 901 J/cm². Bath PUVA: 214.4 J/cm².	N/A	1 melanoma developed in patient receiving 18 mo of UVA1 and bath PUVA.
Calzavara-Pinton et al,[28] 2010	21175855	2	Case report. Italy.	Cumulative doses for each patient: 4900 J/cm² and 6900 J/cm².	N/A	2 immunosuppressed patients (1 on methotrexate and prednisone for eosinophilic fasciitis and chronic lymphocytic leukemia; 1 with myelodysplastic anemia status post bone marrow transplant) developed Merkel cell carcinoma soon after treatment with high-dose UVA1.

Abbreviations: PUVA, psoralen and ultraviolet A; UVA1, ultraviolet A1; N/A = not applicable.

approximately 15 years after initiation of PUVA. There is a paucity of evidence surrounding the risk of photocarcinogenesis in UVB and UVA1. According to available evidence, NBUVB appears to be overall the safest phototherapy modality.

These findings recommend the cautious use of phototherapy, especially PUVA, in high-risk patient populations. The risk of skin cancer should be discussed with patients before PUVA is used, and total number of treatments should be monitored and documented to guide the duration of therapy. Due to unclear and potentially persistent risk, all patients who have received phototherapy should be followed with appropriate skin cancer screenings throughout their lives.

REFERENCES

1. Gallagher RP, Lee TK, Bajdik CD, et al. Ultraviolet radiation. Chronic Dis Can 2010;29(Suppl 1):51–68.
2. Cadet J, Sage E, Douki T. Ultraviolet radiation-mediated damage to cellular DNA. Mutat Res 2005;571(1–2):3–17.
3. Valejo Coelho MM, Matos TR, Apetato M. The dark side of the light: mechanisms of photocarcinogenesis. Clin Dermatol 2016;34(5):563–70.
4. Cadet J, Douki T, Ravanat JL, et al. Sensitized formation of oxidatively generated damage to cellular DNA by UVA radiation. Photochem Photobiol Sci 2009;8(7):903–11.
5. Douki T, Reynaud-Angelin A, Cadet J, et al. Bipyrimidine photoproducts rather than oxidative lesions are the main type of DNA damage involved in the genotoxic effect of solar UVA radiation. Biochemistry 2003;42(30):9221–6.
6. Nishisgori C. Current concept of photocarcinogenesis. Photochem Photobiol Sci 2015;14(9):1713–21.
7. Weichenthal M, Schwarz T. Phototherapy: how does UV work? Photodermatol Photoimmunol Photomed 2005;21(5):260–6.
8. Schwarz T, Beissert S. Milestones in photoimmunology. J Invest Dermatol 2013;133(E1):E7–10.
9. Hart PH, Norval M. Ultraviolet radiation-induced immunosuppression and its relevance for skin carcinogenesis. Photochem Photobiol Sci 2018;17(12):1872–84.
10. Lai C, August S, Albibas A, et al. OX40+ regulatory T cells in cutaneous squamous cell carcinoma suppress effector T-cell responses and associate with metastatic potential. Clin Cancer Res 2016;22(16):4236–48.
11. Euvrard S, Kanitakis J, Claudy A. Skin cancers after organ transplantation. N Engl J Med 2003;348(17):1681–91.
12. Honigsmann H. History of phototherapy in dermatology. Photochem Photobiol Sci 2013;12(1):16–21.
13. Parrish JA, Fitzpatrick TB, Tanenbaum L, et al. Photochemotherapy of psoriasis with oral methoxsalen and longwave ultraviolet light. N Engl J Med 1974;291(23):1207–11.
14. Stern RS. Psoralen and ultraviolet A light therapy for psoriasis. N Engl J Med 2007;357(7):682–90.
15. Stern RS, PUVA Follow Up Study. The risk of melanoma in association with long-term exposure to PUVA. J Am Acad Dermatol 2001;44(5):755–61.
16. Stern RS, PUVA Follow-Up Study. The risk of squamous cell and basal cell cancer associated with psoralen and ultraviolet A therapy: a 30-year prospective study. J Am Acad Dermatol 2012;66(4):553–62.
17. Murase JE, Lee EE, Koo J. Effect of ethnicity on the risk of developing nonmelanoma skin cancer following long-term PUVA therapy. Int J Dermatol 2005;44(12):1016–21.
18. Parrish JA, Jaenicke KF. Action spectrum for phototherapy of psoriasis. J Invest Dermatol 1981;76(5):359–62.
19. Walters IB, Burack LH, Coven TR, et al. Suberythematogenic narrow-band UVB is markedly more effective than conventional UVB in treatment of psoriasis vulgaris. J Am Acad Dermatol 1999;40(6 Pt 1):893–900.
20. Weischer M, Blum A, Eberhard F, et al. No evidence for increased skin cancer risk in psoriasis patients treated with broadband or narrowband UVB phototherapy: a first retrospective study. Acta Derm Venereol 2004;84(5):370–4.
21. Lim JL, Stern RS. High levels of ultraviolet B exposure increase the risk of non-melanoma skin cancer in psoralen and ultraviolet A-treated patients. J Invest Dermatol 2005;124(3):505–13.
22. Hearn RM, Kerr AC, Rahim KF, et al. Incidence of skin cancers in 3867 patients treated with narrowband ultraviolet B phototherapy. Br J Dermatol 2008;159(4):931–5.
23. Krutmann J, Diepgen TL, Luger TA, et al. High-dose UVA1 therapy for atopic dermatitis: results of a multicenter trial. J Am Acad Dermatol 1998;38(4):589–93.
24. Morita A, Werfel T, Stege H, et al. Evidence that singlet oxygen-induced human T helper cell apoptosis is the basic mechanism of ultraviolet-A radiation phototherapy. J Exp Med 1997;186(10):1763–8.
25. Gruss C, Reed JA, Altmeyer P, et al. Induction of interstitial collagenase (MMP-1) by UVA-1 phototherapy in morphea fibroblasts. Lancet 1997;350(9087):1295–6.
26. Sample A, He YY. Mechanisms and prevention of UV-induced melanoma. Photodermatol Photoimmunol Photomed 2018;34(1):13–24.
27. Wallenfang K, Stadler R. Association between UVA1 and PUVA bat therapy and development of malignant melanoma. Hautarzt 2001;52(8):705–7.

28. Calzavara-Pinton P, Monari P, Manganoni AM, et al. Merkel cell carcinoma arising in immunosuppressed patients treated with high-dose ultraviolet A1 (320-400 nm) phototherapy: a report of two cases. Photodermatol Photoimmunol Photomed 2010; 26(5):263–5.

29. Roenigk HH Jr, Caro WA. Skin cancer in the PUVA-48 cooperative study. J Am Acad Dermatol 1981;4(3):319–24.

30. Stern RS, Laird N, Melski J, et al. Cutaneous squamous-cell carcinoma in patients treated with PUVA. N Engl J Med 1984;310(18):1156–61.

31. Forman AB, Roenigk HH Jr, Caro WA, et al. Long-term follow-up of skin cancer in the PUVA-48 cooperative study. Arch Dermatol 1989;125(4):515–9.

32. Lindelof B, Sigurgeirsson B, Tegner E, et al. PUVA and cancer: a large-scale epidemiological study. Lancet 1991;338(8759):91–3.

33. Chuang TY, Heinrich LA, Schultz MD, et al. PUVA and skin cancer. A historical cohort study on 492 patients. J Am Acad Dermatol 1992;26(2 Pt 1): 173–7.

34. McKenna KE, Patterson CC, Handley J, et al. Cutaneous neoplasia following PUVA therapy for psoriasis. Br J Dermatol 1996;134(4):639–42.

35. Stern RS, Nichols KT, Vakeva LH. Malignant melanoma in patients treated for psoriasis with methoxsalen (psoralen) and ultraviolet A radiation (PUVA). The PUVA Follow-Up Study. N Engl J Med 1997; 336(15):1041–5.

36. Stern RS, Vakeva LH, PUVA Follow-Up Study. Noncutaneous malignant tumors in the PUVA follow-up study: 1975-1996. J Invest Dermatol 1997;108(6): 897–900.

37. Cockayne SE, August PJ. PUVA photocarcinogenesis in Cheshire. Clin Exp Dermatol 1997;22(6): 300–1.

38. Lunder EJ, Stern RS. Merkel-cell carcinomas in patients treated with methoxsalen and ultraviolet A radiation. N Engl J Med 1998;339(17):1247–8.

39. Stern RS, Lunder EJ. Risk of squamous cell carcinoma and methoxsalen (psoralen) and UV-A radiation (PUVA). A meta-analysis. Arch Dermatol 1998; 134(12):1582–5.

40. Hannuksela-Svahn A, Sigurgeirsson B, Pukkala E, et al. Trioxsalen bath PUVA did not increase the risk of squamous cell skin carcinoma and cutaneous malignant melanoma in a joint analysis of 944 Swedish and Finnish patients with psoriasis. Br J Dermatol 1999;141(3):497–501.

41. Stern RS, Bagheri S, Nichols K. PUVA Follow-Up Study. The persistent risk of genital tumors among men treated with psoralen plus ultraviolet A (PUVA) for psoriasis. J Am Acad Dermatol 2002;47(1):33–9.

42. Nijsten TE, Stern RS. The increased risk of skin cancer is persistent after discontinuation of psoralen+ultraviolet A: a cohort study. J Invest Dermatol 2003;121(2):252–8.

43. Man I, Crombie IK, Dawe RS, et al. The photocarcinogenic risk of narrowband UVB (TL-01) phototherapy: early follow-up data. Br J Dermatol 2005; 152(4):755–7.

44. Black RJ, Gavin AT. Photocarcinogenic risk of narrowband ultraviolet B (TL-01) phototherapy: early follow-up data. Br J Dermatol 2006;154(3):566–7.

45. Maiorino A, De Simone C, Perino F, et al. Melanoma and non-melanoma skin cancer in psoriatic patients treated with high-dose phototherapy. J Dermatolog Treat 2016;27(5):443–7.

46. Ortiz-Salvador JM, Ferrer DS, Saneleuterio-Temporal M, et al. Photocarcinogenic risk associated with narrowband UV-B phototherapy: an epidemiologic study in a tertiary care hospital. Actas Dermosifiliogr 2018;109(4):340–5.

How It Works
The Immunology Underlying Phototherapy

Zizi Yu, BA[a], Peter Wolf, MD[b],*

KEYWORDS

- Phototherapy • UV radiation • Apoptosis • Immunosuppression • Urocanic acid
- Platelet-activating factor • IL-23/T_H17 axis • Regulatory T cells (Tregs •)

KEY POINTS

- Exposure to UV radiation triggers several initial molecular responses in the skin, including DNA damage (and subsequent apoptosis), damage to self-noncoding RNA, urocanic acid isomerization, platelet-activating factor formation, and aryl hydrocarbon receptor activation.
- Subsequent downstream events leading to UV-induced immunosuppression include decreased number and function of Langerhans cells, induction and activation of immunosuppressive regulatory T cells, and increased release of inhibitory cytokines, such as interleukin (IL)-10.
- Phototherapy (UV-B and UV-A plus psoralen) down-regulates the IL-23/ T-helper 17 (Th17) cell axis, an effect similar to that of current biologic treatment with anti–IL-17 and anti–IL-23 antibodies.
- The mechanisms of UV-induced immunosuppression counteract the immune overactivation and dysregulation underlying many cutaneous diseases, such as psoriasis, atopic dermatitis, chronic pruritus, mastocytosis, vitiligo, and polymorphous light eruption.
- Phototherapy has effects beyond the skin that can be beneficial for conditions, such as graft-versus-host disease with its cutaneous and noncutaneous manifestations.

INTRODUCTION

Despite the introduction of biologics, phototherapy has remained a mainstay for treatment of a large variety of cutaneous diseases, including psoriasis, atopic dermatitis (AD), vitiligo, mastocytosis, pruritus, and early-stage cutaneous T-cell lymphoma (CTCL). Phototherapy treatment is also given prophylactically to prevent occurrence of symptoms in photodermatoses, such as polymorphous light eruption (PLE).[1] Currently, irradiation with broadband UV-B (290–320 nm), narrowband UVB (NBUVB) (311–313 nm), UV-A1 (340–400 nm), and UV-A plus psoralen (PUVA) are used for conventional phototherapeutic purposes. This article provides an up-to-date review on the molecular responses of skin to UV exposure, the physiology of UV-induced immunosuppression, and the current understanding of therapeutic mechanisms for the cutaneous diseases most commonly treated with phototherapy.

On exposure to UV radiation, several initial molecular responses are triggered within the skin. These triggers include the formation of DNA photoproducts, damage to self-noncoding RNA, *trans*-to-*cis* urocanic acid (UCA) isomerization, production of active biophospholipids such as platelet-activating factor (PAF) and PAF-like molecules, and formation of aryl hydrocarbon receptor (AhR) ligands leading to activation of the receptor.[2]

Disclosure Statement: P. Wolf has been a consultant, lecturer, or investigator for AbbVie, Almirall, Amgen, Celgene, Eli Lilly, Leo Pharma, Janssen-Cilag, Merck Sharp & Dohme, Sandoz, Sanofi-Aventis, UCB Pharma, and Pfizer. Z. Yu has nothing to disclose.

[a] Harvard Medical School, 25 Shattuck Street, Boston, MA 02115, USA; [b] Department of Dermatology, Research Unit for Photodermatology, Medical University of Graz, Auenbruggerplatz 8, Graz A-8036, Austria
* Corresponding author.
E-mail address: peter.wolf@medunigraz.at

Dermatol Clin 38 (2020) 37–53
https://doi.org/10.1016/j.det.2019.08.004
0733-8635/20/© 2019 Elsevier Inc. All rights reserved.

These events are responsible for subsequent downstream local and systemic immunomodulatory effects that attempt to counteract the damage and stress caused by exposure to UV radiation. The multiplicity and redundancy of triggers in these chains leading to immunosuppression after UV exposure suggests that suppression of immunologic reactions to UV-altered molecules in the skin may be crucial to preventing unwanted cutaneous manifestations, such as PLE.[3]

For a better understanding of the potential therapeutic mechanisms of phototherapy, this review starts with some background information on the initial molecules involved in the response to UV radiation, in particular their significance in inducing immunosuppression. The effect of UV radiation on the immune system has recently been reviewed in great detail.[4]

INITIAL MOLECULAR RESPONSES TO UV EXPOSURE: FORMATION OF DNA PHOTOPRODUCTS, DAMAGED SELF-NONCODING RNA, CIS-UROCANIC ACID, PLATELET ACTIVATING FACTOR, PLATELET-ACTIVATING FACTOR–LIKE MOLECULES, AND ARYL HYDROCARBON RECEPTOR LIGANDS

UV radiation is absorbed in the skin by major endogenous chromophores, such as nuclear DNA, trans-UCA , and cell membranes. UV-B absorption by nucleotides leads to the formation of DNA photoproducts, primarily cyclobutane pyrimidine dimers (CPDs) and 6-4 photoproducts. Pyrimidine dimers constitute the majority of total UV radiation-induced DNA damage. UV-A also causes DNA damage indirectly through reactive oxygen species (ROS) and through the formation of unstable complexes of cyclobutane monoadducts with pyrimidine bases of native DNA, which can subsequently form in the presence of psoralen interstrand cross-links in the DNA double helix (**Table 1**).[5] UV exposure also reduces DNA synthesis and can impair DNA repair mechanisms in response to DNA damage. Moreover, it up-regulates expression of tumor suppressor gene p53, resulting in either cell-cycle arrest to allow increased time for DNA repair or apoptosis in cases of irreparable DNA damage.[5,6] Insufficient DNA repair after UV radiation exposure leads to the accumulation of CPDs, which in turn induce immunosuppression.[2] This has been discovered by the work of Kripke and colleagues[7] using the natural photoreactivation repair mechanism in the model of Monodelphis domestica or liposomes containing DNA repair enzymes as mechanistic tools to decrease the number of dimers in the skin and abrogate UV-induced immunosuppression.[8–11] UV exposure, however, also induces alterations in the double-stranded domains of some noncoding RNAs, which is sensed as a damage-associated molecular pattern (DAMP) through Toll-like receptor (TLR) 3, thereby mediating solar injury and immunosuppression.[12,13]

Exposure to UV radiation also causes photoisomerization of UCA, another important

---

Table 1
The effects of phototherapy on healthy skin

Type of Phototherapy	Molecular Events	Cellular and Downstream Events
UV-B	CPDs, damage to self-noncoding RNA (DAMP), UCA isomerization, PAF and PAF-like molecules, AhR activation[2,4]	• Induces cell-cycle arrest or keratinocyte apoptosis through up-regulation of p53[5] • Activates NF-κB leading to T-cell apoptosis[153] • Releases immunosuppressive prostaglandins and cytokines[36] • Decreases number and function of APCs[38] • Down-regulates IL-23/T_H17 and induction of Tregs[53]
UV-A1	ROS production	• Induces apoptosis of T cells through DNA damage and cell cycle arrest[93] • Decreases expression of ICAM-1[154]
PUVA	ROS production, PAF and PAF-like molecules, 8-MOP photoadducts[5]	• Induces formation of DNA monoadducts and double helix interstrand cross-links[5] • Inhibits DNA replication, causes cell cycle arrest, induces apoptosis in T cells, APCs, and keratinocytes[4] • Induces immunosuppression (ie, down-regulation of IL-23/T_H17 axis and induction of Tregs)[54] • Stimulates melanogenesis[124]

chromophore in the epidermis. UCA is synthesized as trans-UCA from histidine in a reaction catalyzed by histidase, accumulates in skin at high concentrations, and is isomerized into cis-UCA after UV absorption.[2] cis-UCA binds to the serotonin 2A receptor and exerts immunosuppressive effects by skewing the cutaneous cytokine production profile from T-helper cell (T_H)1 to a T_H2 response.[14] In vitro experiments have shown that treatment of keratinocytes with cis-UCA causes upregulation of a gene profile similar to that induced by UV exposure.[15] Cytokines and proteins that participate in apoptosis, cell-cycle arrest, and oxidative stress are also up-regulated after cis-UCA treatment, particularly nuclear factor (NF)-κB and lipid peroxidation.[15]

PAF is produced by keratinocytes in response to damage, such as UV exposure.[16,17] PAF is necessary for secretion of interleukin (IL)-10, a proregulatory T cell (Treg) cytokine important in suppression of immune responses.[17] PAF has been demonstrated to act on leukocytes to induce cyclooxygenase-2 expression, leading to generation of prostaglandins that induce IL-10 secretion by many epidermal cell types, including OX40L$^+$ antigen-presenting cells (APCs)s.[18] PAF secretion also promotes the migration of mast cells into draining lymph nodes where they play an important role in immunosuppression.[19] After PAF stimulation, mast cells undergo epigenetic modifications that increase their responsiveness to CXCR4 agonists. PAF also disrupts DNA repair mechanisms on UV radiation exposure by decreasing the expression of response elements, such as MCPH1/BRIT-1 and ATR.[20] In mice treated with PUVA, blockade of PAF receptor leads to reduced IL-10 production, less delayed-type immunosuppression in response to Candida albicans, and lower rates of keratinocyte apoptosis.[21] The binding of both cis-UCA and PAF to their respective receptors, serotonin 2A receptor and PAF receptor, contributes to sunburn cell formation, immunosuppression, and skin cancer induction on UV exposure.[21,22] Moreover, serotonin itself has been found to be involved in PUVA-induced systemic immunosuppression, as measured by delayed-type hypersensitivity to C albicans.[23]

AhR is another sensor of UV in the skin. UV generates formylindolo (3,2-b)carbazole (FICZ), a tryptophan derivative in keratinocytes that is a high-affinity ligand for AhR, serving to activate the receptor.[24] This occurs by translocation of the AhR to the nucleus, leading to gene activation.[25] Target genes, such as CYP1A1, a member of the cytochrome P450 superfamily of enzymes, are up-regulated after UV radiation exposure and

are involved in the effects of AhR activation.[26,27] AhR-knockout mice lack UV-induced immunosuppression and AhR plays a role in the induction of Tregs during T-cell differentiation in the thymus.[28–30] Moreover, AhR activation can also decrease the expression of FcεRI, the high-affinity IgE receptor, in Langerhans cells (LCs) and up-regulates immunosuppressive molecules, such as IDO-1.[31] Intriguingly, AhR signaling also can be activated by Staphylococcus epidermidis, leading to the induction of AhR-responsive CYP1A1 and production of IL-1a and human β-defensin-3 in an AhR-dependent manner.[32] Thus, AhR may be activated as a type of pattern recognition receptor but whether directly by small factors released by S epidermidis or by an increase of endogenous AhR ligands, such as FICZ, remains to be determined. Recent work indicates, however, that the microbiome of the skin interferes with UV-induced immunosuppression.[33–35] Germ-free skin shows exaggerated immunosuppression on UV exposure, linked to altered gene expression and an immunosuppressive microenvironment in skin rich in IL-10.[34]

UV-INDUCED SUPPRESSION OF THE ADAPTIVE IMMUNE RESPONSE

Immunosuppression triggered by UV exposure is likely an adaptive response to mitigate the robust immune response to the release of DAMPs in favor of the repair and remodeling of damaged tissue, as seen in animal models of brain injury and other trauma.[2] The predominate mechanisms of UV-induced immunosuppression include decreased number and function of APCs in the skin, induction and activation of immunosuppressive Tregs and increased release of inhibitory cytokines, such as tumor necrosis factor (TNF)-α and IL-10.[36] These events are all involved in complex regulatory loops of local and systemic immunomodulatory effects, with LCs, other dendritic cells (DCs), and Tregs migrating in and out of the skin, coordinating a series of events crucial for the establishment of an immunosuppressive microenvironment.[2,37]

APCs of the skin are crucial modulators of inflammatory disease, surveying the local environment for foreign antigens and pathogens and presenting them to T cells in a 2-signal process to mount an immune response. UV irradiation impairs normal APC function by disrupting dendritic networks and decreasing expression of both major histocompatibility complex molecules (signal 1) and costimulatory molecules (signal 2), weakening interactions with T cells so as to mount an effective immune response against skin-directed antigens and pathogens.[38] LCs are a subset of skin-specific APCs that link the innate and adaptive immune system through cutaneous antigen uptake and priming of T-cell responses.[2,39]

In a process linked to migrating out of the skin to the lymph nodes, LCs undergo specific changes to induce tolerance and immunosuppression. The transitory depletion of LCs from the skin is counteracted by several compensatory mechanisms, including early recruitment of CD14[+] monocytes and subsequent mobilization of 2 inflammatory subsets of DCs, CD1a[low] CD207[-], and CD1[low] CD207[+], from circulating cells in the blood.[40] In particular, CD11b-type Langerin[-] phenotype cells up-regulate CD86 after UV radiation, leading to antigen-free proliferation of Tregs and transcription of genes associated with immunotolerance.[41] Skin CD103[-] DCs also migrate into lymph nodes on UV exposure and induce Treg activation by the production of retinoic acid.[42] Induction and activation of Tregs (ie, FoxP3[+] CD4[+] Cd25[+] helper T cells) after UV exposure suggests that the role of LCs in the skin is not only to promote immune activation but also to desensitize the skin to UV exposure. Tregs inhibit inflammatory T-cell and APC function through secretion of suppressive cytokines, such as IL-10 and transforming growth factor (TGF)-β, as well as through Fas ligand–mediated apoptosis of effector T cells. UV exposure not only drives expansion of Tregs but also restores suppressive function by inducing demethylation of the Treg genome and promoting gene transcription that counteracts inflammation.[43,44] This effect is not restricted to the skin, because Tregs isolated from the blood of UV-exposed animals have a cytosine-phosphate-guanine (CpG) hypomethylation fingerprint, indicating exposure to light, and CPD-positive cells (LCs) have been found in the lymph nodes of mice exposed to UV radiation.[45]

UV exposure also induces the release of prostaglandins and cytokines. After UV exposure, keratinocytes synthesize important proinflammatory mediators such as IL-1 and TNF-α, which suppress LCs and thereby induce immunosuppression. Several cytokines with important roles in immunosuppression, such as IL-6, IL-8, IL-10, IL-12, IL-15, granulocyte-macrophage colony-stimulating factor, and prostaglandins, are released from UV-irradiated keratinocytes.[46] Prostaglandin E2 is another potent, UV-induced mediator that inhibits the expression of costimulatory molecules on the surface of APCs and thereby prevents the activation of T cells. PGE also may be responsible for effects of UV far beyond the skin, because it may have a long-lasting effect on DC progenitors in the bone marrow.[47,48]

THERAPEUTIC MECHANISMS OF PHOTOTHERAPY

The exact mechanisms behind the therapeutic benefit of phototherapy have not been fully clarified and certainly depend on both the pathophysiology of the disease as well as the modality of phototherapy prescribed. Extensive research over the years, particularly in the field of photoimmunology, has paved the way to a better understanding of how the different phototherapeutic modalities act.[4,37] Recent reviews have addressed the immunoregulatory effects of phototherapy.[2,49,50] This article elucidate the therapeutic mechanism of phototherapy in the diseases most commonly treated with it (Table 2).

Psoriasis

Psoriasis is a chronic, T$_H$17-driven inflammatory condition characterized by keratinocyte hyperproliferation and underlying dysregulation of the immune system. The therapeutic benefit of phototherapy for psoriasis is thought to derive primarily from the induction of apoptosis and promotion of immunosuppression.[49–52] Compared with normal skin, psoriatic lesions are characterized by a relative increase in T$_H$1 and T$_H$17 cytokines and a decrease in T$_H$2 cytokines.[43,53–57]

NBUVB and, in particular, PUVA, one of the most powerful antipsoriatic treatments,[58] have been found to cause apoptosis in several skin cell types in psoriasis, including epidermal T cells, dermal T cells, keratinocytes, and, to a lesser degree, LCs.[4] This apoptotic effect is predominantly mediated by DNA damage and by injury to cellular, mitochondrial, and nuclear membranes through generation of ROS.[59,60] Specifically, UV light is believed to increase cell-surface Fas-ligand expression, clustering and internalization of TNF, IL-1, and epidermal growth factor receptors on cell surfaces, and activation of CD95 surface molecules, triggering pathways that lead to apoptosis and programmed cell death.[61,62] Psoriatic lesions also were found to have lower levels of p53, a cell-cycle suppressor protein, and higher levels of cyclin D1, a cell-cycle promoter protein, than normal skin does.[63] PUVA and NBUVB–mediated normalization of both p53 and cyclin D1 in psoriatic skin may contribute to stabilization of epidermal cell turnover in psoriatic lesions. Psoriatic lesions have also been shown to have increased double-stranded RNA receptor level and activity, and exposure to NBUVB irradiation is thought to inhibit both mRNA expression and double-stranded RNA receptor synthesis.[64] Additionally, the insulinlike growth factor-binding protein 7 (IGFBP7) gene has been shown to be

Table 2
The effects of phototherapy in cutaneous disease

Disease	Therapeutic Impact of UV Radiation
Psoriasis	• Reduces DNA synthesis and cell turnover in epidermal cells[49–51] • Induces apoptosis through up-regulation of p53, DNA damage, ROS damage[5] • Causes shift away from T_H1/T_H17 inflammatory axis toward T_H2 axis[73,155,156] • Decreases epidermal/dermal T cells, keratinocytes,[67] and LCs • Increases FOXP3$^+$ cells Tregs, increases expression of IGFBP7 gene[65]
AD	• Reduces LC number and antigen-presenting function[2] • Suppresses *S aureus* colonization, reduces skin surface bacteria, reduces superantigen production, alters mRNA levels of AMPs[87] • Suppresses mast cell degranulation and histamine release[99] • Inhibits T_H1 immune responses and skews toward T_H2, can also suppress T_H2 and T22 axes[2,88] • Reduces epidermal proliferation, suppresses inflammation and inflammatory cell infiltrates, normalizes barrier proteins[87,89]
Mastocytosis and pruritus	• Suppresses mast cell degranulation and histamine release[99] • Directs mast cell cytotoxicity[2] • Induces apoptosis in skin-infiltrating mast cells[99] • Reduces propruritic IL-31[82,92] • Inhibits itch mediators in sensory/cutaneous nerves[92]
CTCL	• Damages DNA, impairs DNA repair mechanisms, and induces apoptosis to suppress malignant uncontrolled cell growth[112] • Depletes LCs and impairs LC function[112] • Alters cytokine production and adhesion molecule expression by keratinocytes[108] • Induces shift in benign T cell populations from a T_H2 to a T_H1 profile, down-regulates IL-9[114–116] • Restores natural antitumor responses lost in MF disease progression, resulting in regression of clinical disease[116] • Induces a shift of chemokines from T_H2-recruiting chemokine CCL18 to T_H1-recruiting chemokines CXCL9, CXCL10, and CXCL11[116] • Down-regulates OX40L and CD40L gene expression[116]
Vitiligo	• Enhances transcription of tyrosinase gene, up-regulates expression of proopiomelanocortin and its derivative peptides[117] • Increases proliferation of melanocytes through growth factors, such as bFGF and endothelin-1[121] • Increases melanocyte migration through expression of phosphorylated focal adhesion kinase and matrix metalloproteinase-2[121] • Increases formation and melanization of melanosomes, augments anterograde transport from melanosomes to keratinocytes[118] • Promotes Treg differentiation and activity through increased IL-10 and FoxP3 and decreased IL-17 and IL-22[123]
PLE	• Induces melanization in the skin, thickening of the stratum corneum, and immunodulation[3] • Induces UV susceptibility to LC migration from epidermis to skin-draining lymph nodes[126] • Decreases density of epidermal LCs and increases low baseline of mast cell density in the papillary dermis[129] • Increases IL-10 release, induces maturation and induction of Tregs[127–129] • Restores susceptibility to UV-induced neutrophil skin infiltration[126,133] • Increases serum vitamin D levels[134]

underexpressed in psoriatic epidermis, and increased expression levels after NBUVB suggest that IGFBP7 may be a key antiproliferative protein that controls cell migration, angiogenesis, and inflammation.[65]

Phototherapy and PUVA in particular can cause apoptosis of keratinocytes, involving p53 and Fas/Fas ligand interaction.[66] Although some studies indicate that direct keratinocyte apoptosis after UV exposure may be sufficient to clear lesional skin,[67] cleared psoriatic lesions still contain residual tissue resident memory T-cell–like populations capable of producing IL-17.[68] Memory T cells are likely responsible for recurrent psoriatic flares at the same body locations, implying that clinical resolution does not depend on complete depletion of a specific population of dysregulated cells and that there may be additional direct proapoptotic effects on keratinocytes or immunomodulatory effects playing a crucial role in clinical response.[68]

Phototherapy reverses the cytokine profile typically seen in psoriasis by shifting the immune response toward the counter-regulatory T_H2 axis and away from the T_H17 inflammatory axis.[43,53–55,69,70] NBUVB has been shown to suppress the IL-23/T_H17 axis both in animal models and in patients, with many studies showing increased IL-10 in UV-B–irradiated skin.[71,72] Administration of recombinant IL-10 into psoriatic plaques has also been shown to result in increased T_H2 cytokine expression of IL-4, IL-5, and IL-10, and decreased T_H1 cytokine expression of IL-12, TNF-α, IL-17, IL-18, IL-20, IL-22, IL-23, and interferon (IFN)-γ.[73] This is consistent with the observation that along with down-regulation of the T_H17 axis, PUVA-induced induction of Tregs in the TGF-β transgenic mouse model and blockade of Tregs by a cytotoxic T-lymphocyte–associated antigen-4 antibody entirely abrogated PUVA's antipsoriatic effect.[54] The viewpoint of investigators of several recent reviews stress the potential role of Tregs in the antipsoriatic activity of phototherapy, although clinical data are still lacking to confirm this.[49,50] As in CTCL, the therapeutic effect of phototherapy in psoriasis is limited to the site of UV exposure,[74–77] indicating that local factors, such as direct elimination of keratinocytes and/or immunocytes, are involved in the therapeutic response, in addition to systemic induction of regulatory immune cells, such as Tregs. The role of LCs in the pathophysiology of psoriasis is controversial; as in the skin of healthy subjects, UV irradiation was found to deplete LCs in nonlesional skin of psoriasis patients, possibly contributing to the therapeutic effect of phototherapy.[78,79]

Phototherapy-induced senescence involving the mammalian target of rapamycin pathway also may be involved in the therapeutic response in psoriasis.[80] There is also evidence that UV-B and PUVA irradiation leads to decreased mast cell degranulation and histamine release, which may be associated with reduction of erythema and pruritus in psoriatic lesions.[81] Moreover, the itch cytokine IL-31 has been found to be down-regulated in the serum of psoriasis patients after NBUVB phototherapy.[82]

Under certain conditions and on a particular genetic background, however, phototherapy may aggravate psoriasis through propsoriatic activity, including increased DAMP/pathogen-associated molecular pattern response; activation of TLRs; inflammasome activation; microRNA dysregulation; induction of certain antimicrobial peptides (AMPs), such as HBD2, HBD3, S100A7, and cathelicidin peptide LL-37; and production and release of inflammatory cytokines, such as TNF-α and IL-6, as well as prostaglandins.[52] It remains to be determined whether certain polymorphisms in the IL-10 gene may play a role in the susceptibility of skin diseases to respond to phototherapy.[83,84] Other polymorphisms, such as at the TNF-α locus, IL-1β, or glutathione S-transferase genotype, may determine sensitivity to UV as well.[4,85]

Atopic Dermatitis

AD is a common inflammatory skin disease characterized by immune activation, marked epidermal hyperplasia, and a defective barrier function, reflecting underlying changes in keratinocyte differentiation. AD is predominantly a T_H2/T22-polarized disease with a component of T_H1 polarization in the chronic phase, along with a relative impairment of the T_H17 pathway.[86–89] Theories for AD pathogenesis include the outside-in hypothesis, in which primary barrier dysfunction (with low expression of filaggrin as well as aberrant regulation of other barrier proteins, such as loricrin and involucrin) leads to immune polarization, and the inside-out hypothesis, in which epidermal abnormalities arise secondary to underlying immune dysregulation.[87,89,90]

Acute AD lesions are characterized by profound increases in T_H2 cytokine levels (IL-4, IL-5, IL-13, IL-31, and CCL18) and T_H22 (IL-22 and S100A proteins) responses, and the T22 cytokine IL-22 has been found to induce epidermal hyperplasia and inhibit keratinocyte terminal differentiation.[89] Chronic lesions are characterized by even more intensified T_H2 and T_H22 responses with parallel activation of the T_H1 axis (IFN-γ, CXCL9, and CXCL10 cytokines) rather than a complete switch to a T_H1-only signature.[91] T_H2 polarization also facilitates S aureus colonization, and IL-4 and IL-13 inhibit skin production of AMPs, both of which contribute to and exacerbate the impaired barrier function of the skin.[87] Phototherapy functions to inhibit inflammation, induce release of immunosuppressive cytokines and normalize the skin barrier in AD. Intriguingly, AhR activation (by UV radiation) also may lead to the up-regulation of barrier proteins, such as filaggrin.[90]

UV-B creates an immunosuppressive effect by decreasing APC number and function, reducing inflammatory cell infiltrates, and inducing release of immunosuppressive cytokines. UV radiation is known to inhibit T_H1 immune responses and skew immune reactions toward a T_H2 phenotype.[2] Although atopy generally is regarded as a T_H2-driven disease, chronic AD exhibits a significant T_H1 reaction that resembles a delayed-type hypersensitivity response.[88] For this reason most likely, chronic AD lesions have been shown to respond to the immunomodulationg effects of UV-B.[88] NBUVB has been shown to suppress inflammatory cell infiltrates in AD skin, with significant reductions in $CD3^+$ and $CD8^+$ T cells as well as numerous DC subsets.[89] Lower numbers of eosinophils and mast cells also have been detected after NBUVB. Reversal of disease activity with NBUVB has been shown to be most strongly associated with elimination of $CD8^+$ T cells and several DC subsets as well as reduction of the cytokine IL-22 and the T_H2 chemokines CCL17, CCL18, and CCL22.[89] The fact that NBUVB induces strong suppression of the T_H2 and T22 axes in AD suggests that NBUVB can suppress activated or polarized T-cell immune pathways in a nonselective manner, as evidenced by its utility in a wide variety of inflammatory cutaneous diseases.

Similarly, PUVA and UV-A1 may act through immunosuppression by inhibiting inflammation and inflammatory cell infiltrates. Although long-term use for AD is discouraged, PUVA induces photoadducts (mainly monoadducts and DNA crosslinks) that inhibit cell proliferation and cause T-cell apoptosis and necrosis (at higher doses). It also reduces epidermal hyperinnervation in AD and may target pruritus.[92] UV-A1 also causes T-cell apoptosis, depletion of T cells from cutaneous lesions, and reduction in TNF-α, IL-12, INF-γ, and intercellular adhesion molecule-1 (ICAM-1).[93] Intriguingly, in some patients, NBUVB phototherapy is more effective than UV-A1 in diminishing the severity of the skin changes of AD, whereas in other patients the latter treatment modality is more effective.[94] Currently, however, predictive markers for the differential response to the different types of phototherapy are lacking. In patients with severe AD, treatment with oral PUVA using 5-methoxypsoralen (MOP), a less erythematogenic treatment than 8-MOP, seems to produce the most satisfactory results in this condition.[95] This indicates that the erythema component of phototherapy and the molecular mechanisms linked to it are dispensable for the efficacy of the treatment, at least in AD.

As discussed previously, phototherapy also plays a critical role in restoring epidermal barrier homeostasis in AD. Mechanistic studies have found that NBUVB induces genomic reversal of epidermal hyperplasia, reduction of pathologic epidermal proliferation, and normalization of barrier proteins.[89] Many of the overexpressed T_H2 cytokines and mediators have been demonstrated to down-regulate terminal differentiation genes and tight junction products, such as claudins, contributing to the barrier defect in patients with AD.[87] Histologic evaluation has revealed increased granular layer expression of lorocrin, filaggrin, and involucrin after NBUVB therapy.[89] NBUVB also may reduce skin surface bacteria and superantigen production and alter mRNA levels of AMPs, all of which have been shown to be involved in AD.[87] Importantly, UV irradiation has been shown to induce AMPs (such as BD3, a homologue to the human BD2, and cathelicidin-related AMP).[4,96,97] Such UV-induced AMPs may play a role in modifying the skin microbiome (eg, through reduction of colonization by S aureus) and thereby diminish skin manifestation of AD.[98]

Mastocytosis and Pruritus

Mastocytosis represents a group of rare disorders characterized by an abnormal proliferation of abnormal mast cells in one or more tissues, involving mainly the skin, bone marrow, gastrointestinal tract, and liver.[99] Urticaria pigmentosa, the most common cutaneous form of the disease, is most often treated by phototherapy. Both cutaneous and systemic symptoms of mastocytosis (such as wheals) are caused by the local accumulation and release of secretory products from activated and hyperproliferating mast cells.[99]

NBUVB, UV-A1, and PUVA may allow for direct cytotoxicity against activated mast cells and stabilize mast cells, inhibiting them from releasing soluble proinflammatory mediators, such as histamine.[2] Mast cells can be driven toward apoptosis in response to irradiation with UV-B or UV-A1, an effect that occurs in a dose-dependent manner. There is also evidence of decreased mast cell degranulation and histamine release from UV-B irradiated skin in animal models.[99] This may occur through altered membrane function and changes in intracellular Ca^+ content as well as through noncytotoxic damage to membrane phospholipid metabolism, which is tied to the degranulation mechanism.[100,101] Additionally, PUVA can affect not only epidermal cells but also resident mast cells and circulating cells, such as basophils. PUVA inhibits the in vitro release of histamine from human skin mast cells, and 8-MOP alone not followed by UV-A irradiation can inhibit mediator release from skin mast cells and basophils.[102]

Overall, PUVA has been shown to reduce the histamine content of the skin.[103]

Phototherapy's mechanism of action in pruritus is unknown but may be at least comediated through UV-B-induced reduction of levels of propruritic IL-31.[92] Systemic IL-31 levels were found to be down-regulated after NBUVB treatment in psoriasis, a condition often accompanied by itch.[82] Another hypothesis is that UV irradiation affects multiple mediators from the sensory nerves as well as resident and infiltrating cells. These mediators interact extensively with the cutaneous nerves and cells, eventually leading to an inhibition of itch perception and signaling to the brain.[92] In addition, a yet unknown UV-induced soluble antipruritic factor from the skin may reach the peripheral as well as the central nervous system and contribute to the inhibition of itch signaling and perception.[92] Regardless of the exact mechanism, the antipruritic effect of phototherapy is likely systemic, because even nonirradiated areas have been found to respond to an equal degree.[2]

Cutaneous T-cell Lymphoma

CTCL is a heterogeneous group of non-Hodgkin lymphomas characterized by malignant clonal proliferation of T cells in the skin. The pathogenesis of mycosis fungoides (MF), the most common form of CTCL, and Sézary syndrome, the leukemic form of CTCL, is thought to relate to a combination of genetic and environmental factors interplaying with the immune response. Constitutive activation of the NF-κB pathway has been observed in MF, leading to increased transcription of DNA, cytokine production, and cell survival.[104,105] MF is also believed to result at least in part from chronic antigenic stimulation leading to uncontrolled clonal expansion and accumulation of memory helper T cells in the skin. Although increased numbers of DCs and up-regulation of APC ligands B7 and CD40 and their respective T-cell costimulatory ligands CD28 and CD40L have been found in MF lesions, no specific antigen or pathogen has been identified to play a decisive role in the pathogenesis of the disease.[105,106] S aureus colonization of the skin has been linked, however, to erythrodermic CTCL.[107] With regard to immunopathology, keratinocyte expression of the adhesion molecule ICAM-1 has been shown to be up-regulated in epidermotropic areas and down-regulated in loss of epidermotropism.[108] Neoplastic T cells in CTCL are derived from CD4+ T cells with a T_H2 cytokine profile characterized by production of IL-4, IL-5, and IL-10.[105,106,109] A shift from a predominantly T_H1 cytokine profile to a T_H2 cytokine profile with progression of MF has been suggested, with increased levels of T_H2 cytokines impairing the T_H1 cell-mediated antitumor response.[105,106,109]

Treatment options for CTCL are diverse, ranging from skin-directed treatments to systemic therapy, and depend on the severity of disease and the type of lesions. UV-B has a high success rate in patients with early patch-stage lesions, whereas PUVA can also be effective in patients with plaque-stage and even early tumor-stage lesions, presumably due to the deeper penetration of UV-A into the dermis.[2,110,111] The clinical benefit of phototherapy in CTCL has been thought to be due to direct tumor cell apoptosis, inhibition of APC function, depletion of LCs from the skin, and suppression of cytokine production.[112] As demonstrated recently, PUVA can affect systemic levels of certain cytokines and chemokines in MF patients; soluble chemotactic factors, such as CXCL9, CXCL11 to 13, TNFSF13, and TWEAK, can serve as potential biomarkers for therapeutic response to PUVA.[113] PUVA has also been shown to down-regulate IL-9 in lesional MF skin, and anti–IL-9 treatment successfully reduced tumor growth in a skin lymphoma mouse model.[114] By weakening APC–T-cell interactions and depleting LCs from the skin, phototherapy may decrease cutaneous inflammation and suppress immune responses to antigens in the skin of CTCL. NBUVB also has been shown to decrease expression of ICAM-1, potentially inhibiting the epidermotropic tendencies of malignant T cells.[45] Moreover, it also may kill S aureus and hereby diminish stimulation of inflammatory and/or malignant T cells.[98]

Recent work showed that PUVA induces a shift in benign T-cell populations from a T_H2 to a T_H1 profile, potentially restoring natural antitumor responses lost in MF disease progression and resulting in regression of clinical disease.[115,116] Intriguingly, benign T cells were found to be associated with the T_H2-recruiting chemokine CCL18 before therapy and with the T_H1-recruiting chemokines CXCL9, CXCL10, and CXCL11 after therapy, suggesting a switch from T_H2 to T_H1 phenotype.[116] Moreover, skin inflammation correlated with OX40L and CD40L gene expression, and these receptors localized to CCL18-expressing c-Kit+ DCs that clustered together with CD40+ OX40+ benign and CD40+ CD40L+ malignant T cells.[116] Together, this suggests a proinflammatory synapse in skin between malignant T cells, benign T cells, and c-Kit–expressing DCs. Visible inflammation in MF likely results from the recruitment and activation of benign T cells by c-Kit+ OX40L+ CD40 L+ DCs, which may provide tumorigenic signals.[116] Targeting c-Kit, OX40, and

CD40 signaling may thus be novel therapeutic avenues for the treatment of MF.

Vitiligo

The pathogenesis of vitiligo is complex and multifactorial, including genetic components. Theories on the pathophysiology of vitiligo implicate nervous system dysfunction and intrinsic melanocyte deficiencies in morphology, adhesive properties, and growth factors.[117–119] The most commonly accepted prevailing theory is that of autoimmune-related destruction of melanocytes, which can be mediated by cellular immunity through CD8[+] T cells directed against melanocytic antigens, linked to the action of increased expression of TNF-α and IFN-γ, suggesting a T_H1 response, and/or humoral antibody-mediated immunity against tyrosinase, tyrosine hydroxylase, pigment cell surface antigens, and thyroid antigens.[117]

Proliferation of melanocytes is induced by increased release of melanocyte growth factors, such as basic fibroblast growth factor (bFGF) and endothelin-1 from keratinocytes after NBUVB therapy.[120] Vitiliginous lesions have been shown to have lower levels of bFGF.[121] Melanocyte migration is also stimulated by expression of phosphorylated focal adhesion kinase and matrix metalloproteinase-2.[120] NBUVB induces transcription of tyrosinase via micropthalmia-associated transcription factor, up-regulates expression of proopiomelanocortin and its derivative peptides within keratinocytes and melanocytes, and stimulates melanocyte dendricity and melanosome transport to keratinocytes.[118] In addition, NBUVB enhances melanosome transport to keratinocytes in a process mediated by increased Rac1 activity, augmented anterograde transport due to increased kinesin-to-dynein ratio, and up-regulation of protease-activated receptor-2.[119,122]

With regard to immunomodulation, phototherapy induces production of IL-10 in the epidermis, which promotes differentiation of Tregs that subsequently suppress autoreactive T cells. Restoration of the balance between T_H17 cells and Tregs has been proposed as one potential pathway for the clinical improvement seen in vitiligo patients after NBUVB, because treatment with NBUVB can significantly reduce IL-17 and IL-22 levels and increase FoxP3 levels in lesional and perilesional skin of vitiligo patients.[123]

PUVA also stimulates proliferation of melanocytes that repopulate the epidermis, increases synthesis of tyrosinase via stimulation of cAMP activity, enhances formation and melanization of melanosomes, and enhances transfer of melanosomes to keratinocytes.[124]

Polymorphous Light Eruption

PLE is a photosensitive disorder characterized by an intermittent eruption of nonscarring erythematous papules, vesicles, or plaques that develop within hours of UV exposure of the skin.[3,125] The immunologic mechanisms underlying PLE share features with those of allergic contact dermatitis and delayed-type hypersensitivity reactions.[125] The pathophysiology of PLE is thought to relate to a failure of apoptosis and a failure of immunosuppression linked to LC resistance and impaired neutrophil infiltration of the skin on UV exposure. Lower expression of genes associated with apoptotic cell clearance, such as complement 1s subunit, scavenger receptor B1, fibronectin, immunoglobulin superfamily member 3, caspase-1, and paraoxonase 2, have been found in PLE patients.[125] Both photoinduced neoantigens and autoantigens deriving from inefficient clearance of apoptotic cells may be taken up by DCs and presented to naïve T cells, resulting in autoreactive T cells.

Phototherapy, most often with NBUVB, is administered prophylactically in the early spring to protect patients against PLE during the summer season. The mechanisms underlying the photohardening effect most likely include melanization in the skin, thickening of the stratum corneum, and, most importantly, immunodulation.[3] Prophylactic UV photohardening in PLE patients restores susceptibility to UV-induced LC migration from the epidermis to the skin-draining lymph nodes as well as neutrophilic skin infiltration, key cellular events in UV-induced immunosuppression.[126] Furthermore, an immunosuppressive microenvironment may be induced by the release of cytokines, such as IL-10 and by the maturation and induction of Tregs.[127,128]

Moreover, photohardening has been shown to transiently decrease the density of epidermal LCs and significantly increase a low baseline of mast cell density in the papillary dermis of PLE patients.[129] Although traditionally associated with atopy, mast cells accumulate at sites of acute and chronic sun exposure and also have the capacity to induce immunologic tolerance. This suggests that LC suppression and recruitment of mast cells into photohardened skin may be the key cellular events underlying the mechanism by which phototherapy protects from PLE.[2,3,129] That mast cells may indeed play a crucial role in the pathophysiology of PLE is consistent with findings from a mouse model in which they were required to suppress itch on UV exposure.[130,131] Photohardening can also induce normalization of systemic cytokine levels (in particular IL-1β) and neutrophil chemotactic responsiveness.[132,133]

PLE patients also have demonstrated low levels of vitamin D, and prophylactic UV-B can induce increased vitamin D serum levels.[134] Intriguingly, a clinical trial has shown that one week of topical treatment with calcipotriol, a vitamin D analog, can reduce the photoprovocative effect of simulated sun exposure and decrease PLE disease severity.[135] Topical vitamin D_3 has multiple effects, however, including modulation of adaptive and acquired immunity as well as potential influences on the local microbiome that may be involved in triggering or aggravating the symptoms of PLE.[136,137] Furthermore, it remains to be investigated whether photohardening in PLE may exert at least some of its effects by down-regulating the itch cytokine IL-31.[138]

Other Phototherapy-responsive Cutaneous and Systemic Disorders

The list of phototherapy-responsive diseases is long and contains much more than the most commonly treated model disorders covered in this. The phototherapeutic armamentarium not only offers treatment of many other diseases, such as lichen planus, prurigo, chronic urticaria, granuloma annulare, sarcoid, lymphomatoid papulosis, pityriasis lichenoides chronica, and graft-versus-host disease (GVHD), but also stretches in particular with UV-A1 into the area of fibrotic skin conditions, including lichen sclerosus, localized scleroderma, systemic sclerosis, and nephrogenic fibrosis.[139–142] In all those diseases, the therapeutic action may rely on the phototherapy's proapoptotic and/or immunosuppressive properties, alone or in combination, depending on the disease. In the fibrotic conditions, a direct effect of UV-A1 on fibroblasts and collagen may be responsible for therapeutic efficacy.[143] UV-A1 can induce changes in fibroblast cytokine production, such as TGF-β/Smad signaling and IL-6, leading to up-regulation of collagenase activity and thus resulting in reduced tissue fibrosis.[143]

The effects of phototherapy, however, go far beyond the skin. For instance, phototherapy-induced prostaglandins may affect myeloid and progenitor DCs in the bone marrow,[47,48] an effect that may be useful to treat certain systemic diseases through immunomodulation. Although extracorporeal photopheresis has long been used in the treatment of the cutaneous and extracutaneous symptoms of GVHD,[144] recent experimental evidence suggests that NBUVB exposure of the skin alone also may be a therapeutic option for systemic symptoms of GVHD, particularly in the presence of intestinal involvement.[145] Moreover, experimental evidence and clinical data indicate that UV-B phototherapy may be beneficial for the treatment of clinically isolated syndromes or multiple sclerosis.[146,147]

DUAL ACTION OF PHOTOTHERAPY: MOST LIKELY RESPONSIBLE FOR LONG-LASTING EFFECTS

Poriasis and CTCL, 2 model diseases responding to phototherapy, are characterized by long lasting remission after stopping phototherapy. For instance, a study by Yones and colleagues[148] revealed that the median time to recurrence after stopping PUVA treatment in chronic plaque-type psoriasis was 8 months, a favorable outcome in comparison to recurrence after stopping treatment with anti–IL-17 or anti–IL-23 antibody, the latest generation of biologics (in contrast to anti-TNF agents).[149–152] Most likely, as in the case of anti-IL-17 and anti-IL-23 treatment, the dual action of phototherapy (in particular PUVA) on keratinocytes and immune cells may be responsible for the sustained resolution of psoriatic disease after stopping treatment (**Fig. 1**). This is in line with the fact that the effect of phototherapy in psoriasis is limited to the site of exposure, indicating that a direct effect on keratinocytes (eg, apoptosis)[67] may work in synergy with a systemic effect of the treatment on immune cells.

SUMMARY AND PERSPECTIVES

Phototherapy in its many forms has maintained a prominent place in the therapeutic armamentarium of dermatology as a powerful and suitably safe first-line therapy for a wide variety of both inflammatory and malignant skin diseases. Initial UV exposure triggers several molecular responses that lead to apoptosis[67] and subsequent downstream local and systemic immunomodulatory effects.[2,49,50] The diverse mechanisms of UV-induced immunosuppression counteract the immune overactivation and dysregulation underlying many cutaneous diseases, such as psoriasis, AD, mastocytosis, and vitiligo. Only recently have the therapeutic mechanisms of PUVA in CTCL been unraveled through the discovery that visible inflammation in CTCL results from the recruitment and activation of benign T cells by c-Kit+ OX40L+ CD40L+ DCs and that this activation may provide tumorigenic signals.[116] Further research on phototherapeutic mechanisms will help to advance, optimize, and refine treatment strategies in the field of dermatology and beyond.

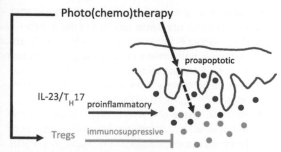

Fig. 1. Schematic presentation of psoriasis as a model for photo(chemo)therapy-responsive disease. Dual action of phototherapy on lesions leads to apoptosis of keratinocytes and immune cells and induces Tregs and an immune-suppressive microenvironment. In turn, IL-23/T$_H$17 axis is down-regulated, resulting in long-lasting lesion clearance.

ACKNOWLEDGMENTS

The authors would like to thank Dr Honnovara N. Ananthaswamy, Houston, Texas, for critical reading and Jude Richard, Austin, Texas, for editing the article.

REFERENCES

1. Richard EG, Hönigsmann H. Phototherapy, psoriasis, and the age of biologics. Photodermatol Photoimmunol Photomed 2014. https://doi.org/10.1111/phpp.12088.
2. Vieyra-Garcia PA, Wolf P. From early immunomodulatory triggers to immunosuppressive outcome: therapeutic implications of the complex interplay between the wavebands of sunlight and the skin. Front Med (Lausanne) 2018;5. https://doi.org/10.3389/fmed.2018.00232.
3. Gruber-Wackernagel A, Byrne SN, Wolf P. Polymorphous light eruption: clinic aspects and pathogenesis. Dermatol Clin 2014. https://doi.org/10.1016/j.det.2014.03.012.
4. Bernard JJ, Gallo RL, Krutmann J. Photoimmunology: how ultraviolet radiation affects the immune system. Nat Rev Immunol 2019. https://doi.org/10.1038/s41577-019-0185-9.
5. Hönigsmann H. Phototherapy for psoriasis. Clin Exp Dermatol 2001;26(4):343–50. https://doi.org/10.1046/j.1365-2230.2001.00828.x.
6. Bäckvall H, Asplund A, Gustafsson A, et al. Genetic tumor archeology: microdissection and genetic heterogeneity in squamous and basal cell carcinoma. Mutat Res 2005. https://doi.org/10.1016/j.mrfmmm.2004.10.011.
7. Kripke ML, Cox PA, Alas LG, et al. Pyrimidine dimers in DNA initiate systemic immunosuppression in UV-irradiated mice. Proc Natl Acad Sci U S A 2006. https://doi.org/10.1073/pnas.89.16.7516.
8. Applegate LA, Ley RD, Alcalay J, et al. Identification of the molecular target for the suppression of contact hypersensitivity by ultraviolet radiation. J Exp Med 1989. https://doi.org/10.1084/jem.170.4.1117.
9. Wolf P, Cox P, Yarosh DB, et al. Sunscreens and T4N5 liposomes differ in their ability to protect against ultraviolet-induced sunburn cell formation, alterations of dendritic epidermal cells, and local suppression of contact hypersensitivity. J Invest Dermatol 1995. https://doi.org/10.1111/1523-1747.ep12612828.
10. Wolf P, Yarosh DB, Kripke ML. Effects of sunscreens and a DNA excision repair enzyme on ultraviolet radiation-induced inflammation, immune suppression, and cyclobutane pyrimidine dimer formation in mice. J Invest Dermatol 1993. https://doi.org/10.1111/1523-1747.ep12365902.
11. Stege H, Roza L, Vink AA, et al. Enzyme plus light therapy to repair DNA damage in ultraviolet-Birradiated human skin. Proc Natl Acad Sci U S A 2000. https://doi.org/10.1073/pnas.030528897.
12. Bernard JJ, Cowing-Zitron C, Nakatsuji T, et al. Ultraviolet radiation damages self noncoding RNA and is detected by TLR3. Nat Med 2012. https://doi.org/10.1038/nm.2861.
13. Duthie MS, Kimber I, Norval M. The effects of ultraviolet radiation on the human immune system. Br J Dermatol 1999. https://doi.org/10.1046/j.1365-2133.1999.02898.x.
14. Walterscheid JP, Nghiem DX, Kazimi N, et al. Cis-urocanic acid, a sunlight-induced immunosuppressive factor, activates immune suppression via the 5-HT2A receptor. Proc Natl Acad Sci U S A 2006. https://doi.org/10.1073/pnas.0603119103.
15. Kaneko K, Smetana-Just U, Matsui M, et al. cis-urocanic acid initiates gene transcription in primary human keratinocytes. J Immunol 2014. https://doi.org/10.4049/jimmunol.181.1.217.
16. Marathe GK, Johnson C, Billings SD, et al. Ultraviolet B radiation generates platelet-activating factor-like phospholipids underlying cutaneous damage. J Biol Chem 2005. https://doi.org/10.1074/jbc.M503811200.
17. Walterscheid JP, Ullrich SE, Nghiem DX. Platelet-activating Factor, a Molecular Sensor for Cellular Damage, Activates Systemic Immune Suppression. J Exp Med 2002. https://doi.org/10.1084/jem.20011450.
18. Shreedhar V, Giese T, Sung VW, et al. A cytokine cascade including prostaglandin E2, IL-4, and IL-10 is responsible for UV-induced systemic immune suppression. J Immunol 1998.
19. Chacon-Salinas R, Chen L, Chavez-Blanco AD, et al. An essential role for platelet-activating factor in activating mast cell migration following ultraviolet irradiation. J Leukoc Biol 2013. https://doi.org/10.1189/jlb.0811409.

20. Puebla-Osorio N, Damiani E, Bover L, et al. Platelet-activating factor induces cell cycle arrest and disrupts the DNA damage response in mast cells. Cell Death Dis 2015. https://doi.org/10.1038/cddis.2015.115.

21. Wolf P, Nghiem DX, Walterscheid JP, et al. Platelet-activating factor is crucial in psoralen and ultraviolet A-induced immune suppression, inflammation, and apoptosis. Am J Pathol 2006. https://doi.org/10.2353/ajpath.2006.060079.

22. Sreevidya CS, Khaskhely NM, Fukunaga A, et al. Inhibition of photocarcinogenesis by platelet-activating factor or serotonin receptor antagonists. Cancer Res 2008. https://doi.org/10.1158/0008-5472.CAN-07-6132.

23. Wolf P, Byrne SN, Limon-Flores AY, et al. Serotonin signalling is crucial in the induction of PUVA-induced systemic suppression of delayed-type hypersensitivity but not local apoptosis or inflammation of the skin. Exp Dermatol 2016. https://doi.org/10.1111/exd.12990.

24. Fritsche E, Schafer C, Calles C, et al. Lightning up the UV response by identification of the arylhydrocarbon receptor as a cytoplasmatic target for ultraviolet B radiation. Proc Natl Acad Sci U S A 2007. https://doi.org/10.1073/pnas.0701764104.

25. Memari B, Nguyen-Yamamoto L, Salehi-Tabar R, et al. Endocrine aryl hydrocarbon receptor signaling is induced by moderate cutaneous exposure to ultraviolet light. Sci Rep 2019;9(1):8486. https://doi.org/10.1038/s41598-019-44862-4.

26. Navid F, Bruhs A, Schuller W, et al. The aryl hydrocarbon receptor is involved in UVR-Induced immunosuppression. J Invest Dermatol 2013. https://doi.org/10.1038/jid.2013.221.

27. Park SL, Justiniano R, Williams JD, et al. The tryptophan-derived endogenous aryl hydrocarbon receptor ligand 6-formylindolo[3,2-b]carbazole is a nanomolar UVA photosensitizer in epidermal keratinocytes. J Invest Dermatol 2015;135(6):1649–58. https://doi.org/10.1038/jid.2014.503.

28. Jux B, Kadow S, Esser C. Langerhans cell maturation and contact hypersensitivity are impaired in aryl hydrocarbon receptor-null mice. J Immunol 2009. https://doi.org/10.4049/jimmunol.0713344.

29. Quintana FJ, Basso AS, Iglesias AH, et al. Control of Treg and TH17 cell differentiation by the aryl hydrocarbon receptor. Nature 2008. https://doi.org/10.1038/nature06880.

30. Ye J, Qiu J, Bostick JW, et al. The aryl hydrocarbon receptor preferentially marks and promotes gut regulatory T cells. Cell Rep 2017. https://doi.org/10.1016/j.celrep.2017.10.114.

31. Koch S, Stroisch TJ, Vorac J, et al. AhR mediates an anti-inflammatory feedback mechanism in human Langerhans cells involving FcεRI and IDO. Allergy 2017. https://doi.org/10.1111/all.13170.

32. Rademacher F, Simanski M, Hesse B, et al. Staphylococcus epidermidis activates aryl hydrocarbon receptor signaling in human keratinocytes: implications for cutaneous defense. J Innate Immun 2019. https://doi.org/10.1159/000492162.

33. Patra VK, Byrne SN, Wolf P. The skin microbiome: Is it affected by UV-induced immune suppression? Front Microbiol 2016;7:1–11. https://doi.org/10.3389/fmicb.2016.01235.

34. Patra V, Wagner K, Arulampalam V, et al. Skin microbiome modulates the effect of ultraviolet radiation on cellular response and immune function. iScience 2019. https://doi.org/10.1016/j.isci.2019.04.026.

35. Patra V, Laoubi L, Nicolas J-F, et al. A perspective on the interplay of ultraviolet-radiation, skin microbiome and skin resident memory TCRαβ+ cells. Front Med 2018. https://doi.org/10.3389/fmed.2018.00166.

36. Wolf P, Maier H, Müllegger RR, et al. Topical treatment with liposomes containing T4 endonuclease V protects human skin in vivo from ultraviolet-induced upregulation of interleukin-10 and tumor necrosis factor-α. J Invest Dermatol 2000. https://doi.org/10.1046/j.1523-1747.2000.00839.x.

37. Gibbs NK, Norval M. Photoimmunosuppression: A brief overview. Photodermatol Photoimmunol Photomed 2013. https://doi.org/10.1111/phpp.12021.

38. Aubin F. Mechanisms involved in ultraviolet light-induced immunosuppression. Eur J Dermatol 2003;13(6):515–23.

39. Singh TP, Zhang HH, Borek I, et al. Monocyte-derived inflammatory Langerhans cells and dermal dendritic cells mediate psoriasis-like inflammation. Nat Commun 2016. https://doi.org/10.1038/ncomms13581.

40. Achachi A, Vocanson M, Bastien P, et al. UV radiation induces the epidermal recruitment of dendritic cells that compensate for the depletion of Langerhans cells in human skin. J Invest Dermatol 2015. https://doi.org/10.1038/jid.2015.118.

41. Yamazaki S, Odanaka M, Nishioka A, et al. Ultraviolet B–induced maturation of CD11b-type Langerin⁻ dendritic cells controls the expansion of Foxp3+ regulatory T cells in the skin. J Immunol 2018;200(1):119–29. https://doi.org/10.4049/jimmunol.1701056.

42. Guilliams M, Crozat K, Henri S, et al. Skin-draining lymph nodes contain dermis-derived CD103. Blood 2010;115(10):1–3. https://doi.org/10.1182/blood-2009-09-245274.

43. Furuhashi T, Saito C, Torii K, et al. Photo(chemo) therapy reduces circulating Th17 cells and restores circulating regulatory T cells in psoriasis. PLoS One 2013. https://doi.org/10.1371/journal.pone.0054895.

44. Yamazaki S, Nishioka A, Kasuya S, et al. Homeostasis of thymus-derived Foxp3 + regulatory T cells is controlled by ultraviolet B exposure in the skin. J Immunol 2014. https://doi.org/10.4049/jimmunol. 1400985.

45. Vink AA. Localization of DNA damage and its role in altered antigen-presenting cell function in ultraviolet-irradiated mice. J Exp Med 2004. https://doi.org/10.1084/jem.183.4.1491.

46. Bulat V, Situm M, Dediol I. The mechanisms of action of phototherapy in the treatment of the most common dermatoses. Coll Antropol 2011;35 Suppl 2:147–51.

47. Ng RLX, Scott NM, Bisley JL, et al. Characterization of regulatory dendritic cells differentiated from the bone marrow of UV-irradiated mice. Immunology 2013. https://doi.org/10.1111/imm.12145.

48. Scott NM, Ng RLX, Gorman S, et al. Prostaglandin E 2 imprints a long-lasting effect on dendritic cell progenitors in the bone marrow. J Leukoc Biol 2014. https://doi.org/10.1189/jlb.0513294.

49. Buhl T, Schön MP. Peeking into immunoregulatory effects of phototherapy. Exp Dermatol 2016. https://doi.org/10.1111/exd.13020.

50. Morita A. Current developments in phototherapy for psoriasis. J Dermatol 2018. https://doi.org/10. 1111/1346-8138.14213.

51. Stern RS. Psoralen and ultraviolet A light therapy for psoriasis. N Engl J Med 2007. https://doi.org/ 10.1056/NEJMct072317.

52. Wolf P, Weger W, Patra VK, et al. Desired response to phototherapy vs photoaggravation in psoriasis: what makes the difference? Exp Dermatol 2016. https://doi.org/10.1111/exd.13137.

53. Singh TP, Schön MP, Wallbrecht K, et al. Involvement of IL-9 in Th17-associated inflammation and angiogenesis of psoriasis. PLoS One 2013. https://doi.org/10.1371/journal.pone.0051752.

54. Singh TP, Schon MP, Wallbrecht K, et al. 8-Methoxypsoralen plus Ultraviolet A therapy acts via inhibition of the IL-23/Th17 axis and induction of Foxp3+ regulatory T cells involving CTLA4 signaling in a psoriasis-like skin disorder. J Immunol 2010; 184(12):7257–67. https://doi.org/10.4049/ jimmunol.0903719.

55. Rácz E, Prens EP, Kurek D, et al. Effective treatment of psoriasis with narrow-band UVB phototherapy is linked to suppression of the IFN and Th17 pathways. J Invest Dermatol 2011. https://doi.org/ 10.1038/jid.2011.53.

56. Zaba LC, Fuentes-Duculan J, Eungdamrong NJ, et al. Psoriasis is characterized by accumulation of immunostimulatory and Th1/Th17 cell-polarizing myeloid dendritic cells. J Invest Dermatol 2009. https://doi.org/10.1038/jid.2008.194.

57. Krueger JG, Fretzin S, Suárez-Fariñas M, et al. IL-17A is essential for cell activation and inflammatory gene circuits in subjects with psoriasis. J Allergy Clin Immunol 2012. https://doi.org/ 10.1016/j.jaci.2012.04.024.

58. Wolf P. Psoralen-ultraviolet A endures as one of the most powerful treatments in dermatology: reinforcement of this 'triple-product therapy' by the 2016 British guidelines. Br J Dermatol 2016. https://doi.org/10.1111/bjd.14341.

59. Kulms D, Poppelmann B, Yarosh D, et al. Nuclear and cell membrane effects contribute independently to the induction of apoptosis in human cells exposed to UVB radiation. Proc Natl Acad Sci U S A 2002. https://doi.org/10.1073/pnas.96. 14.7974.

60. Kulms D, Zeise E, Pöppelmann B, et al. DNA damage, death receptor activation and reactive oxygen species contribute to ultraviolet radiation-induced apoptosis in an essential and independent way. Oncogene 2002. https://doi.org/10.1038/sj.onc. 1205743.

61. Rosette C, Karin M. Ultraviolet light and osmotic stress: activation of the JNK cascade through multiple growth factor and cytokine receptors. Science 1996;(80). https://doi.org/10.1126/science. 274.5290.1194.

62. Aragane Y, Kulms D, Metze D, et al. Ultraviolet light induces apoptosis via direct activation of CD95 (Fas/APO-1) independently of its ligand CD95L. J Cell Biol 1998. https://doi.org/10.1083/jcb.140.1. 171.

63. Abou El-Ela M, Nagui N, Mahgoub D, et al. Expression of cyclin D1 and p16 in psoriasis before and after phototherapy. Clin Exp Dermatol 2010. https://doi.org/10.1111/j.1365-2230.2009.03774.x.

64. Rácz E, Prens EP, Kant M, et al. Narrowband ultraviolet B inhibits innate cytosolic double-stranded RNA receptors in psoriatic skin and keratinocytes. Br J Dermatol 2011. https://doi.org/10.1111/j. 1365-2133.2010.10169.x.

65. Hochberg M, Zeligson S, Amariglio N, et al. Genomic-scale analysis of psoriatic skin reveals differentially expressed insulin-like growth factor-binding protein-7 after phototherapy. Br J Dermatol 2007. https://doi.org/10.1111/j.1365-2133.2006. 07628.x.

66. Santamaria AB, Davis DW, Nghiem DX, et al. p53 and Fas ligand are required for psoralen and UVA-inducedapoptosis in mouse epidermal cells. Cell Death Differ 2002. https://doi.org/10.1038/sj. cdd.4401007.

67. Weatherhead SC, Farr PM, Jamieson D, et al. Keratinocyte apoptosis in epidermal remodeling and clearance of psoriasis induced by UV radiation. J Invest Dermatol 2011. https://doi.org/10.1038/ jid.2011.134.

68. Matos TR, O'Malley JT, Lowry EL, et al. Clinically resolved psoriatic lesions contain psoriasis-

specific IL-17-producing αβ T cell clones. J Clin Invest 2017. https://doi.org/10.1172/JCI93396.

69. Coimbra S, Oliveira H, Reis F, et al. Interleukin (IL)-22, IL-17, IL-23, IL-8, vascular endothelial growth factor and tumour necrosis factor-α levels in patients with psoriasis before, during and after psoralen-ultraviolet A and narrowband ultraviolet B therapy. Br J Dermatol 2010;163(6):1282–90. https://doi.org/10.1111/j.1365-2133.2010.09992.x.

70. Ravić-Nikolić A, Radosavljević G, Jovanović I, et al. Systemic photochemotherapy decreases the expression of IFN-γ, IL-12p40 and IL-23p19 in psoriatic plaques. Eur J Dermatol 2011. https://doi.org/10.1684/ejd.2010.1199.

71. Barr RM, Walker SL, Tsang W, et al. Suppressed alloantigen presentation, increased TNF-α, IL-1, IL-1Ra, IL- 10, and modulation of TNF-R in UV-irradiated human skin. J Invest Dermatol 1999. https://doi.org/10.1046/j.1523-1747.1999.00570.x.

72. Skov L, Hansen H, Allen M, et al. Contrasting effects of ultraviolet A1 and ultraviolet B exposure on the induction of tumour necrosis factor-α in human skin. Br J Dermatol 1998. https://doi.org/10.1046/j.1365-2133.1998.02063.x.

73. Asadullah K, Sterry W, Stephanek K, et al. IL-10 is a key cytokine in psoriasis: Proof of principle by IL-10 therapy: A new therapeutic approach. J Clin Invest 1998. https://doi.org/10.1172/JCI1476.

74. Gilchrest BA. Methoxsalen photochemotherapy for mycosis fungoides. Cancer Treat Rep 1979;63(4):663–7.

75. Gilchrest BA, Parrish JA, Tanenbaum L, et al. Oral methoxsalen photochemotherapy of mycosis fungoides. Cancer 1976. https://doi.org/10.1002/1097-0142(197608)38:2<683::AID-CNCR2820380210>3.0.CO;2-V.

76. Legat FJ, Hofer A, Quehenberger F, et al. Reduction of treatment frequency and UVA dose does not substantially compromise the antipsoriatic effect of oral psoralen-UVA. J Am Acad Dermatol 2004. https://doi.org/10.1016/j.jaad.2004.04.029.

77. Legat FJ, Hofer A, Wackernagel A, et al. Narrowband UV-B phototherapy, alefacept, and clearance of psoriasis. Arch Dermatol 2007. https://doi.org/10.1001/archderm.143.8.1016.

78. Eidsmo L, Martini E. Human Langerhans cells with pro-inflammatory features relocate within psoriasis lesions. Front Immunol 2018. https://doi.org/10.3389/fimmu.2018.00300.

79. Desilva B, McKenzie RC, Hunter JAA, et al. Local effects of TL01 phototherapy in psoriasis. Photodermatol Photoimmunol Photomed 2008. https://doi.org/10.1111/j.1600-0781.2008.00366.x.

80. Shirsath N, Mayer G, Singh TP, et al. 8-methoxypsoralen plus UVA (PUVA) therapy normalizes signalling of phosphorylated component of mTOR pathway in psoriatic skin of K5.hTGF β 1 transgenic mice. Exp Dermatol 2015. https://doi.org/10.1111/exd.12779.

81. Horio T. Indications and action mechanisms of phototherapy. J Dermatol Sci 2000. https://doi.org/10.1016/S0923-1811(99)00069-9.

82. Narbutt J, Olejniczak I, Sobolewska-Sztychny D, et al. Narrow band ultraviolet B irradiations cause alteration in interleukin-31 serum level in psoriatic patients. Arch Dermatol Res 2013. https://doi.org/10.1007/s00403-012-1293-6.

83. Alamartine E, Berthoux P, Mariat C, et al. Interleukin-10 promoter polymorphisms and susceptibility to skin squamous cell carcinoma after renal transplantation. J Invest Dermatol 2003. https://doi.org/10.1046/j.1523-1747.2003.12016.x.

84. Nagano T, Kunisada M, Yu X, et al. Involvement of interleukin-10 promoter polymorphisms in nonmelanoma skin cancers - A case study in non-Caucasian skin cancer patients. Photochem Photobiol 2008. https://doi.org/10.1111/j.1751-1097.2007.00245.x.

85. Ibbotson SH, Dawe RS, Dinkova-Kostova AT, et al. Glutathione S-transferase genotype is associated with sensitivity to psoralen-ultraviolet A photochemotherapy. Br J Dermatol 2012. https://doi.org/10.1111/j.1365-2133.2011.10661.x.

86. Patrizi A, Raone B, Ravaioli GM. Management of atopic dermatitis: safety and efficacy of phototherapy. Clin Cosmet Investig Dermatol 2015;511–20. https://doi.org/10.2147/CCID.S87987.

87. Brunner PM, Guttman-yassky E, Leung DYM. The immunology of atopic dermatitis and its reversibility with broad-spectrum and targeted therapies. J Allergy Clin Immunol 2018;139(4):S65–76. https://doi.org/10.1016/j.jaci.2017.01.011.

88. Grundmann SA, Beissert S. Modern aspects of phototherapy for atopic dermatitis. J Allergy (Cairo) 2012;2012. https://doi.org/10.1155/2012/121797.

89. Tintle S, Shemer A, Suárez-Fariñas M, et al. Reversal of atopic dermatitis with narrow-band UVB phototherapy and biomarkers for therapeutic response. J Allergy Clin Immunol 2011. https://doi.org/10.1016/j.jaci.2011.05.042.

90. Furue M, Tsuji G, Mitoma C, et al. Gene regulation of filaggrin and other skin barrier proteins via aryl hydrocarbon receptor. J Dermatol Sci 2015. https://doi.org/10.1016/j.jdermsci.2015.07.011.

91. Thepen T, Langeveld-Wildschut EG, Bihari IC, et al. Biphasic response against aeroallergen in atopic dermatitis showing a switch from an initial T(H2) response to a T(H1) response in situ: an immunocytochemical study. J Allergy Clin Immunol 1996. https://doi.org/10.1016/S0091-6749(96)80161-8.

92. Legat FJ. The antipruritic effect of phototherapy. Front Med (Lausanne) 2018;5:1–9. https://doi.org/10.3389/fmed.2018.00333.

93. Edström DW, Porwit A, Ros AM. Effects on human skin of repetitive ultraviolet-A1 (UVA1) irradiation and visible light. Photodermatol Photoimmunol Photomed 2001. https://doi.org/10.1034/j.1600-0781.2001.017002066.x.

94. Legat FJ, Hofer A, Brabek E, et al. Narrowband UV-B vs medium-dose UV-A1 phototherapy in chronic atopic dermatitis. Arch Dermatol 2003. https://doi.org/10.1001/archderm.139.2.223.

95. Tzaneva S, Kittler H, Holzer G, et al. 5-Methoxypsoralen plus ultraviolet (UV) A is superior to medium-dose UVA1 in the treatment of severe atopic dermatitis: a randomized crossover trial. Br J Dermatol 2010. https://doi.org/10.1111/j.1365-2133.2009.09514.x.

96. Gallo RL, Bernard JJ. Innate immune sensors stimulate inflammatory and immunosuppressive responses to UVB radiation. J Invest Dermatol 2014. https://doi.org/10.1038/jid.2014.32.

97. Gläser R, Navid F, Schuller W, et al. UV-B radiation induces the expression of antimicrobial peptides in human keratinocytes in vitro and in vivo. J Allergy Clin Immunol 2009. https://doi.org/10.1016/j.jaci.2009.01.043.

98. Bernard JJ, Gallo RL. Cyclooxygenase-2 enhances antimicrobial peptide expression and killing of Staphylococcus aureus. J Immunol 2010. https://doi.org/10.4049/jimmunol.1002009.

99. Brazzelli V, Grassi S, Merante S, et al. Narrow-band UVB phototherapy and psoralen – ultraviolet A photochemotherapy in the treatment of cutaneous mastocytosis : a study in 20 patients. Photodermatol Photoimmunol Photomed 2016. https://doi.org/10.1111/phpp.12248.

100. Danno K, Fujii K, Tachibana T, et al. Suppressed histamine release from rat peritoneal mast cells by ultraviolet B irradiation: decreased diacylglycerol formation as a possible mechanism. J Invest Dermatol 1988. https://doi.org/10.1111/1523-1747.ep12462027.

101. Krönauer C, Eberlein-König B, Ring J, et al. Influence of UVB, UVA and UVA1 irradiation on histamine release from human basophils and mast cells in vitro in the presence and absence of antioxidants. Photochem Photobiol 2004. https://doi.org/10.1562/0031-8655(2003)077<0531:iouuau>2.0.co;2.

102. de Paulis A, Monfrecola G, Casula L, et al. 8-Methoxypsoralen and long-wave ultraviolet A inhibit the release of proinflammatory mediators and cytokines from human FcERI+ cells: An in vitro study. J Photochem Photobiol B Biol 2003. https://doi.org/10.1016/S1011-1344(03)00019-8.

103. Kolde G, Frosch PJ, Czarnetzki BM. Response of cutaneous mast cells to PUVA in patients with urticaria pigmentosa: Histomorphometric, ultrastructural, and biochemical investigations. J Invest Dermatol 1984. https://doi.org/10.1111/1523-1747.ep12263520.

104. Contassot E, French LE. Targeting apoptosis defects in cutaneous T-cell lymphoma. J Invest Dermatol 2009. https://doi.org/10.1038/jid.2009.14.

105. Willemze R. 120 - cutaneous T-cell lymphoma. Bolognia's Dermatology.. 4th edition. Elsevier Ltd; 2017. https://doi.org/10.1016/B978-0-7020-6275-9.00120-3.

106. Querfeld C, Zain J, Rosen ST. Primary cutaneous T-Cell lymphomas: mycosis fungoides and sezary syndrome. Cancer Treat Res 2019; 176(2):225–48. https://doi.org/10.1007/978-3-319-99716-2_11.

107. Jackow CM, Cather JC, Hearne V, et al. Association of erythrodermic cutaneous T cell lymphoma, superantigen-positive staphylococcus aureus, and oligoclonal T cell receptor Vbeta gene expansion. Blood 1997. https://doi.org/10.1016/j.urology.2007.10.001.

108. López-Lerma I, Estrach MT. A distinct profile of serum levels of soluble intercellular adhesion molecule-1 and intercellular adhesion molecule-3 in mycosis fungoides and Sézary syndrome. J Am Acad Dermatol 2009. https://doi.org/10.1016/j.jaad.2009.03.041.

109. Kim EJ, Hess S, Richardson SK, et al. Immunopathogenesis and therapy of cutaneous T cell lymphoma. J Clin Invest 2005. https://doi.org/10.1172/JCI200524826.

110. Hofer A, Cerroni L, Kerl H, et al. Narrowband (311-nm) UV-B therapy for small plaque parapsoriasis and early-stage mycosis fungoides. Arch Dermatol 1999. https://doi.org/10.1001/archderm.135.11.1377.

111. Phan K, Ramachandran V, Fassihi H, et al. Comparison of narrowband UV-B with Psoralen-UV-A phototherapy for patients with early-stage mycosis fungoides: a systematic review and meta-analysis. JAMA Dermatol 2019. https://doi.org/10.1001/jamadermatol.2018.5204.

112. Trautinger F. Phototherapy of cutaneous T-cell lymphomas. Photochem Photobiol Sci 2018; 1904–12. https://doi.org/10.1039/c8pp00170g.

113. Vieyra-Garcia P, Fink-Puches R, Porkert S, et al. Evaluation of low-dose, low-frequency oral psoralen-UV-A treatment with or without maintenance on early-stage mycosis fungoides: a randomized clinical trial. JAMA Dermatol 2019. https://doi.org/10.1001/jamadermatol.2018.5905.

114. Vieyra-Garcia PA, Wei T, Naym DG, et al. STAT3/5-dependent IL9 overexpression contributes to neoplastic cell survival in mycosis fungoides. Clin Cancer Res 2016;22(13):3328–39. https://doi.org/10.1158/1078-0432.CCR-15-1784.

115. De Masson A, O'Malley JT, Elco CP, et al. High-throughput sequencing of the T cell receptor b

gene identifies aggressive early-stage mycosis fungoides. Sci Transl Med 2018. https://doi.org/10.1126/scitranslmed.aar5894.

116. Vieyra-Garcia P, Crouch JD, O'Malley JT, et al. Benign T cells drive clinical skin inflammation in cutaneous T cell lymphoma. JCI Insight 2019. https://doi.org/10.1172/jci.insight.124233.

117. Cláudia A, Abreu G, Duarte GG, et al. Immunological parameters associated with vitiligo treatments : a literature review based on clinical studies. Autoimmune Dis 2015;2015:196537. https://doi.org/10.1155/2015/196537.

118. Speeckaert R. Vitiligo: an update on pathophysiology and treatment options. Am J Clin Dermatol 2017;18(6):733–44. https://doi.org/10.1007/s40257-017-0298-5.

119. Abyaneh MY, Grif RD, Nouri K. Narrowband ultraviolet B phototherapy in combination with other therapies for vitiligo: mechanisms and efficacies. J Eur Acad Dermatol Venereol 2014;1610–22. https://doi.org/10.1111/jdv.12619.

120. Wu CS, Yu CL, Wu CS, et al. Narrow-band ultraviolet-B stimulates proliferation and migration of cultured melanocytes. Exp Dermatol 2004. https://doi.org/10.1111/j.0906-6705.2004.00221.x.

121. Moretti S, Spallanzani A, Amato L, et al. New insights into the pathogenesis of vitiligo: imbalance of epidermal cytokines at sites of lesions. Pigment Cell Res 2002. https://doi.org/10.1034/j.1600-0749.2002.1o049.x.

122. Hara M, Yaar M, Byers HR, et al. Kinesin participates in melanosomal movement along melanocyte dendrites. J Invest Dermatol 2000. https://doi.org/10.1046/j.1523-1747.2000.00894.x.

123. Hegazy RA, Fawzy MM, Gawdat HI, et al. T helper 17 and Tregs: a novel proposed mechanism for NB-UVB in vitiligo. Exp Dermatol 2014. https://doi.org/10.1111/exd.12369.

124. Westerhof W, Nieuweboer-Krobotova L. Treatment of vitiligo with UV-B radiation vs topical psoralen plus UV-A. Arch Dermatol 1997. https://doi.org/10.1001/archderm.1997.03890480045006.

125. Lembo S, Raimondo A. Polymorphic light eruption: what's new in pathogenesis and management. Front Med 2018. https://doi.org/10.3389/fmed.2018.00252.

126. Janssens AS, Pavel S, Out-Luiting JJ, et al. Normalized ultraviolet (UV) induction of Langerhans cell depletion and neutrophil infiltrates after artificial UVB hardening of patients with polymorphic light eruption. Br J Dermatol 2005. https://doi.org/10.1111/j.1365-2133.2005.06690.x.

127. Schweintzger N, Gruber-Wackernagel A, Reginato E, et al. Levels and function of regulatory T cells in patients with polymorphic light eruption: Relation to photohardening. Br J Dermatol 2015. https://doi.org/10.1111/bjd.13930.

128. Schweintzger NA, Gruber-Wackernagel A, Shirsath N, et al. Influence of the season on vitamin D levels and regulatory T cells in patients with polymorphic light eruption. Photochem Photobiol Sci 2016. https://doi.org/10.1039/c5pp00398a.

129. Wolf P, Gruber-Wackernagel A, Bambach I, et al. Photohardening of polymorphic light eruption patients decreases baseline epidermal Langerhans cell density while increasing mast cell numbers in the papillary dermis. Exp Dermatol 2014. https://doi.org/10.1111/exd.12427.

130. Schweintzger NA, Bambach I, Reginato E, et al. Mast cells are required for phototolerance induction and scratching abatement. Exp Dermatol 2015. https://doi.org/10.1111/exd.12687.

131. de Gruijl FR. The mastocyte: the off switch of UV itch. Exp Dermatol 2015. https://doi.org/10.1111/exd.12742.

132. Wolf P, Gruber-Wackernagel A, Rinner B, et al. Phototherapeutic hardening modulates systemic cytokine levels in patients with polymorphic light eruption. Photochem Photobiol Sci 2013. https://doi.org/10.1039/c2pp25187f.

133. Gruber-Wackernagel A, Heinemann A, Konya V, et al. Photohardening restores the impaired neutrophil responsiveness to chemoattractants leukotriene B4 and formyl-methionyl-leucyl-phenylalanin in patients with polymorphic light eruption. Exp Dermatol 2011. https://doi.org/10.1111/j.1600-0625.2011.01264.x.

134. Gruber-Wackernagel A, Obermayer-Pietsch B, Byrne SN, et al. Patients with polymorphic light eruption have decreased serum levels of 25-hydroxyvitamin-D$_3$ that increase upon 311 nm UVB photohardening. Photochem Photobiol Sci 2012. https://doi.org/10.1039/c2pp25188d.

135. Gruber-Wackernagel A, Bambach I, Legat FJ, et al. Randomized double-blinded placebo-controlled intra-individual trial on topical treatment with a 1,25-dihydroxyvitamin D 3 analogue in polymorphic light eruption. Br J Dermatol 2011. https://doi.org/10.1111/j.1365-2133.2011.10333.x.

136. Patra VK, Mayer G, Gruber-Wackernagel A, et al. Unique profile of antimicrobial peptide expression in polymorphic light eruption lesions compared to healthy skin, atopic dermatitis, and psoriasis. Photodermatol Photoimmunol Photomed 2018. https://doi.org/10.1111/phpp.12355.

137. Patra VK, Wolf P. Microbial elements as the initial triggers in the pathogenesis of polymorphic light eruption? Exp Dermatol 2016. https://doi.org/10.1111/exd.13162.

138. Patra V, Strobl J, Gruber-Wackernagel A, et al. CD 11b+ cells markedly express the itch cytokine interleukin 31 in polymorphic light eruption. Br J Dermatol 2019. https://doi.org/10.1111/bjd.18092.

139. Schlaak M, Schwind S, Wetzig T, et al. UVA (UVA-1) therapy for the treatment of acute GVHD of the skin. Bone Marrow Transplant 2010. https://doi.org/10.1038/bmt.2010.230.

140. Garbutcheon-Singh KB, Fernández-Peñas P. Phototherapy for the treatment of cutaneous graft versus host disease. Australas J Dermatol 2015. https://doi.org/10.1111/ajd.12191.

141. Knobler R, Moinzadeh P, Hunzelmann N, et al. European dermatology forum S1-guideline on the diagnosis and treatment of sclerosing diseases of the skin, part 1: localized scleroderma, systemic sclerosis and overlap syndromes. J Eur Acad Dermatol Venereol 2017. https://doi.org/10.1111/jdv.14458.

142. Knobler R, Moinzadeh P, Hunzelmann N, et al. European dermatology forum S1-guideline on the diagnosis and treatment of sclerosing diseases of the skin, Part 2: Scleromyxedema, scleredema and nephrogenic systemic fibrosis. J Eur Acad Dermatol Venereol 2017. https://doi.org/10.1111/jdv.14466.

143. Gambichler T, Schmitz L. Ultraviolet A1 phototherapy for fibrosing conditions. Front Med 2018. https://doi.org/10.3389/fmed.2018.00237.

144. Knobler R, Berlin G, Calzavara-Pinton P, et al. Guidelines on the use of extracorporeal photopheresis. J Eur Acad Dermatol Venereol 2014. https://doi.org/10.1111/jdv.12311.

145. Hashimoto A, Sato T, Iyama S, et al. Narrow-band ultraviolet B phototherapy ameliorates acute graft-versus-host disease of the intestine by expansion of regulatory T cells. PLoS One 2016. https://doi.org/10.1371/journal.pone.0152823.

146. Breuer J, Schwab N, Schneider-Hohendorf T, et al. Ultraviolet B light attenuates the systemic immune response in central nervous system autoimmunity. Ann Neurol 2014. https://doi.org/10.1002/ana.24165.

147. Hart PH, Jones AP, Trend S, et al. A randomised, controlled clinical trial of narrowband UVB phototherapy for clinically isolated syndrome: the PhoCIS study. Mult Scler J Exp Transl Clin 2018. https://doi.org/10.1177/2055217318773112.

148. Yones SS, Palmer RA, Garibaldinos TT, et al. Randomized double-blind trial of the treatment of chronic plaque psoriasis. Arch Dermatol 2006. https://doi.org/10.1001/archderm.142.7.836.

149. Reich K, Papp KA, Blauvelt A, et al. Tildrakizumab versus placebo or etanercept for chronic plaque psoriasis (reSURFACE 1 and reSURFACE 2): results from two randomised controlled, phase 3 trials. Lancet 2017. https://doi.org/10.1016/S0140-6736(17)31279-5.

150. Mrowietz U, Leonardi CL, Girolomoni G, et al. Secukinumab retreatment-as-needed versus fixed-interval maintenance regimen for moderate to severe plaque psoriasis: a randomized, double-blind, noninferiority trial (SCULPTURE). J Am Acad Dermatol 2015. https://doi.org/10.1016/j.jaad.2015.04.011.

151. Blauvelt A, Papp KA, Sofen H, et al. Continuous dosing versus interrupted therapy with ixekizumab: an integrated analysis of two phase 3 trials in psoriasis. J Eur Acad Dermatol Venereol 2017. https://doi.org/10.1111/jdv.14163.

152. Nakamura M, Lee K, Jeon C, et al. Guselkumab for the treatment of psoriasis: a review of phase III trials. Dermatol Ther (Heidelb) 2017. https://doi.org/10.1007/s13555-017-0187-0.

153. Kasibhatla S, Brunner T, Genestier L, et al. DNA damaging agents induce expression of Fas ligand and subsequent apoptosis in T lymphocytes via the activation of NF-κB and AP-1. Mol Cell 1998. https://doi.org/10.1016/S1097-2765(00)80054-4.

154. Treina G, Scaletta C, Fourtanier A, et al. Expression of intercellular adhesion molecule-1 in UVA-irradiated human skin cells in vitro and in vivo. Br J Dermatol 1996. https://doi.org/10.1111/j.1365-2133.1996.tb01154.x.

155. Schlaak JF, Buslau M, Jochum W, et al. T cells involved in psoriasis vulgaris belong to the Th1 subset. J Invest Dermatol 1994. https://doi.org/10.1111/1523-1747.ep12371752.

156. Uyemura K, Yamamura M, Fivenson DF, et al. The cytokine network in lesional and lesion-free psoriatic skin is characterized by a t-helper type 1 cell-mediated response. J Invest Dermatol 1993. https://doi.org/10.1111/1523-1747.ep12371679.

Phototherapy for Vitiligo

Raheel Zubair, MD, MHS[a], Iltefat H. Hamzavi, MD[b],*

KEYWORDS

- Phototherapy • Vitiligo • NBUVB • Afamelanotide • Topical calcineurin inhibitors • JAK inhibitors

KEY POINTS

- Narrowband UVB (NBUVB) has supplanted psoralen UVA as a first-line treatment of vitiligo due to its superior safety and efficacy.
- Initiate phototherapy early in active vitiligo in order to halt disease progression and to stimulate repigmentation in stable vitiligo.
- Expert recommendations simplify phototherapy regimens by using erythema to guide dosing and by forgoing minimal erythema dose calculation.
- Excimer is preferred for small areas, whereas NBUVB is more useful for widespread vitiligo.
- Phototherapy can be combined with various medications to enhance vitiligo treatment.

INTRODUCTION

Vitiligo is an incurable acquired autoimmune disorder resulting in white, hypopigmented macules and patches caused by the progressive destruction of functional melanocytes (**Fig. 1**). It is a common disorder that has a worldwide prevalence between 0.5% and 2%.[1] Vitiligo is not life threatening. Nonetheless, it decreases quality of life, causes psychological distress, is associated with multiple autoimmune diseases, and should not be considered a cosmetic problem.[2]

Phototherapy has been used to treat vitiligo for more than 3000 years, dating back to the use of sun exposure in combination with extracts of *Psoralea corylifolia* and *Ammi majus* in ancient India and Egypt.[3,4]

Today dermatologists continue to use phototherapy in a variety of forms to treat vitiligo, including psoralen ultraviolet A (PUVA), excimer lamp and laser, and narrowband UVB (NBUVB). PUVA was previously the most common treatment but has been supplanted by NBUVB in recent years as the treatment modality of choice.[5,6] Excimer is a targeted therapy that works well for localized disease, but NBUVB is preferable for widespread vitiligo (greater than 5% of the body surface area). NBUVB will be the focus of this article, as excimer is discussed in Karen Ly and colleagues' article, "Beyond the Booth: Excimer Laser for Cutaneous Conditions," elsewhere in this issue.

Vitiligo pathogenesis and repigmentation are illustrated by FM. Strickland and modified by I. Hamzavi.

Stressors cause keratinocytes to release CXCL9 and CXCL10 contributing to an inflammatory environment. These molecules recruit CD8+ T cells that subsequently destroy melanocytes resulting in depigmentation. Repigmentation occurs when melanocytes from hair follicles migrate and proliferate.

NARROWBAND ULTRAVIOLET B OR PSORALEN ULTRAVIOLET A?

In 1997, Westerhof and Nieuweboer-Krobotova compared twice-weekly NBUVB with topical PUVA for the treatment of vitiligo. The NBUVB group had 67% of patients repigmented after 4 months compared with 46% of the PUVA group.[5] A 2015 Cochrane review also showed

Disclosure: Dr I.H. Hamzavi is an investigator for Incyte and Pfizer. Dr R. Zubair is a subinvestigator for Incyte.
[a] Broward Health Medical Center, Graduate Medical Education, 1600 S Andrews Avenue, Fort Lauderdale, FL 33301, USA; [b] Department of Dermatology, Henry Ford Health System, 3031 West Grand Boulevard, Suite 800, Detroit, MI, USA
* Corresponding author.
E-mail address: IHAMZAV1@hfhs.org

Dermatol Clin 38 (2020) 55–62
https://doi.org/10.1016/j.det.2019.08.005
0733-8635/20/© 2019 Elsevier Inc. All rights reserved.

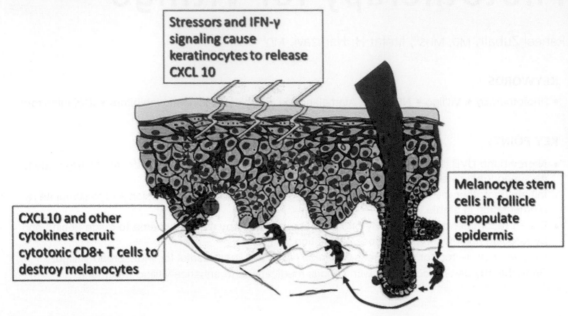

Stressors and IFN-γ signaling cause keratinocytes to release CXCL 10

Melanocyte stem cells in follicle repopulate epidermis

CXCL10 and other cytokines recruit cytotoxic CD8+ T cells to destroy melanocytes

Fig. 1. Vitiligo pathogenesis.

that NBUVB is marginally more effective at achieving repigmentation than PUVA and has more favorable side-effect profile.[7]

MECHANISM

Vitiligo pathogenesis involves the destruction of melanocytes by cytotoxic CD8+ T cells, which are recruited through an interferon gamma (IFNγ), CXCL9, and CXCL10 pathway (**Fig. 2**).[8–10] Phototherapy is a critical tool for halting the progression of active, rapidly depigmenting vitiligo early in the disease course. This may be because the immunosuppressive effects of NBUVB reduce autoimmune melanocyte destruction. NBUVB induces apoptosis in T cells, downregulation of inflammatory cytokines, and upregulation of interleukin (IL)-10, which induces regulatory T cells.[3,11–13] In addition, NBUVB depletes epidermal Langerhans cells, thereby reducing antigen presentation.[13] Patients with stable disease also benefit from NBUVB due to its stimulation of melanocyte proliferation and migration from the outer root sheath of follicles to the epidermis resulting in the freckled appearance of islands of repigmentation.[10,14,15] Lastly, NBUVB upregulates tyrosinase to increase melanin synthesis.[16,17]

IFNγ signaling via the Janus kinase /single transducers and activators of transcription (JAK/STAT) pathway in keratinocytes increases the expression of CXLCL9 and CXCL10. These cytokines recruit cytotoxic CD8+ T cells to destroy melanocytes. Phototherapy, steroids, calcineurin inhibitors, and JAK inhibitors suppress the autoimmune component of vitiligo. In addition to this immunomodulatory effect, phototherapy stimulates melanocyte proliferation and migration from reservoirs such as the hair follicle.

NARROWBAND ULTRAVIOLET B PROTOCOL

There are vitiligo guidelines published in Japan and Europe that discuss phototherapy.[18,19] The Vitiligo Working Group (VWG), now known as the Global Vitiligo Foundation published expert recommendations for NBUVB in 2017.[20] These recommendations are summarized in **Table 1**.

Dosing, Frequency, and Length of Treatment

NBUVB phototherapy is typically performed 2 or 3 times a week. The latter induces earlier repigmentation, whereas less-frequent dosing may be easier for the schedules of patients and phototherapy centers. The VWG recommends an initial dose of 200 mJ/cm^2 with dose increases of 10% to 20% in the absence of erythema. In the presence of bright red or symptomatic erythema, treatment should be held until the erythema fades, then the last tolerated dose can be resumed. It can be difficult to establish when phototherapy should be stopped for treatment failure/lack of response. Some patients may not respond until more than 72 exposures, so early discontinuation should be avoided.[20] There is insufficient data to recommend a maximum number of exposures and it is unclear when phototherapy should be terminated.[21] In

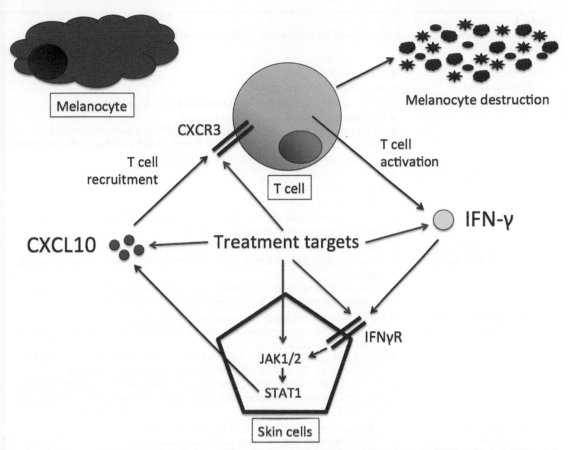

Fig. 2. Therapeutic targets. (*Reprinted from* New discoveries in the pathogenesis and classification of vitiligo." by Rodrigues M, Ezzedine K, Hamzavi I, Pandya AG, Harris JE in the Journal of the American Academy of Dermatology 2017;77(1):1–13; with permission.)

general, 35.7% patients can expect a greater than 75% degree of repigmentation at 12 months. This long-term nature of therapy must be explained to the patient when therapy is initiated.[22]

COMBINATION THERAPIES
Steroids

Systemic steroids combined with phototherapy are a common strategy to arrest the progression of depigmentation in active vitiligo. Oral mini-pulse (OMP) regimens of dexamethasone on 2 consecutive days a week are an option to achieve stability while minimizing side effects.[23,24] Although systemic corticosteroids can be a useful adjunct to phototherapy, alone they are not as effective for repigmentation.[25] Perhaps steroids are able to halt the loss of melanocytes, but without phototherapy there is no stimulus for their replacement (see **Fig. 2**). Topical steroids are also popularly used in early, localized vitiligo.[26] A randomized control trial demonstrated that the combination of NBUVB and clobetasol ointment resulted in earlier repigmentation than NBUVB and placebo, although other measures such as final overall pigmentation were comparable.[27]

Afamelanotide

Afamelanotide is a synthetic analogue of the endogenous peptide α-melanocyte stimulating hormone. This hormone stimulates both melanin synthesis and melanocyte proliferation. A randomized clinical trial compared the combination of NBUVB and afamelanotide against NBUVB monotherapy.[28] The combination therapy[21] group received 1 month of NBUVB phototherapy followed by 4 months of NBUVB combined with monthly subcutaneous afamelanotide implants. This combination achieved repigmentation in a significantly higher percentage of patients in the face and upper extremities as compared with NBUVB alone. The median time to the onset of repigmentation in these areas was 20 days earlier in the combination therapy group as well.[28] These results are meaningful given that the face and

Table 1
The Vitiligo Working Group (now known as the Global Vitiligo Foundation) phototherapy expert recommendations

Frequency of administration	• Optimal: 3 times per wk • Acceptable: 2 times per wk
Dosing protocol	• Initial dose of 200 mJ/cm^2 regardless of skin type • Increase by 10% to 20% per treatment • Fixed dosing based on skin phototype (SPT) is another acceptable dosing strategy that considers the inherent differences in the minimal erythema dose (MED) of various skin types
Maximum acceptable dose	• Face: 1500 mJ/cm^2 • Body: 3000 mJ/cm^2
Maximum number of exposures	• SPT IV–VI: no limit • SPT I–III: more data on the risk of cutaneous malignancy is needed before a recommendation can be made
Course of narrowband ultraviolet B (NBUVB)	• Assess treatment response after 18–36 exposures • Minimum number of doses needed to determine lack of response: 48 exposures • Because of the existence of slow responders, up to 72 exposures may be needed to determine lack of response to phototherapy
Dose adjustment based on degree of erythema	• No erythema: increase next dose by 10% to 20% • Pink asymptomatic erythema: hold at current dose until erythema disappears then increase by 10% to 20% • Bright red asymptomatic erythema: stop phototherapy until affected areas become light pink, then resume at last tolerated dose • Symptomatic erythema (includes pain and blistering): stop phototherapy until the skin heals and erythema fades to a light pink, then resume at last tolerated dose
Dose adjustment following missed doses	• 4–7 d between treatments: hold dose constant • 8–14 d between treatments: decrease dose by 25% • 15–21 d between treatments: decrease dose by 50% • More than 3 wk between treatments: restart at initial dose
Device calibration or bulb replacement	• Decrease dose by 10% to 20%
Outcome measures to evaluate response	• Serial photography to establish baseline severity, disease stability, and response to treatment • Validated scoring systems, such as the Vitiligo Area Scoring Index or Vitiligo European Task Force, to quantify degree of response
Posttreatment recommendations	• Application of sunscreen • Avoidance of sunlight
Topical products before phototherapy	• Avoid all topical products for 4 h EXCEPT mineral oil • Mineral oil can be used to enhance light penetration in areas of dry, thickened skin, such as the elbows and knees
Tapering NBUVB after complete repigmentation achieved	• First month: phototherapy twice weekly • Second month: phototherapy once weekly • Third and fourth months: phototherapy every other week • After 4 mo, discontinue phototherapy
Follow-up	• SPT I–III: yearly follow-up for total body skin examination to monitor for adverse effects of phototherapy, including cutaneous malignancy • SPT IV–VI: no need to return for safety monitoring, as no reports of malignancy exist with this group • All patients: return on relapse for treatment
Minimum age for NBUVB in children	• Minimum age is when children are able to reliably stand in the booth with either their eyes closed or wearing goggles • Typically, those aged approximately 7–10 y depending on the child
Treatment of eyelid lesions	• Keep eyes closed during treatment, use adhesive tape if necessary

Continued	
Special sites	• Cover face during phototherapy if uninvolved • Shield male genitalia • Protect female areola with sunscreen before treatment, especially in SPT I–III
Combination treatment of stabilization	• Oral antioxidants • Topical treatments • Oral pulse corticosteroids
Treatment of NBUVB-induced skin changes	• Xerosis: emollient or mineral oil • Skin thickening: topical corticosteroids or keratolytics

Abbreviation: SPT, skin phototype.

Adapted from The Vitiligo Working Group recommendations for narrowband ultraviolet B light phototherapy treatment of vitiligo by Mohammad TF, Al-Jamal M, Hamzavi IH, et al. in the Journal of the American Academy of Dermatology 2017;76(5):879-888; with permission.

upper extremities are the most exposed and apparent areas of skin. More studies are needed to discover the optimal dose and frequency of afamelanotide administration, the long-term response to afamelanotide, and the effect of afamelanotide in people with skin phototypes I and II.

Topical Calcineurin Inhibitors

Topical calcineurin inhibitors (TCI) include tacrolimus and pimecrolimus. These medications inhibit the activation and proliferation of T cells and suppress the production of the proinflammatory cytokines, IFN-γ, IL-2, and tumor necrosis factor alpha (see **Fig. 1**). They are used in atopic dermatitis, psoriasis, and vitiligo where they can spare patients the effects of long-term steroid use.[26] The results of several studies combining tacrolimus 0.1% ointment with NBUVB have been variable. Some have not shown the combination to be significantly more efficacious than placebo ointment and NVUVB, although this may be due to small sample sizes of 15 or fewer patients and underpowered study designs.[29-31] Nordal, Guleng, and Ronnevig reported a larger randomized control trial in which 27 out of 40 patients had better repigmentation on the tacrolimus 0.1% ointment and NBUVB side compared with placebo and NBUVB and this result did reach significance ($P = .005$).[32] Esfandiarpour and colleagues[33] reported a randomized clinical trial of pimecrolimus 1% cream and NBUVB with placebo and found greater facial repigmentation in the pimecrolimus group (64.3 vs 25.1%, $P<.05\%$). Overall, combining TCIs with NBUVB has had mixed results and it is questionable whether it is superior to NBUVB alone. In addition, the long-term safety of this combination has not been established. There is evidence that the combination of systemic corticosteroids, topical tacrolimus, and excimer can improve repigmentation. This triad may be

especially useful for UV-resistant areas such as acral sites and bony prominences.[34]

Janus Kinase Inhibitors

The JAK-STAT pathway is involved in IFNγ signaling, which is a major element of vitiligo pathogenesis. There are reports showing the benefit of topical and oral JAK inhibitors for vitiligo.[35,36] Most commonly used are the JAK1/3 inhibitor, tofacitinib, and the JAK 1/2 inhibitor, ruxolitinib. A case series of patients treated with tofacitinib found repigmentation only in sun-exposed areas or areas undergoing NBUVB phototherapy. These results support a model in which the JAK inhibitor suppresses inflammation and autoimmunity, whereas a low dose of NBUVB is sufficient to stimulate melanocytes (see **Fig. 1**). There are ongoing clinical trials that will further test the potential synergy between JAK inhibitors and NBUVB[37,38] (**Table 2**).

SAFETY

NBUVB is a well-tolerated and safe treatment compared with other therapies. UVB light is an established carcinogen and, although data are limited, it seems the patients with psoriasis and vitiligo undergoing NBUVB therapy may be at an increased risk for cutaneous malignancies, most frequently superficial basal cell carcinoma.[39] There does not seem to be an increase in the risk of melanoma. Photocarcinogenesis is discussed in greater detail in Katherine G. Thompson and Noori Kim's article, "Distinguishing Myth from Fact: Photocarcinogenesis and Phototherapy," in this issue. Phototherapy patients with skin phototypes (SPT) I–III should have annual total body skin examinations for early detection of cutaneous malignancy. The most common acute adverse effects of NBUVB are pruritus, erythema, and xerosis. The VWG recommends a maximum dose of 3000 mJ/cm^2 for the body and 1500 mJ/cm^2 for

Table 2
NBUVB combination therapies

Category	Effect of Combination	Specific Product	Study	Recommended
Topical steroids	Earlier repigmentation	Clobetasol	Lim-Ong et al[27]	Yes
Oral steroids	Arrest disease progression	Dexamethasone	Rath et al,[25] 2008	Yes
Topical calcineurin inhibitors	Improved repigmentation	Tacrolimus Pimecrolimus	Satyanarayan et al,[29] 2013 Klahan & Asawanoda,[30] 2009 Mehrabi & Pandya,[31] 2006 Nodal et al,[32] 2011 Esfandiarpour et al,[33] 2009	Mixed results
Afamelanotide	Earlier and greater repigmentation on face and upper extremities	Subcutaneous Afamelanotide implant	Lim et al,[28] 2015	Experimental, not clinically available
JAK inhibitors	Repigmentation in light-exposed areas with lower NBUVB dose	Tofacitinib Ruxolitinib	Rothstein et al,[35] 2017	Further study required

the face.[20] There is no recommended ceiling for the number of treatments in patients with SPT IV–VI and insufficient data to make a recommendation for SPT I–III. Before phototherapy, patients should not apply any sunscreen or other topical products, including the medications discussed in the combination therapies section. Patients undergoing phototherapy should be cautious about sun exposure so that they do not inadvertently increase their cumulative dose of UVB.

Regarding shielding, eyes should remain closed during phototherapy. Encouragingly, patients are not at increased risk for cataracts or the loss of visual acuity after a year of NBUVB.[40] Male genitalia be shielded to reduce the risk of genital malignancy and female areola may be protected with sunscreen to prevent burns in lighter skin phototypes.[20]

Vitiligo can start at an early age, and it is safe for children to undergo phototherapy if they are able to keep their eyes closed during phototherapy or wear goggles. This is typically at the age of 7 to 10 years.[20] NBUVB is also regarded as safe for pregnant and nursing women, unlike PUVA.

SUMMARY

Phototherapy, especially NBUVB, is an effective and well-tolerated first-line treatment of vitiligo. Technological advances are likely to decrease costs and lead to the creation of new devices such as those now available for home

phototherapy. Simultaneously, drug development is producing new medications to improve and speed repigmentation when combined with phototherapy. Large-scale and longer follow-up studies of all these treatments are required if we hope to better understand their safety and the longevity of the repigmentation they cause. It will also be up to clinicians to rise to the challenge of learning and mastering these therapies in order to provide the best care for patients with vitiligo.

REFERENCES

1. Krüger C, Schallreuter KU. A review of the worldwide prevalence of vitiligo in children/adolescents and adults. Int J Dermatol 2012;51(10):1206–12.
2. Ongenae K, Van Geel N, De Schepper S, et al. Effect of vitiligo on self-reported health-related quality of life. Br J Dermatol 2005;152(6):1165–72.
3. Colin Theng TS, Tan ES. Pigmentary skin disorders. Cham (Switzerland): Springer; 2018.
4. Pacifico A, Leone G. Photo(chemo)therapy for vitiligo. Photodermatol Photoimmunol Photomed 2011; 27(5):261–77.
5. Westerhof W, Nieuweboer-Krobotova L. Treatment of vitiligo with UV-B radiation vs topical psoralen plus UV-A. Arch Dermatol 1997;133(12):1525–8.
6. Yones SS, Palmer RA, Garibaldinos TM, et al. Randomized double-blind trial of treatment of vitiligo: efficacy of psoralen-UV-A therapy vs Narrowband-UV-B therapy. Arch Dermatol 2007;143(5):578–84.

7. Whitton ME, Pinart M, Batchelor J, et al. Interventions for vitiligo. Cochrane Database Syst Rev 2015;(2):CD003263.

8. van den Boorn JG, Konijnenberg D, Dellemijn TA, et al. Autoimmune destruction of skin melanocytes by perilesional T cells from vitiligo patients. J Invest Dermatol 2009;129(9):2220–32.

9. Wang XX, Wang QQ, Wu JQ, et al. Increased expression of CXCR3 and its ligands in patients with vitiligo and CXCL10 as a potential clinical marker for vitiligo. Br J Dermatol 2016;174(6):1318–26.

10. Liu LY, Strassner JP, Refat MA, et al. Repigmentation in vitiligo using the Janus kinase inhibitor tofacitinib may require concomitant light exposure. J Am Acad Dermatol 2017;77(4):675–82.e1.

11. Ozawa M, Ferenczi K, Kikuchi T, et al. 312-nanometer ultraviolet B light (Narrow-Band UVB) induces apoptosis of T cells within psoriatic lesions. J Exp Med 1999;189(4):711–8.

12. Hegazy RA, Fawzy MM, Gawdat HI, et al. T helper 17 and Tregs: a novel proposed mechanism for NB-UVB in vitiligo. Exp Dermatol 2014;23(4):283–6.

13. El-Ghorr AA, Norval M. Biological effects of narrowband (311 nm TL01) UVB irradiation: a review. J Photochem Photobiol B 1997;38(2–3):99–106.

14. Wu C-S, Yu C-L, Wu C-S, et al. Narrow-band ultraviolet-B stimulates proliferation and migration of cultured melanocytes. Exp Dermatol 2004; 13(12):755–63.

15. Cui J, Shen L-Y, Wang G-C. Role of hair follicles in the repigmentation of vitiligo. J Invest Dermatol 1991;97(3):410–6.

16. Wu CS, Lan CC, Yu HS. Narrow-band UVB irradiation stimulates the migration and functional development of vitiligo-IgG antibodies-treated pigment cells. J Eur Acad Dermatol Venereol 2012;26(4):456–64.

17. Rodrigues M, Ezzedine K, Hamzavi I, et al. New discoveries in the pathogenesis and classification of vitiligo. J Am Acad Dermatol 2017;77(1):1–13.

18. Oiso N, Suzuki T, Wataya-kaneda M, et al. Guidelines for the diagnosis and treatment of vitiligo in Japan. J Dermatol 2013;40(5):344–54.

19. Taieb A, Alomar A, Böhm M, et al. Guidelines for the management of vitiligo: the European Dermatology Forum consensus. Br J Dermatol 2013;168(1):5–19.

20. Mohammad TF, Al-Jamal M, Hamzavi IH, et al. The Vitiligo Working Group recommendations for narrowband ultraviolet B light phototherapy treatment of vitiligo. J Am Acad Dermatol 2017;76(5):879–88.

21. Cabrera R, Hojman L, Recule F, et al. Predictive model for response rate to narrowband ultraviolet B phototherapy in vitiligo: a retrospective cohort study of 579 patients. Acta Derm Venereol 2018; 98(3–4):416–20.

22. Bae JM, Jung HM, Hong BY, et al. Phototherapy for vitiligo: a systematic review and meta-analysis. JAMA Dermatol 2017;153(7):666–74.

23. Kanwar AJ, Mahajan R, Parsad D. Low-dose oral mini-pulse dexamethasone therapy in progressive unstable vitiligo. J Cutan Med Surg 2013;17(4): 259–68.

24. Radakovic-Fijan S, Fürnsinn-Friedl AM, Hönigsmann H, et al. Oral dexamethasone pulse treatment for vitiligo. J Am Acad Dermatol 2001; 44(5):814–7.

25. Rath N, Kar H, Sabhnani S. An open labeled, comparative clinical study on efficacy and tolerability of oral minipulse of steroid (OMP) alone, OMP with PUVA and broad/narrow band UVB phototherapy in progressive vitiligo. Indian J Dermatol Venereol Leprol 2008;74(4):357.

26. Rodrigues M, Ezzedine K, Hamzavi I, et al. Current and emerging treatments for vitiligo. J Am Acad Dermatol 2017;77(1):17–29.

27. Lim-Ong M, Leveriza RMS, Ong BET, et al. Comparison between narrow-band UVB with topical corticosteroid and narrow-band UVB with placebo in the treatment of vitiligo: a randomized controlled trial. J Phillipine Dermatol Soc 2005;14:17–25.

28. Lim HW, Grimes PE, Agbai O, et al. Afamelanotide and narrowband UV-B phototherapy for the treatment of vitiligo: a randomized multicenter trial. JAMA Dermatol 2015;151(1):42–50.

29. Satyanarayan HS, Kanwar AJ, Parsad D, et al. Efficacy and tolerability of combined treatment with NB-UVB and topical tacrolimus versus NB-UVB alone in patients with vitiligo vulgaris: a randomized intra-individual open comparative trial. Indian J Dermatol Venereol Leprol 2013;79(4):525–7.

30. Klahan S, Asawanonda P. Topical tacrolimus may enhance repigmentation with targeted narrowband ultraviolet B to treat vitiligo: a randomized, controlled study. Clin Exp Dermatol 2009;34(8): e1029–30.

31. Mehrabi D, Pandya AG. A randomized, placebo-controlled, double-blind trial comparing narrowband UV-B plus 0.1% Tacrolimus ointment with narrowband UV-B plus placebo in the treatment of generalized vitiligo. JAMA Dermatol 2006;142(7):927–47.

32. Nordal EJ, Guleng GE, Ronnevig JR. Treatment of vitiligo with narrowband-UVB (TL01) combined with tacrolimus ointment (0.1%) vs. placebo ointment, a randomized right/left double-blind comparative study. J Eur Acad Dermatol Venereol 2011;25(12): 1440–3.

33. Esfandiarpour I, Ekhlasi A, Farajzadeh S, et al. The efficacy of pimecrolimus 1% cream plus narrowband ultraviolet B in the treatment of vitiligo: a double-blind, placebo-controlled clinical trial. J Dermatolog Treat 2009;20(1):14–8.

34. Le Duff F, Fontas E, Giacchero D, et al. 308-nm excimer lamp vs. 308-nm excimer laser for treating vitiligo: a randomized study. Br J Dermatol 2010; 163(1):188–92.

35. Rothstein B, Joshipura D, Saraiya A, et al. Treatment of vitiligo with the topical Janus kinase inhibitor ruxolitinib. J Am Acad Dermatol 2017;76(6):1054–60. e1.

36. Damsky W, King BA. JAK inhibitors in dermatology: the promise of a new drug class. J Am Acad Dermatol 2017;76(4):736–44.

37. A Study of INCB018424 Phosphate Cream in Subjects With Vitiligo. Bethesda (MD): National Library of Medicine; 2014. Available at: https://clinicaltrials.gov/ct2/show/NCT03099304. Accessed March 27, 2019.

38. A Phase 2b study to evaluate the efficacy and safety profile of PF-06651600 and PF-06700841 in active non-segmental vitiligo subjects. Bethesda (MD): National Library of Medicine; 2018. Available at: https://clinicaltrials.gov/ct2/show/NCT03715829?cond=vitiligo&cntry=US&draw=3&rank=26. Accessed May 1, 2019.

39. Raone B, Patrizi A, Gurioli C, et al. Cutaneous carcinogenic risk evaluation in 375 patients treated with narrowband-UVB phototherapy: A 15-year experience from our Institute. Photodermatol Photoimmunol Photomed 2018;34(5):302–6.

40. El-fattah MAA, Esmat SM, El-hadidi HH, et al. The effect of phototherapy and photochemotherapy on the eye. Med J Cairo Univ 2011;79(2):55–9.

Phototherapy in Skin of Color

Olivia R. Ware, BA[a],*, Jonathan Guiyab, BSN, RN[b], Ginette A. Okoye, MD[c]

KEYWORDS

- Phototherapy • Skin of color • Ethnic skin • Ultraviolet radiation • PUVA • NBUVB

KEY POINTS

- Phototherapy in skin of color poses unique challenges and special considerations.
- Skin of color is defined as a person with pigmented skin from diverse racial and ethnic backgrounds, frequently represented as Fitzpatrick skin types IV to VI.
- Administering phototherapy solely based on Fitzpatrick skin type can lead to undertreatment or overdosing.
- Patients with skin of color can exhibit photosensitivity despite the presence of larger amount of epidermal melanin.

Ultraviolet (UV) radiation has been used to treat skin disease in skin of color for centuries. Dating back to 2000 BC, residents of the Nile Delta used phototherapy to treat vitiligo by ingesting crude plant extracts containing psoralen.[1] In addition, Hindu scripture from 1000 BC notes the use of black seeds containing psoralen (likely from the plant *Psoralea corylifolia*) to treat uneven skin tone.[2] Currently, phototherapy is widely used for the management of inflammatory and neoplastic dermatologic disorders in all skin types. Given the inexorable link between epidermal melanin and the skin's response to UV radiation, there are important differences in the dosing, efficacy, and safety of phototherapy in skin of color compared with white skin. Yet, there is a dearth of literature on this subject. Most of these data on phototherapy in nonwhite skin involves patients of East Asian ancestry (eg, Korean, Japanese, Chinese, Thai), with few studies involving patients with Fitzpatrick skin type (FST) V or VI.[3] Herein the authors summarize the known literature and discuss some of the issues unique to the management of phototherapy in skin of color.

SKIN OF COLOR

The term "skin of color" represents people from a wide range of racial and ethnic backgrounds: people from the African and Asian diasporas, Hispanics/Latinos, Pacific Islanders, Native Americans, and other Indigenous groups. The term "skin of color," often used as a euphemism for nonwhite skin, represents people with a wide range of constitutive skin pigmentation, including lightly pigmented nonwhite individuals. Thus, an individual's race or ethnicity, or classification as a person of skin of color, does not provide enough information to determine their propensity for sunburning or their phototherapy dosing regimen. Instead, all patients should be assessed individually regarding their propensity for sunburning. Historically, this assessment has been done using the FST classification system. Developed in 1975, the FST classification system

Disclosure Statement: The authors have nothing to disclose.
[a] Howard University College of Medicine, 2041 Georgia Avenue Northwest, Towers Building, Suite 4300, Washington, DC 20060, USA; [b] Department of Dermatology, Johns Hopkins University School of Medicine, 601 North Caroline Street, Baltimore, MD 21287, USA; [c] Department of Dermatology, Howard University Hospital, 2041 Georgia Avenue Northwest, Towers Building, Suite 4300, Washington, DC 20060, USA
* Corresponding author.
E-mail address: olivia.ware@bison.howard.edu

Dermatol Clin 38 (2020) 63–69
https://doi.org/10.1016/j.det.2019.08.006
0733-8635/20/© 2019 Elsevier Inc. All rights reserved.

assesses the propensity of the skin to burn during phototherapy.[4] The original FST classification included only skin types I to IV and was initially based on skin and eye color. When people with brown eyes and hair were identified as "sun-reactive" type I, the classification evolved to include patients' self-reported response to sun exposure. Skin types V and VI were later added to the classification to represent individuals of Asian, Indian, and African descent.[4] Currently, skin of color is frequently represented as FST IV to VI. However, individuals with skin of color possess a wide range of responses to UV exposure and can be classified anywhere on the FST I to VI scale.

Skin of Color: Response to Ultraviolet Radiation

Individuals with skin of color tend to have larger, more numerous melanosomes that contain more melanin and are distributed throughout the epidermis, including the upper layers.[5] Therefore, pigmented skin is a very efficient UV filter and more effective at preventing UV-induced DNA damage in the lower epidermis (including keratinocyte stem cells and melanocytes). Because of the relative dearth of melanin in the epidermis of white skin, up to 5 times as much UV radiation reaches the upper dermis of white skin compared with darker skin.[6,7] In addition, apoptosis to remove cells with UV-induced DNA damage is significantly greater in darker skin. These factors decrease the risk of skin cancer in people with skin of color, particularly those with darker skin pigmentation. However, data suggest that, in people with skin of color with lighter pigmentation, more UV radiation reaches the basal layer of the epidermis, producing DNA damage in both keratinocytes and melanocytes.[8] Hence, although higher doses of UV radiation are generally more effective and well tolerated in darker skin, this may not necessarily be true of skin of color patients with lighter skin.

Despite the protective effect of melanin, idiosyncratic patterns of photosensitivity exist in patients with skin of color. In the United States, sunburns and melanoma are more common in Native Americans than in any other nonwhite racial group.[9,10] Patients with skin of color are more likely than Caucasians to develop certain photodermatoses, including polymorphous light eruption, recalcitrant chronic actinic dermatitis, actinic prurigo, and diltiazem-induced photo-mediated reaction.[11] The pathophysiology of this paradox has not yet been determined but may be related to the contribution of melanin to the production of UV-induced reactive oxygen species.

In darker skin, UVA exposure produces more pronounced immediate pigment darkening, persistent pigment darkening, and long-lasting delated tanning (DT).[12] This UVA-induced skin darkening attenuates the response to subsequent UVA exposure in a dose-dependent manner and can decrease the efficacy of UVA therapy.[13] UVB is more erythemogenic than melanogenic.[12] However, UVB exposure is less likely to cause erythema in darker skin but induces pigment darkening through DT.[12] Both UVA and UVB light induce relative immunosuppression in the skin but differences between lighter and darker skin have not been studied.[12]

PHOTOTHERAPY DOSING IN SKIN OF COLOR
The Limitations of Fitzpatrick Skin Type and Minimal Erythema Dose

In the United States, the overall approach to phototherapy dosing is fixed and cautious,[14] and there is no universally acceptable protocol for initiation of phototherapy in various skin diseases. Clinicians usually determine the initial phototherapy dose using FST or by starting at 70% of the patients minimal erythema dose (MED), with subsequent dosage increases by predetermined increments.[15] Determination of the patient's UV sensitivity via MED phototesting is the more accurate of these approaches but is often impractical in the clinical setting.[14] In addition, the clinical challenge of perceiving erythema in darker skin tones may make MED testing less valid in skin of color. Clinicians therefore most commonly use the patient's FST when determining initial phototherapy dose, but this may be problematic in skin of color. Data suggest that administering phototherapy solely based on FST may lead to under- or overdosing in skin of color.[16–18] Although it is a good clinical predictor of skin cancer risk, FST is not a good predictor of UV sensitivity and MED.[16,18] Objective measurement of skin color (via colorimetry) is often more reliable than FST to predict UV sensitivity and erythema due to UV radiation but may be impractical in daily practice.[17,19]

More studies are needed to inform alternative ways to determine the initial dose of phototherapy in skin of color, such as colorimetry or validated skin-type identification scales based on constitutive skin color.[20,21] However, in the meantime, MED testing should be used when possible, to allow for detection of unexpectedly photosensitive patients. If MED is impractical, and FST is being used to determine the initial dose, practitioners should not make assumptions about a patient's FST based on their race. Instead, the FST-typing questions should be deliberately asked of every patient.

When treating skin of color with phototherapy, the key is finding the right balance between treating conservatively to avoid adverse effects and treating assertively to overcome the natural UV filter of pigmented skin. Clinical pearls and considerations for phototherapy in skin of color are summarized in **Box 1**.

SAFETY OF PHOTOTHERAPY IN SKIN OF COLOR

In skin of color there is decreased risk of sunburn and skin cancer, making phototherapy a relatively safe modality in these patients. The known short-term side effects of phototherapy include erythema, burning, stinging, xerosis, pruritus, and blistering.[22] The long-term side effects include photoaging and carcinogenesis. These side effects are less likely in darker skin. When it occurs, UVB-induced erythema in darker skin lasts less than 3 days (vs 1–2 weeks in lighter skin).[14] Oral psoralen ultraviolet A (PUVA) is associated with nausea and vomiting as well as PUVA itch and lentigines. An analysis of predisposing factors to PUVA lentiginosis found patients with skin types V and VI were significantly less likely to have moderate or severe lentigines after phototherapy.[23]

In skin of color, additional potential side effects should be addressed when consenting patients for phototherapy. Tanning due to narrowband ultraviolet B in patients with psoriasis has been shown to negatively affect patient compliance, particularly in dark-skinned individuals.[24] Patients should be informed that increased pigmentation (tanning) will occur in all exposed areas, and that this tanning may persist for weeks to months after treatment is discontinued. In addition, darker-skinned individuals are at higher risk for prolonged postinflammatory hyperpigmentation (PIH) from inflammatory disorders, and although phototherapy will likely improve the disorder it is being used to treat, it may prolong PIH.

UVA radiation is more likely to cause hair damage in patients of African descent, compared with Caucasians and Asians.[25] Hair damage may be a significant concern for black patients, likely related to cultural beliefs and attitudes toward hair and could affect overall compliance with treatment. Hair damage in patients of African descent should be included in the consenting process, and patients should be encouraged to wear head scarves or other protective devices.

Consideration should also be given to specific photosensitivity concerns that are unique to skin of color. People of Native American ancestry may be more photosensitive than their constitutive skin color suggests. Among nonwhite groups, people of Native American ancestry are the most likely to sunburn.[9] Inquiring about potential Native American ethnicity should be a part of the history for all phototherapy patients, especially because the presence of Native American ancestry cannot necessarily be gleaned from an individual's appearance or skin color. Other important considerations are that African-Americans are more susceptible to hypertension than Caucasians and are more likely to be prescribed hydrochlorothiazide, a potentially photosensitizing drug, and that photosensitivity related to human immunodeficiency virus (HIV) infection is more common in African American patients.[26–29]

HEALTH DISPARITIES IN DERMATOLOGIC DISEASES IN SKIN OF COLOR: A POTENTIAL ROLE FOR PHOTOTHERAPY

Compared with white patients, there are differences in the prevalence, quality of life impact, and/or outcomes in skin of color patients with psoriasis,[30,31] atopic dermatitis,[32,33] mycosis fungoides,[34–37] pruritus (eg, renal and HIV-related pruritus),[38–41] and vitiligo.[42] Phototherapy is a relatively safe and inexpensive treatment modality that has been shown to be effective in the disorders noted earlier and can be used in our attempts to reduce these disparities.[22,40,43–48]

ACCESS TO PHOTOTHERAPY: BARRIERS AND PROPOSED SOLUTIONS

When considering the use of phototherapy in skin of color, issues surrounding health disparities become apparent. Patients with skin of color who are of lower socioeconomic status are at risk for poorer outcomes and may have underappreciated barriers to access to phototherapy. Phototherapy often requires frequent treatment visits and long treatment durations for the management of chronic dermatologic disorders such as vitiligo, psoriasis, and mycosis fungoides. This time-intensive therapy results in lost time from work or school, increased childcare needs, increased transportation and/or parking costs, and multiple insurance copayments per week. These costs may be prohibitive for some patients, and likely disproportionately affect those of lower socioeconomic status (SES). Potential solutions to ameliorate the impact of these issues include the following:

- Flexible scheduling, that is, patient given a window of time to present for treatment instead of a defined appointment time

Box 1
Practical recommendations for phototherapy in skin of color

Patients should be consented before initiating phototherapy, including an overview of how phototherapy works, expected outcomes, and potential adverse effects. Emphasis should be placed on the importance of consistent compliance with the treatment schedule in order to increase efficacy and decrease the risk of burning.

Skin of color patients are often concerned about hyperpigmentation. It is important to explain that this is both a temporary and anticipated effect of phototherapy. Skin color will eventually return to baseline once treatment is discontinued.

Patients of African descent are more likely to have hair damage from ultraviolet (UV) radiation. This should be included in the consenting process and a head scarf or other protective headwear should be encouraged.

Minimal erythema dose (MED) testing is the most accurate way to ascertain the initial phototherapy dose. However, if it is not practical, then Fitzpatrick skin type (FST) can be used. More studies are needed, but objectively measuring constitutive skin pigmentation using colorimetry may be another option for determining phototherapy dosing for skin of color.

Patients with skin of color should be asked specifically about their prior responses to ultraviolet light. Asking about erythema and "tanning" may not be the best way to ascertain UV reactions in this patient population. These questions can be supplemented by asking open-ended questions such as the following:

- "How does your skin react to sun exposure?"
- "Have you ever had redness, pain, or peeling of your skin after spending time in the sun?"

In the absence of MED testing, consider starting patients with skin of color with a conservative initial dose, and if tolerated, use larger incremental dosage increases than would be used on FST I and -II.

Consider more conservative initial dosing in patients with Native American ancestry.

Because erythema may be subtle in skin of color, dose adjustments should be made according to patient feedback regarding skin pain, pruritus, or other side effects before each treatment session.

Obtain a thorough medical history. Ask specifically about systemic lupus erythematosus (SLE) and human immunodeficiency virus (HIV) infection. SLE would be a contraindication to phototherapy. For patients with HIV, consider performing MED testing or decreasing the initial phototherapy dose by 25% to 50% of that used for their baseline FST.

Obtain a detailed list of the patient's current medications. If the patient is on a photosensitizing drug (eg, doxycycline, hydrochlorothiazide), decrease their phototherapy dose by 25% to 50%.

If the patient is erythrodermic (eg, atopic dermatitis), consider a starting dose appropriate for FST I and II, regardless of the patient's baseline FST.

When treating vitiligo, use a treatment protocol appropriate for FST I, regardless of the patient's baseline FST.

- Availability of appointments outside work hours or on weekends
- Subsidized parking for phototherapy patients
- Enhanced efficiency of phototherapy appointments to decrease time spent in the visit, for example, an expedited patient registration process

Another potential barrier to access to phototherapy is the availability of phototherapy centers. Phototherapy is not offered by all dermatology practices, and especially in rural areas, patients may have to travel long distances to receive treatment. A potential solution to this issue is the use of home UVB phototherapy devices.[49,50] The cost of

these devices is often covered by the patient's health insurance for certain diagnoses but involves the submission of prior authorizations, letters of necessity and advocacy on the part of the provider. Unfortunately, for patients from a lower SES, who may not have a consistently stable living situation or adequate space for portable UV units, home phototherapy is not a practical option. Building relationships and a safe space for patients to openly discuss their living situation is the key to ascertaining the impact of this issue on an individual patient.

Patient-derived factors are not the only barriers to care. Provider perception of an individual's overall health and need for aggressive treatment is another potential barrier for skin of color patients. Race and ethnicity are significant predictors of the quality of health care received.[51] Black patients are less likely to receive equal medical treatments when compared with whites, even when controlling for factors such as insurance, age, and place of treatment.[51] Physician-derived factors such as assumptions made about patients (eg, patient reliability, self-control, compliance with medical advice, social support) and clinical uncertainty when providing care for patients from minority backgrounds may exacerbate these disparities.[51] Provider training in implicit bias and culturally competent care, as well as improving racial/ethnic diversity in dermatology providers may contribute to improving these issues.

OTHER CONSIDERATIONS IN SKIN OF COLOR

UV radiation has been used to treat disease in skin of color for centuries, long before the advent of modern-day phototherapy. The role of holistic, naturopathic, and/or alternative medicines, such as Ayurvedic medicine, in the treatment of chronic skin disorders should be addressed during the clinical encounter. Ayurvedic medicine originated in India and remains one of the world's oldest medical systems. Ayurvedic treatment combines natural elements (mainly derived from plants) and lifestyle modifications to treat physical and mental illness. The World Health Organization estimates that 75% to 80% of the world's population relies on herbal medicine as their primary form of health care. In the United States, approximately 9.2% of all out-of-pocket health care costs go toward alternative medicine.[52] Providers should demonstrate cultural competency by adopting behaviors that allow them to provide effective cross-cultural care. This requires respect for health beliefs and cultural practices of diverse patients.[53] There are numerous reasons why an individual might eschew Western medicine in favor of Ayurvedic treatments, including perceived health benefits, cost, prior failure of physician-guided treatment due to under- or overdosing, a lack of awareness about the risks that alternative products may carry, cultural norms, and desperation born of the psychosocial burden of one's disease.

Topically and systemically administered psoralen-containing products for the treatment of skin disease are widely available without a prescription from major Internet retailers. These products are affordable and use suggestive packaging to tout their benefits without mention of their risks. Products are available in formulations intended for ingestion, such as tablets or powders, or as topical creams, ointments, and oils. It is important for physicians to specifically ask about products that patients have acquired over the counter or online to determine their risk of additional phototoxicity before starting phototherapy.

SUMMARY

In summary, phototherapy in skin of color necessitates special considerations. Pigmented skin is an efficient UV filter that significantly decreases UV-induced DNA damage. Thus, higher doses of UV radiation are generally more effective and well tolerated in darker skin. However, an objective and practical system has not yet been established to consistently predict the response to UV light in skin of color and thus determine optimal phototherapy dosing for these patients. In the interim, the authors recommend deliberately eliciting a history of each individual patient's response to sun exposure before assigning an FST, inquiring regarding Native American ancestry, obtaining a careful medical history, particularly seeking the presence of systemic lupus erythematosus and HIV infection, and obtaining a medication history including over-the-counter drugs and herbal medications. In addition, providers should be cognizant of SES factors that may affect patients' phototherapy-related outcomes, including barriers to compliance and access.

REFERENCES

1. Couperus M. Ammoidin (xanthotoxin) in the treatment of vitiligo. Calif Med 1954;81:402–6.
2. Nordlund JJ. The medical treatment of Vitiligo: a historical review. Dermatol Clin 2017;35(2):107.
3. Alexis AF. Lasers and light-based therapies in ethnic skin: treatment options and recommendations for Fitzpatrick skin types V and VI. Br J Dermatol 2013;169(Suppl 3):91–7.
4. Reddy KK, Lenzy YM, Brown KL, et al. Chapter 9. Racial considerations: skin of color. In: Goldsmith LA, editor. Fitzpatrick's dermatology in general medicine. 8th edition. New York: McGraw-Hill; 2012. Available at: http://accessmedicine.mhmedical.com/content.aspx?bookid=392&sectionid=41138702.
5. Bolognia J, Schaffer J, Cerroni L, editors. Dermatology. 4th edition. Philadelphia: Elsevier; 2018.
6. Yamaguchi Y, Beer JZ, Hearing VJ. Melanin mediated apoptosis of epidermal cells damaged by ultraviolet radiation: factors influencing the incidence of skin cancer. Arch Dermatol Res 2008; 300(Suppl 1):S43–50.
7. Kaidbey KH, Agin PP, Sayre RM, et al. Photo protection by melanin – a comparison of black and Caucasian skin. J Am Acad Dermatol 1979;1(3): 249–60.

8. Del Bino S, Duval C, Bernerd F. Clinical and biological characterization of skin pigmentation diversity and its consequences on UV impact. Int J Mol Sci 2018;19(9) [pii:E2668].

9. Hall I, Saraiya M, Thompson T. Correlates of sunburn experiences among U.S. adults: results of the 2000 national health interview survey. Public Health Rep 2003;118:540–8.

10. Howlader N, Noone AM, Krapcho M, et al. SEER cancer statistics review, 1975-2004. National Cancer Institute; 2017.

11. Gutierrez D, Gaulding JV, Motta Beltran AF, et al. Photodermatoses in skin of colour. J Eur Acad Dermatol Venereol 2018;32(11):1879–86.

12. Sklar LR, Almutawa F, Lim HW, et al. Effects of ultraviolet radiation, visible light, and infrared radiation on erythema and pigmentation: a review. Photochem Photobiol Sci 2013;12:54–64.

13. Wang F, Garza L, Cho S, et al. Effect of increased pigmentation on the antifibrotic response of human skin to UV-A1 phototherapy. Arch Dermatol 2008; 144(7):851–8.

14. Hönigsmann H, Schwarz T. Ultraviolet therapy. In: Bolognia J, Schaffer J, Cerroni L, editors. Dermatology. 4th edition. Elsevier Limited; 2018. p. 2325–40.

15. Madigan LM, Al-Jamal M, Hamzavi I. Exploring the gaps in the evidence-based application of narrowband UVB for the treatment of vitiligo. Photodermatol Photoimmunol Photomed 2016;32: 66–80.

16. Stern RS, Momtaz K. Skin typing for assessment of skin cancer risk and acute response to UV-B and oral methoxsalen photochemotherapy. Arch Dermatol 1984;120:869–73.

17. Leenutaphong V. Relationship between skin color and cutaneous response to ultraviolet radiation in Thai. Photodermatol Photoimmunol Photomed 1996;11:198–203.

18. Venkataram MN, Haitham AA. Correlating skin phototype and minimum erythema dose in Arab skin. Int J Dermatol 2003;42:191–2.

19. Westerhof W, Estevez-Uscanga O, Meens J, et al. The relation between constitutional skin color and photosensitivity estimated from UV-induced erythema and pigmentation dose-response curves. J Invest Dermatol 1990;94:812–6.

20. Ho BK, Robinson J. Color bar tool for skin type self-identification: a cross sectional study. J Am Acad Dermatol 2015;73(2):312–3.

21. Taylor SC, Arsonnaud S, Czernielewski J, et al. The Taylor Hyperpigmentation Scale: a new visual assessment tool for the evaluation of skin color and pigmentation. Cutis 2005;76(4):270–4.

22. Syed ZU, Hamzavi IH. Photomedicine and phototherapy considerations for patients with skin of color. Photodermatol Photoimmunol Photomed 2011;27: 10–6.

23. Rhodes AR, Stern RS, Melski JW. The PUVA lentigo: an analysis of predisposing factors. J Invest Dermatol 1983;81(5):459–63.

24. Kwon IH, Woo SM, Choi JW, et al. Recovery from tanning induced by narrow-band UVB phototherapy in brown-skinned individuals with psoriasis: twelve-month follow-up. J Dermatol Sci 2010;57: 12–8.

25. Ji JH, Park TS, Lee HJ, et al. The ethnic differences of the damage of hair and integral hair lipid after ultra violet radiation. Ann Dermatol 2013;25:54–60.

26. Rosenthal A, Herrmann J. Hydrochlorothiazide-induced photosensitivity in psoriasis patient following exposure to narrow-band UVB excimer therapy. Photodermatol Photoimmunol Photomed 2019. https://doi.org/10.1111/phpp.12471.

27. Harman J, Walker ER, Charbonneau V, et al. Treatment of hypertension among African Americans: the Jackson Heart Study. J Clin Hypertens (Greenwich) 2013;15(6):367–74.

28. Williams SK, Ravenell J, Seyedali S, et al. Hypertension in blacks: discussion of the U.S. clinical practice guidelines. Prog Cardiovasc Dis 2016;59(3): 282–8.

29. Bilu D, Mamelak A, Nguyen R, et al. Clinical and epidemiologic characterization of photosensitivity in HIV-positive individuals. Photodermatol Photoimmunol Photomed 2004;20(4):175–83.

30. Kaufman BP, Alexis AF. Psoriasis in skin of color: insights into the epidemiology, clinical presentation, genetics, quality-of-life impact, and treatment of psoriasis in non-white racial/ethnic groups. Am J Clin Dermatol 2018;19:405–23.

31. Kaufman BP, Alexis AF. Author correction to: psoriasis in skin of color: insights into the epidemiology, clinical presentation, genetics, quality-of-life impact, and treatment of psoriasis in non-white racial/ethnic groups. Am J Clin Dermatol 2018;19: 425.

32. Shaw TE, Currie GP, Koudelka CW, et al. Eczema prevalence in the United States from the 2003 National Survey of Children's Health. J Invest Dermatol 2011;131:67–73.

33. Moore MM, Rifas-Shiman SL, Rich-Edwards JW, et al. Perinatal predictors of atopic dermatitis occurring in the first six months of life. Pediatrics 2004; 113:468–74.

34. Bradford PT, Devesa SS, Anderson WF, et al. Cutaneous lymphoma incidence patterns in the United States: a population-based study of 3884 cases. Blood 2009;113:5064–73.

35. Criscione VD, Weinstock MA. Incidence of cutaneous T-cell lymphoma in the United States, 1973-2002. Arch Dermatol 2007;143:854–9.

36. Wilson LD, Hinds GA, Yu JB. Age, race, sex, stage, and incidence of cutaneous lymphoma. Clin Lymphoma Myeloma Leuk 2012;12:291–6.

37. Sun G, Berthelot C, Li Y, et al. Poor prognosis in non-Caucasian patients with early-onset mycosis fungoides. J Am Acad Dermatol 2009;60:231–5.

38. Shaw FM, Luk KMH, Chen KH, et al. Racial disparities in the impact of chronic pruritus: a cross-sectional study on quality of life and resource utilization in United States veterans. J Am Acad Dermatol 2017;77(1):63–9.

39. National Institute of Diabetes and Digestive and Kidney Disease. Kidney disease statistics for the United States. Available at: www.niddk.nih.gov. Accessed May 10, 2019.

40. Singh F, Rudikoff D. HIV-associated pruritus: etiology and management. Am J Clin Dermatol 2003; 4(3):177–88.

41. Boozalis E, Tang O, Patel S, et al. Ethnic differences and comorbidities of 909 prurigo nodularis patients. J Am Acad Dermatol 2018;79(4):714–9.e3.

42. Pahwa P, Mehta M, Khaitan BK, et al. The psychosocial impact of vitiligo in Indian patients. Indian J Dermatol Venereol Leprol 2013;79(5):679.

43. Rodenbeck DL, Silverberg JK, Silverberg NB. Phototherapy for atopic dermatitis. Clin Dermatol 2016; 34(5):607–13.

44. Yones SS, Palmer RA, Garibaldinos TM, et al. Randomized double-blind trial of treatment of vitiligo: efficacy of psoralen-UV-A therapy vs Narrowband-UV-B therapy. Arch Dermatol 2007;143:578–84.

45. Honigsmann H. Erythema and pigmentation. Photodermatol Photoimmunol Photomed 2002;18:75–81.

46. Hinds G, Heald P. Cutaneous T-cell lymphoma in skin of color. J Am Acad Dermatol 2008;60:359–75.

47. Agi C, Kuhn D, Chung J, et al. Racial differences in the use of extracorporeal photopheresis for mycosis fungoides. J Dermatolog Treat 2015;26:266–8.

48. Lim HW, Vallurupalli S, Meola T. UVB phototherapy is an effective treatment for pruritus in patients infected with HIV. J Am Acad Dermatol 1997; 37(3 Pt 1):414–7.

49. Anderson KL, Feldman SR. A guide to prescribing home phototherapy for patients with psoriasis: the appropriate patient, the type of unit, the treatment regimen, and the potential obstacles. J Am Acad Dermatol 2015;72:868–78.e1.

50. Mohammad TF, Silpa-Archa N, Griffith JL, et al. Home phototherapy in vitiligo. Photodermatol Photoimmunol Photomed 2017;33:241–52.

51. Smedley BD, Smith AY, Nelson AR, et al, Institute of Medicine. Committee on understanding and eliminating racial and ethnic disparities in health care. Unequal treatment: confronting racial and ethnic disparities in health care. Washington DC: National Academy Press; 2003. p. 764.

52. Americans Spent $30.2 billion out-of-pocket on complementary health approaches. 2017. Available at: https://nccih.nih.gov/news/press/cost-spending-062 22016. Accessed May 1, 2019.

53. Vashi NA, Patzelt N, Wirya S, et al. Dermatoses caused by cultural practices: cosmetic cultural practices. J Am Acad Dermatol 2018;78(1):19.

Phototherapy in the Evaluation and Management of Photodermatoses

Angela J. Jiang, MD, Henry W. Lim, MD*

KEYWORDS

- Phototesting • Phototherapy • Photodermatoses • Polymorphous light eruption
- Chronic actinic dermatitis • Solar urticaria • Erythropoietic porphyria • Actinic prurigo

KEY POINTS

- Phototesting and photopatch testing are multiple-day procedures. Minimal urticarial dose should be determined within 20 minutes after radiation, and minimal erythema dose (MED) should be assessed after 24 hours.
- Narrowband UVB can be used for hardening in many photodermatoses, but UVA1 is preferred in prophylactic therapy for patients with solar urticaria.
- For photosensitive patients, phototesting should be ascertained before initiating phototherapy.

INTRODUCTION

Diagnoses of photodermatoses can be challenging; patients can exhibit a wide variety of symptoms and physical examination findings, and they can present during a disease-free period. In a patient with a suspected photodermatosis, clinical evaluation should always consist of a thorough history and physical examination.

Ultraviolet light (UV) and visible light are important components in the diagnosis of photodermatoses, and UV has the unique ability to also be used to manage photodermatoses. Phototesting may be helpful in confirmation of a photosensitivity disorder, particularly photodermatoses that are immunologically mediated. Once a diagnosis is confirmed, phototherapy can be used in the management of many photodermatoses. This article discusses phototesting protocols and interpretation as well as the management of photodermatoses with phototherapy.

PHOTOTESTING

Following a thorough history and physical examination of a patient with a suspected photodermatosis, phototesting can be pursued. Phototesting is most beneficial in the evaluation of immunologically mediated photodermatoses such as chronic actinic dermatitis (CAD), solar urticaria, and to a lesser extent polymorphous light eruption (PMLE).[1] It is not helpful in the diagnosis of porphyrias because the action spectrum is in the visible light range (Soret band, 400–410 nm); therefore, it is difficult to achieve a positive phototest result. It is of academic interest in genodermatoses because the action spectrum for many has not been well characterized.[2] The objective of

Disclosures: A.J. Jiang has nothing to disclose. H.W. Lim is a Consultant at Pierre Fabre, and an Investigator at Estee Lauder, Ferndale, Unigen, and Incyte.
Department of Dermatology, Henry Ford Health System, 3031 West Grand Boulevard, Suite 800, Detroit, MI 48202, USA
* Corresponding author.
E-mail address: hlim1@hfhs.org

Dermatol Clin 38 (2020) 71–77
https://doi.org/10.1016/j.det.2019.08.007

derm.theclinics.com

phototesting is to determine the action spectrum of the photodermatosis and to better plan for management.

PROTOCOLS

Before phototesting, patients should be instructed to avoid systemic immunosuppressants and topical steroids to the site of phototesting for at least 2 weeks.[1,3] Antihistamines should be avoided in the 2 to 3 days before phototesting.

Phototesting

An opaque template with several windows (2 cm × 2 cm) is placed on unaffected skin, preferably on the back or abdomen. The skin is subsequently exposed to increasing doses of ultraviolet A (UVA), broadband ultraviolet B (UVB), and/or visible light. Broadband UVB is used for phototesting for possible UVB sensitivity. At the Henry Ford Photodermatology Unit, the UVB doses used for phototesting are 6, 12, 24, 36, 48, 72, 96, and 108 mJ/cm^2. A PUVA (psoralen and UVA) booth is used for UVA phototesting, and patients stand in the center of the booth. The UVA doses are 3, 6, 12, and 18 J/cm^2. A slide projector is used as the light source for visible light testing, with the light source placed 30 cm away from the skin surface. To avoid heat-induced urticaria, a water filter is placed in front of the light source. The visible light exposure times are 15, 30, 45, and 60 minutes.

An immediate reading is performed within 20 minutes after the exposures to examine for an urticarial response as seen in patients with solar urticaria. The lowest dose of radiation that induces wheal formation is defined as the minimal urticarial dose (MUD). The patient is then instructed to return in 24 hours to determine the minimal erythema dose (MED). The MED is defined as the dose of UVB, UVA, or visible light that induces a just perceptible erythema covering the entire irradiated area.

Provocative Light Testing

If induction of lesions is desired, provocative light testing can be performed. Provocative light testing can be used in the diagnosis of PMLE, particularly in patients whose MED value is normal. It has also been used in patients with hydroa vacciniforme or erythropoietic porphyria (EPP) with varying degrees of success. The test involves exposure of the same site for 3 to 4 consecutive days.[4,5] The authors usually begin at 80% of the MED and increase it by 10% to 20% on the subsequent days. Lesions typically develop within 24 hours and can be assessed and biopsied. In practice,

owing to the logistical challenge of the patient having to return to the clinic on 4 to 5 consecutive days, difficulty in insurance coverage, and the availability of other diagnostic data (history, morphology, histology, and porphyrin profile), photoprovocative testing is no longer commonly performed.

Photopatch Testing

Photopatch testing should be used for patients in whom photoallergic contact dermatitis is suspected. Photopatch testing is similar to standard patch testing; however, photopatch testing includes irradiation of patches with UVA. Duplicate panels of photoallergen panels are placed on unaffected skin, preferably on the back (**Table 1**). The sites are covered with an opaque material for 24 hours to prevent any UV exposure. After 24 hours, one set of panels is irradiated with UVA, either 10 J/cm^2 of UVA or 50% of the MED-A if the patient has low MED-A. The other panel remains covered by opaque material to serve as the unirradiated control.

INTERPRETATION

Phototesting can confirm the presence of photosensitivity and provide an action spectrum. With the MED-B testing doses used (broadband UVB, 6–108 mJ/cm^2), in the authors' center, the normal range for Fitzpatrick skin phototype (SFT) I to II is 20 to 40 mJ/cm^2, and for those with SFT V to VI, greater than 96 mJ/cm^2. For UVA phototesting, with the dose range used (3–18 J/cm^2), any response at any of these doses is considered positive/abnormal for all skin types. Exposure with visible light (15–60 min) should result in a completely negative response; therefore, any urticarial or erythematous response would be considered positive.

Expected phototesting results can vary (**Table 2**). Phototesting in PMLE may reveal abnormal reactions to UVB, UVA, visible light, or no reaction at all.[6–8] In CAD, patients may have reduced MEDs to UVB and/or UVA and/or visible light exposure. Reports from photodermatology centers from various locations worldwide showed that 10% to 27% of phototested patients had clinically relevant positive photopatch test results.[8–10]

Determination of the precise action spectrum of solar urticaria can present a challenge. Patients with solar urticaria have demonstrated varying sensitivity to UVB, UVA, and visible light.[11–13] One action spectrum, often shorter wavelengths, can result in wheal formation, whereas another, typically longer wavelength, may cause wheal inhibition, leading to the "double action spectrum."[14,15] An

Table 1
Example of photopatch test series

Class of Photoallergen	Allergen	Concentration
Sunscreen ingredients	2-Ethylhexyl-4-methoxycinnamate	7.5% pet
	2-Hydroxy-4-methoxy-benzophenon-5-sulfonic acid (sulisobenzone)	10.0% pet
	Octyl salicylate	5.0% pet
	4-Tertbutyl-4'-methoxydibenzoylmethane (Parsol 1789; avobenzone)	5.0% pet
	Homomenthylsalicylate (homosalate)	5.0% pet
	Methyl anthranilate	5.0% pet
	6-Methylcoumarin	1.0% alc
	4-Aminobenzoic acid (PABA)	1.0% pet
	4-Aminobenzoic acid (PABA)	5.0% alc
	2-Ethylhexyl-4-dimethylaminobenzoate (Padimate O)	5.0% alc
	2-Ethylhexyl-4-dimethylaminobenzoate (Padimate O)	5.0% pet
	2-Hydroxy-4-methoxybenzophenone (benzophenone 3; oxybenzone)	3.0% pet
Microbicides	Dichlorophene	1.0% pet
	Triclosan (Ingasan DP300)	2.0% pet
	Hexachlorophene	1.0% pet
	Chlorhexidine diacetate	0.5% aq
	3,4,5-Tribromosalicylanilide (tribromsalan, TBS)	1.0% pet
	Bithionol	1.0% pet
	Fentichlor (2,2'-thiobis(4-chlorophenol))	1.0% pet
Antipsychotics	Promethazine hydrochloride	1.0% pet
	Chlorpromazine hydrochloride	0.1% pet
Plants	Chamomilla Romana (*Anthemis nobilis*)	1.0% pet
	Diallyldisulfide	1.0% pet
	Arnica montana (mountain tobacco)	0.5% pet
	Taraxacum officinale (dandelion)	2.5% pet
	Achillea millefolium (yarrow)	1.0% pet
	Propolis	10.0% pet
	Chrysanthemum cinerariaefolium (pyrethrum)	1.0% pet
	Sesquiterpene lactone mix	0.1% pet
	α-Methylene-γ-butyrolactone	0.01% pet
	Tanacetum vulgare (tansy)	1.0% pet
	Alantolactone	0.033% pet
	Lichen acid mix	0.3% pet
	Atranorin	0.1% pet
	Usnic acid	0.1% pet
	Evernic acid	0.1% pet
Miscellaneous	White petrolatum (Penreco Snow White)	100.0% pet
	Thiourea	0.1% pet
	Sandalwood oil (Indian)	2.0% pet

Abbreviations: alc, alcohol; aq, water; pet, petrolatum.

augmentation spectrum may also exist.[13,16] Thus, patients with suspected solar urticaria may have different action spectra on repeated phototesting.[13] It should be noted that of all photodermatoses, solar urticaria has the highest probability of having a positive response to visible light testing, manifesting as an urticarial response at immediate to 20 minutes' reading.

In actinic prurigo, patients may demonstrate decreased MED to UVA only, UVA and UVB, or no reaction at all.[17,18] Patients with hydroa vacciniforme can demonstrate a lowered MED to UVA and, rarely, to UVB.[19] Lesions of hydroa vacciniforme have been reproduced on provocative phototesting.[19] Patients with EPP may report development of burning sensations during exposure to visible light, followed by erythema and swelling.[20] Vesicles, bullae, or purpura, though uncommon, may be observed.

Interpretation of photopatch testing results is shown in **Table 3**. Erythema, edema, and/or vesiculation indicate a positive reaction.[1,3,21] If a

Table 2
Expected phototest and photopatch test results

Photodermatosis	MED for UVA	MED for UVB	Visible Light	Photopatch Test
Polymorphous light eruption	Normal/↓	Normal/↓	Normal	Negative
Chronic actinic dermatitis	↓	↓	Normal/↓	Negative/positive
Solar urticaria	Urticaria	Urticaria	Urticaria	Negative
Actinic prurigo	↓	Normal/↓	Normal	Negative
Hydroa vacciniforme	↓	Rarely ↓	Normal	Negative
Phototoxicity	↓	Normal	Normal	Negative
Photoallergy	↓	Normal	Normal	Positive

Data from Refs.[7–22]

positive reaction is noted at the irradiated site only, this would be interpreted as a photoallergic reaction. A positive reaction at both unirradiated and irradiated sites is consistent with an allergic contact dermatitis. Finally, a positive reaction at the unirradiated site with a stronger reaction at an irradiated site indicates the presence of both allergic contact and photoallergic dermatitis.

Although a negative photopatch test could reliably exclude photoallergic response to substances tested, it should be noted that phototesting may not always be positive in patients with suspected photodermatoses. Phototesting should be considered as another data point, together with history, morphology and distribution of lesions, histology, and appropriate laboratory testing (eg, lupus panel, plasma porphyrins) in arriving at the final diagnosis.

PHOTOTHERAPY FOR PHOTODERMATOSES

First-line management for all photodermatoses is sun protection and avoidance. Patients should be educated about a proper photoprotection strategy, which includes seeking shade when outdoors, and wearing photoprotective clothing, a wide-brimmed hat, and sunglasses. On exposed areas, broad-spectrum sunscreen with sun protection factor (SPF) greater than 50 should be

used. Because of the photosensitivity, we recommend broad-spectrum sunscreen with SPF greater than 50 rather than sunscreen with SPF greater than 30 recommended to otherwise healthy individuals.

Before beginning phototherapy, the patient should be evaluated for intake of any medications with photosensitizing potential such as thiazide diuretics, doxycycline, and minocycline. The action spectrum of almost all photosensitizing medications is in the UVA range. Given that a narrowband UVB (NBUVB) light source emits a minimal amount of UVA, photosensitizing medications should be of no concern. However, the appropriate UV dose should be adjusted if PUVA or UVA1 (ie, 340–400 nm) is to be administered. Topical and systemic retinoids would result in thinning of the epidermis, resulting in greater penetration of UV; therefore, a dose decrease (usually 30%) of all forms of phototherapy should be initiated.

In practice, the most common photodermatoses treated with phototherapy are PMLE and solar urticaria, although the use of phototherapy has been described in other photodermatoses in anecdotal reports.[22,23]

Protocols

For patients with photodermatoses, their degree of photosensitivity, as determined by phototesting, would dictate the phototherapy protocol. Although broadband UVB is used as a light source of UVB phototesting to obtain an assessment of photosensitivity across the UVB spectrum, the result does serve as a guide in NBUVB phototherapy for the same patient.

Protocols outlined here for NBUVB and UVA1 should serve as a general guide. Adjustment of starting dose and rate of dose increase should be made based on clinical judgment. In patients who are exquisitely photosensitive, prednisone at 0.6 to 0.8 mg/kg for a total of 5 to 10 days can

Table 3
Expected photopatch test results

Diagnosis	Unirradiated	Irradiated (UVA)
Photoallergy	Normal	+
Contact allergy	+	+
Both contact allergy and photoallergy	+	++

Data from Refs.[1,3,22]

be administered, starting 1 day before initial exposure to phototherapy.

For those with normal broadband UVB MED values, a starting dose of NBUVB for PMLE hardening is based on Fitzpatrick skin phototype (**Table 4**); the dose is increased by 10% to 15% each session, and treatment takes place 2 to 3 times weekly.

Patients receiving UVA1 therapy should be informed that the treatment time in a standing unit is in the range of 8 to 10 minutes, which may be a limiting factor for some patients. The MUD to UVA1 should ideally be administered; treatment should start with 50% of MUD. If MUD is not performed, one can start at 10 J/cm^2, with an increase of 5 to 10 J/cm^2 per treatment as tolerated, until 20 J/cm^2 is reached. To minimize the risk of anaphylaxis, only body sites that would normally be exposed to sunlight should be treated; there is no need to treat the entire body surface. Furthermore, patients should be informed that tanning response would occur with UVA1 phototherapy.

If phototherapy booths have a new bulb, it is prudent to decrease the dose by 20%, followed by an increase of 10% to 15% per treatment until the initial dose is reached.

Polymorphous Light Eruption

While PUVA and broadband UVB have been used for PMLE in the past, NBUVB is currently the phototherapy of choice for hardening in PMLE.[24] Patients with PMLE have been shown to have relative resistance to UV-induced localized immunosuppression, resulting in an immunologic response to as yet uncharacterized neoantigens on the skin formed following sunlight exposure; this results in the development of lesions. Sunlight-induced or NBUVB-induced hardening would overcome this relative resistance, hence downregulating the immune response to the neoantigens.[25]

The starting dose of NBUVB is shown in **Table 4**. In the authors' center, patients are treated 2 to 3 times weekly for a total of 15 treatments; treatment is then discontinued. For patients who are exquisitely photosensitive by history, prednisone (0.6–0.8 mg/kg) should be administered for 7 to 10 days, starting on the day before treatment, to minimize flaring induced by the hardening procedure. Patients are then instructed to acquire 20 to 30 minutes weekly of midday sun exposure (without sunscreen) to maintain the state of hardening; these 20 to 30 minutes reflect the average MED for patients with SFT I to II at that setting. All patients should begin treatment at the start of spring. For patients living in a temperate climate, hardening treatment can be discontinued during the winter months.

PUVA therapy can be considered if patients relapse frequently despite NBUVB phototherapy. Roelandts[24] has reported success with a UVA starting dose of 1.5 J/cm^2, 3 times weekly. The dosage may be gradually increased by 20%. This regimen is recommended for 4 to 8 weeks.

Chronic Actinic Dermatitis

Although NBUVB phototherapy is not often used for patients with CAD, one report demonstrated the efficacy of prophylactic NBUVB in Chinese patients with CAD.[26] NBUVB treatments were performed 3 times weekly with 10% increase in dose until patients achieved clearance or improvement of clinical symptoms. The frequency of phototherapy was then reduced to twice weekly for 3 to 4 additional weeks. Of the 19 Chinese patients who underwent this regimen, 87.5% of previously UVB-sensitive patients and 75% of previously UVA-sensitive patients had normal or improved MEDs following treatment. Patients required an average of 27 treatments in total to achieve this response.

PUVA therapy can be used for CAD.[24,27] It is prudent to start at 0.5 to 1 J/cm^2 and even lower for patients with exquisite photosensitivity. Prednisone (0.6–0.8 mg/kg) should be administered for 10 to 14 days, starting on the day before treatment. Treatment should be administered 2 to 3 times weekly. Although evidence-based data are lacking, it is reasonable to continue PUVA for 15 to 20 treatments.[24,27]

The effects of PUVA and UVB in CAD may be mediated by suppression of abnormal immune response, either through disruption of antigen presentation or by secretion of inhibitory cytokines.[28]

Solar Urticaria

Solar urticaria can be very difficult to treat because symptoms are limited in time, making topical

Table 4			
Narrowband ultraviolet B dosage for polymorphous light eruption hardening based on skin type			
Skin Type	Starting Dose (mJ/cm^2)	Dose Increase	Maximum
I	100	10%–15%	3 J/cm^2 body,
II	100	per session	1 J/cm^2
III	200	as tolerated	face
IV	200		
V	300		
VI	300		

medications limited in utility. Patients often demonstrate sensitivity to the UVA or visible light spectrum; the latter is not effectively filtered by broad-spectrum sunscreens.[29] First-line treatment of solar urticaria includes antihistamines and photoprotection. If these treatments do not suppress the disease, phototherapy is indicated. For those patients who have access to omalizumab, it can be considered as the next line of treatment after phototherapy.[30,31]

Different types of phototherapy have been used, such as UVA1, PUVA, broadband UVB, NBUVB, and visible light.[29] UVA phototherapy is considered the standard treatment for UVA-sensitive solar urticaria but is not effective for patients with UVB-sensitive solar urticaria because tolerance usually lasts only for a few days.[29,32] Photoprophylaxis is hypothesized to result in hardening in solar urticaria by competitive binding of altered photoallergens on immunoglobulin E (IgE) binding sites on skin mast cells. It is also hypothesized to downregulate IgE production and inhibit histamine release from mast cells.[33]

The authors' preferred regimen for solar urticaria is the use of low-dose UVA1 ($<$40 J/cm^2) for hardening.[23,34] Starting at 5 J/cm^2, the dose is increased by 5 J/cm^2 with a maximum dose of 20 J/cm^2. If a patient is exceptionally photosensitive, the MUD should be determined at 1, 2, 4, and 5 J/cm^2, followed by an immediate reading. The patient can then be started at 50% to 70% of MUD and increased by 10% to 15%. This regimen is recommended 3 times weekly. Patients should be evaluated for response after 15 to 20 treatments.[34]

Systemic psoralen UVA photochemotherapy has been used to control solar urticaria, with long-lasting results. Roelandts[29] reported using 0.6 mg/kg of 8-methoxypsoralen (8-MOP) given orally 2 hours before UVA irradiation. Three sessions should be provided each week with a starting UVA dose less than the MUD.

Patients who demonstrated sensitivity to visible light and UVA have been successfully treated with NBUVB. Calzavara-Pinton and colleagues[32] reported success with the same prophylactic phototherapy protocol used for PMLE.

Actinic Prurigo

The mechanism of the preventative use of phototherapy in actinic prurigo is unclear. It is hypothesized to have a mechanism similar to that of phototherapy in the management of PMLE.[28] Some reports have shown limited improvement with NBUVB therapy.[17,18,35] Initial dose typically begins at 50% of MED with 20% increases at each visit. The authors recommend a regimen similar to the PMLE desensitization regimen with a 3-times weekly treatment for 5 weeks.[18]

A few reports have shown limited success with the use of PUVA, with temporary improvement and recurrence a few months following treatment.[17,36,37]

Hydroa Vacciniforme

Phototherapy has been used with success in some patients with hydroa vacciniforme. NBUVB treatment 3 times weekly for 5 weeks is most often recommended.[19,35] PUVA photochemotherapy has been used in the past but is not recommended for younger populations.[38,39]

Erythropoietic Porphyria

NBUVB has been reported to be beneficial in some patients with EPP.[24,40] Sivaramakrishnan and colleagues[40] suggested starting NBUVB at 50% to 70% of MED-B with increases of 10% to 20% each treatment. This was typically done for up to 15 treatments. If NBUVB does not provide sufficient control, PUVA can be considered. A starting dose at 1.5 J/cm^2 and increase by 20% on alternate treatments has been suggested.[24]

SUMMARY

Light has the unique potential to be both the inciting and suppressing modality for patients with photodermatoses. This article discussed the protocols for phototesting, provocative light testing, and photopatch testing. The treatment of photodermatoses with phototherapy and the hypothesized underlying mechanisms were reviewed. NBUVB is the preferred therapy for most photodermatoses, although UVA1 therapy should be considered for patients with solar urticaria.

REFERENCES

1. Choi D, Kannan S, Lim HW. Evaluation of patients with photodermatoses. Dermatol Clin 2014;32(3): 267–75, vii.
2. Kim JJ, Lim HW. Evaluation of the photosensitive patient. Semin Cutan Med Surg 1999;18(4):253–6.
3. Bylaite M, Grigaitiene J, Lapinskaite GS. Photodermatoses: classification, evaluation and management. Br J Dermatol 2009;161(Suppl 3):61–8.
4. Hölzle E, Plewig G, Lehmann P. Photodermatoses—diagnostic procedures and their interpretation. Photodermatol 1987;4(2):109–14.
5. Hölzle E, Plewig G, Hofmann C, et al. Polymorphous light eruption. Experimental reproduction of skin lesions. J Am Acad Dermatol 1982;7(1):111–25.

6. Paek SY, Lim HW. Chronic actinic dermatitis. Dermatol Clin 2014;32(3):355–61, viii–ix.

7. Harkins CP, Waters AJ, Dawe RS, et al. Polymorphic light eruption with severe abnormal phototesting sensitivity (PLESAPS). Photodermatol Photoimmunol Photomed 2017;33(6):326–8.

8. Yap LM, Foley P, Crouch R, et al. Chronic actinic dermatitis: a retrospective analysis of 44 cases referred to an Australian photobiology clinic. Australas J Dermatol 2003;44(4):256–62.

9. Tan K-W, Haylett AK, Ling TC, et al. Comparison of demographic and photobiological features of chronic actinic dermatitis in patients with lighter vs darker skin types. JAMA Dermatol 2017;153(5): 427–35.

10. Menagé H, Ross JS, Norris PG, et al. Contact and photocontact sensitization in chronic actinic dermatitis: sesquiterpene lactone mix is an important allergen. Br J Dermatol 1995;132(4):543–7.

11. Beattie PE, Dawe RS, Ibbotson SH, et al. Characteristics and prognosis of idiopathic solar urticaria: a cohort of 87 cases. Arch Dermatol 2003;139(9): 1149–54.

12. Farr PM. Solar urticaria. Br J Dermatol 2000;142(1): 4–5.

13. Uetsu N, Miyauchi-Hashimoto H, Okamoto H, et al. The clinical and photobiological characteristics of solar urticaria in 40 patients. Br J Dermatol 2000; 142(1):32–8.

14. Hasei K, Ichihashi M. Solar urticaria. Determinations of action and inhibition spectra. Arch Dermatol 1982; 118(5):346–50.

15. Kapoor R. Phototesting in solar urticaria. J Am Acad Dermatol 2009;60(5):877.

16. Kogame T, Uetsu N, Nguyen CTH, et al. Solar urticaria with an augmentation spectrum in a child. J Dermatol 2017;44(9):e214–5.

17. Crouch R, Foley P, Baker C. Actinic prurigo: a retrospective analysis of 21 cases referred to an Australian photobiology clinic. Australas J Dermatol 2002; 43(2):128–32.

18. Valbuena MC, Muvdi S, Lim HW. Actinic prurigo. Dermatol Clin 2014;32(3):335–44, viii.

19. Gupta G, Man I, Kemmett D. Hydroa vacciniforme: a clinical and follow-up study of 17 cases. J Am Acad Dermatol 2000;42(2 Pt 1):208–13.

20. Berge ten O, Sigurdsson V, Bruijnzeel-Koomen CA, et al. Photosensitivity testing in children. J Am Acad Dermatol 2010;63(6):1019–25.

21. DeLeo V, Gonzalez E, Kim J, et al. Phototesting and photopatch testing: when to do it and when not to do it. Am J Contact Dermatitis 2000;11(1):57–61.

22. Aslam A, Fullerton L, Ibbotson SH. Phototherapy and photochemotherapy for polymorphic light eruption desensitization: a five-year case series review from a university teaching hospital. Photodermatol Photoimmunol Photomed 2017;33(4):225–7.

23. Lyons AB, Peacock A, Zubair R, et al. Successful treatment of solar urticaria with UVA1 hardening in three patients. Photodermatol Photoimmunol Photomed 2018;34(4):262.

24. Roelandts R. Phototherapy of photodermatoses. J Dermatolog Treat 2002;13(4):157–60.

25. Gruber-Wackernagel A, Byrne SN, Wolf P. Polymorphous light eruption: clinic aspects and pathogenesis. Dermatol Clin 2014;32(3):315–34, viii.

26. Ma L, Zhang Q, Hu Y, et al. Evaluation of narrow band ultraviolet B phototherapy in the treatment of chronic actinic dermatitis in Chinese patients. Dermatol Ther 2017;30(6):e12528.

27. Millard TP, Hawk JLM. Photosensitivity disorders: cause, effect and management. Am J Clin Dermatol 2002;3(4):239–46.

28. Hönigsmann H. Mechanisms of phototherapy and photochemotherapy for photodermatoses. Dermatol Ther 2003;16(1):23–7.

29. Roelandts R. Diagnosis and treatment of solar urticaria. Dermatol Ther 2003;16(1):52–6.

30. Griffin LL, Haylett AK, Rhodes LE. Evaluating patient responses to omalizumab in solar urticaria. Photodermatol Photoimmunol Photomed 2019;35(1): 57–65.

31. Snast I, Kremer N, Lapidoth M, et al. Omalizumab for the treatment of solar urticaria: case series and systematic review of the literature. J Allergy Clin Immunol Pract 2018;6(4):1198–204.e3.

32. Calzavara-Pinton P, Zane C, Rossi M, et al. Narrowband ultraviolet B phototherapy is a suitable treatment option for solar urticaria. J Am Acad Dermatol 2012;67(1):e5–9.

33. Leenutaphong V, Hölzle E, Plewig G. Solar urticaria: studies on mechanisms of tolerance. Br J Dermatol 1990;122(5):601–6.

34. Dawe RS, Ferguson J. Prolonged benefit following ultraviolet A phototherapy for solar urticaria. Br J Dermatol 1997;137(1):144–8.

35. Collins P, Ferguson J. Narrow-band UVB (TL-01) phototherapy: an effective preventative treatment for the photodermatoses. Br J Dermatol 1995; 132(6):956–63.

36. Las DY, Youn JI, Park MH, et al. Actinic prurigo: limited effect of PUVA. Br J Dermatol 1997;136(6):972–3.

37. Farr PM, Diffey BL. Treatment of actinic prurigo with PUVA: mechanism of action. Br J Dermatol 1989; 120(3):411–8.

38. Sonnex TS, Hawk JL. Hydroa vacciniforme: a review of ten cases. Br J Dermatol 1988;118(1):101–8.

39. Halasz CL, Leach EE, Walther RR, et al. Hydroa vacciniforme: induction of lesions with ultraviolet A. J Am Acad Dermatol 1983;8(2):171–6.

40. Sivaramakrishnan M, Woods J, Dawe R. Narrowband ultraviolet B phototherapy in erythropoietic protoporphyria: case series. Br J Dermatol 2014; 170(4):987–8.

Utilizing UVA-1 Phototherapy

Smriti Prasad, BSA, Jennifer Coias, BA, Henry W. Chen, BS, Heidi Jacobe, MD, MSCS*

KEYWORDS

- Phototherapy • UVA-1 phototherapy • UVA phototherapy • Morphea • Systemic sclerosis
- Lichen sclerosus

KEY POINTS

- UVA1 radiation has a longer wavelength, enabling it to penetrate into the dermis and subcutis.
- Immunomodulating mechanisms of UVA1 result in depletion of T and B cells and down regulation of proinflammatory and profibrotic cytokines.
- UVA1 has shown potential efficacy for morphea, skin manifestations of systemic sclerosis, graft versus host disease, lIchen sclerosus, atopic dermatitis, mycosis fungoides, dyshidrosis, urticaria pigmentosa, lupus erythematosus, and other skin conditions.
- Acute adverse effects of UVA1 therapy are rare (hyperpigmentation, erythema, xerosis, and pruritus), while long term sequalae such as photocarcinogenesis and photoaging are poorly understood.

INTRODUCTION

The ultraviolet radiation (UVR) spectrum ranges from 10 nm at its highest energy to 400 nm at the lowest energy and is subdivided based on the biological effects of a given wavelength. In dermatology, UVR in the UVB (290–320) to UVA (320–400) range is used for the treatment of many inflammatory skin conditions. Within the UVA spectrum, there are phototherapy devices that emit across the whole 320 to 400 nm range, broad band UVA, that are used with topical or oral psoralen pretreatment. A more recent development in this armamentarium are UVA1-emitting sources (340–400 nm range) that are widely available in Europe and increasingly available in the United States. Unlike UVB (290–320 nm), which produces sunburn erythema more efficiently, UVA1 encompasses the longest and least erythemogenic wavelengths in the UV spectrum (**Table 1**). Also, because as wavelength increases depth of penetration also increases, UVA1 is able to penetrate beyond the papillary dermis into the subcutis and target those cells residing in these deeper layers, including fibroblasts, mast cells, lymphocytes, and dendritic cells.[1] Because of these properties, there has been substantial interest in the use of UVA1 phototherapy for the treatment of sclerosing and other inflammatory skin conditions.

HISTORY OF UVA1 PHOTOTHERAPY

Ultraviolet light, or light that exists beyond (*ultra* in Latin) violet, was first discovered in the 1800s, but there is evidence of its therapeutic use long before then. In the historic period (2000 BC to 1930 AD), there are anecdotal accounts of naturally occurring plants containing psoralens being used in combination with sunlight to treat vitiligo.[2] In 1925, UV radiation from mercury quartz lamps was combined with crude tar oil as a treatment for psoriasis, and in 1953, the combination of tar, UV radiation, and dithranol was described as standard treatment for psoriasis in the United Kingdom.[3,4] Parrish and colleagues[5] described a novel high-intensity UVA therapy to be used in combination with an oral psoralen as a treatment of psoriasis, marking the development and introduction of psoralen UV therapy (PUVA). In 1978,

University of Texas at Southwestern Medical Center, 5323 Harry Hines Boulevard, Dallas, TX 75390-9069, USA
* Corresponding author.
E-mail address: Heidi.jacobe@utsouthwestern.edu

Dermatol Clin 38 (2020) 79–90
https://doi.org/10.1016/j.det.2019.08.011

Table 1
Evidence levels according to disease

Disease	Level of Evidence
Morphea	I, II, III
Systemic sclerosis	II, III
Lichen sclerosus	I, II, III
Chronic graft vs host disease	II, III
Atopic dermatitis	I, II, III
Dyshydrosis	I, II, III
Mycosis fungoides	II, III
Urticaria pigmentosa	II, III
Lupus erythematosus	I, II, III

I: Evidence obtained from well-designed controlled trials with or without randomization.

II: Evidence obtained from well-designed cohort or case–control analytical studies or evidence obtained from multiple time series with or without the intervention.

III: Opinions of respected authorities, based on clinical experience, descriptive studies, case reports/series, or reports of expert committees.

Adapted from Force UPST. Guide to clinical preventive services: report of the U.S. Preventive Services Task Force. 1989; with permission.

Plewig and colleagues[6] described a new super pressure mercury lamp that emitted UV at wavelengths of 340 to 400 nm. They inserted a filter platelet to cut off the UVB portion of the spectrum, and thereby created a lamp limited to only the UVA1 range and described its clinical effects. Although initial studies of UVA1 on acne and vitiligo were disappointing, it was later introduced as a potential treatment for atopic dermatitis.[7] This study demonstrated therapeutic potential for the treatment of atopic dermatitis and laid the foundation for expanding UVA1 use to other conditions including sclerosing skin conditions, mycosis fungoides, and mastocytosis.

MECHANISM OF ACTION

UVR exists from 10 to 400 nm (**Fig. 1**). Below 200 nm, the UVR is absorbed strongly by the oxygen in the air and is therefore termed vacuum UV. After this, the shortest wavelength is UVC at 200 to 290 nm, followed by UVB at 290 to 320 nm, and UVA at 320 to 400 nm. UVA, or black light, is further broken down into UVA2 at 320 to 340 nm and UVA1 at 340 to 400 nm. It is generally thought that the biologic effects of UVA2 mirror those of UVB, including the potential for sunburn erythema, while UVA1 is distinguished by unique effects on tissue different from UVB and UVA2. UVA is the only type of UVR that is not filtered by glass, and comprises the majority of ambient human outdoor exposure. Owing to its long wavelength, it has the ability to penetrate into the deep dermis.[1]

Activation of Apoptosis

UVA1 induces apoptosis of cells.[8] Apoptosis is a programmed cell death that produces fragments of cell bodies that can then be engulfed by resident phagocytic cells. One way this is accomplished is via the production of superoxide anions, which damage the cellular mitochondria. This causes cytochrome *c* release from the mitochondria, activating the caspase-dependent apoptotic pathway.[8,9] UVA1 also produces singlet oxygen species, depolarizing the mitochondrial membrane, resulting in the release of apoptosis-initiating factor into the cell, activating the FAS/FAS ligand system.[8] This second method is unique to UVA1 and has not been observed in other forms of UVR. It occurs immediately (<20 minutes) and does not require the accumulation of new proteins, but rather is able to use inherent intracellular proteins.[8] Via these 2 methods, UVA1 can activate apoptosis of T and B lymphocytes and is thought to be particulary effective in inducing apoptosis in CTCL lymphocytes.[8,10] This is thought to be the underlying mechanism for the therapeutic potential of UVA1 in treating T-cell mediated inflammatory and neoplastic disorders, including atopic dermatitis, localized scleroderma, and mycosis fungoides.[11,12]

Cytokine Modulation

UVA1 has also been shown to downregulate the expression of profibrotic and proinflammatory cytokines. For instance, it decreases the production of profibrotic tumor growth factor-beta (TGF-β) proteins in vivo.[13] It also suppresses proinflammatory cytokines such as tumor necrosis factor-alpha and interleukin-12 (IL-12), involved in activation of antibody-dependent cell-mediated cytotoxicity and eosinophils.[14] However, unlike UVB, UVA1 does not increase the production of IL-10.[15] UVA1 leads to photoisomerization of transurocanic acid, increasing the levels of cis-urocanic acid, which is thought to be immunoregulatory.[14] UVA1 also decreases the levels of intracellular adhesion molecule-1 and interferon-gamma, which are involved in lymphocyte trafficking and activation, respectively.[15,16] These effects are thought to modulate the effect of UVA1 phototherapy on inflammatory skin conditions, as well as the inflammation associated with early morphea and systemic sclerosis.

Collagen Metabolism

MMPs such as collagenase-1 are responsible for collagen breakdown. In vivo experiments demonstrate that collagenase-1 is upregulated in

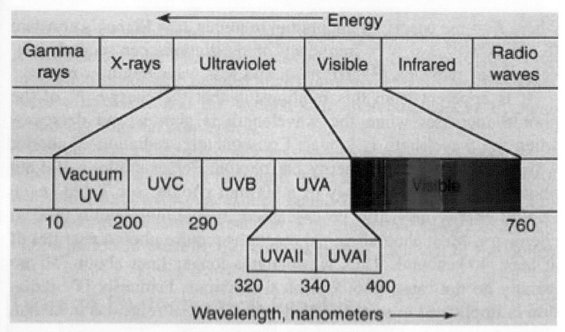

Fig. 1. Electromagnetic spectrum. (*From* York NR, Jacobe HT. UVA1 phototherapy: a review of mechanism and therapeutic application. Int J Dermatol 2010;49:623-630; with permission.)

fibroblasts from patients who were previously treated with UVA1.[17] Wang and colleagues[18] found a decrease in type I and type III collagen with an upregulation in mRNA of MMP-1,-3,-9 that lasted for 3 to 7 days after exposure to a single high dose of UVA1. Another study found increased levels of collagen I and collagen III metabolites in the serum and urine in patients with morphea who were treated with UVA1 5 times weekly for 3 to 6 weeks.[19] UVA1 induces singlet oxygen species and hydrogen peroxide, leading to increased production of matrix metalloproteinases (MMPs). UVA1 has also been shown to induce autocrine stimulation of fibroblast-derived collagenase by interrelated loops of IL-1 and IL-6.[20] IL-1 is thought to stimulate the production of IL-6, which upregulates collagenase production by fibroblasts. There is evidence that UVA1 stimulates synthesis of α-melanocyte-stimulating hormone receptor which increases MMP production.[21] A similar upregulation of MMPs production in endothelial cells, melanocytes, and keratinocytes was seen in patients with morphea.[22] Skin phototype, as determined by melanin content, is thought to impact the efficacy of UVA1 phototherapy. It was previously thought that individuals with higher melanin content do not experience the same beneficial effects of UVA1. However, in a study of 101 patients with morphea, there was no statistically significant difference in response to treatment according to skin phototype.[23] This departs from the findings of

Wang and colleagues,[18] which demonstrated that there was no substantial induction of MMPs at any dose of UVA1 In addition to a poorer treatment response in individuals with darker skin types. These mechanisms of upregulating MMPs make UVA1 an ideal therapeutic modality for treating sclerosing skin conditions.

EQUIPMENT AND DOSING
Equipment

UVA1 treatment units consists of either a fluorescent tube or a filtered metal halide lamp that filters out UVA2. Fluorescent lamps are less expensive but have lower energy output (20 mW/cm^2), whereas metal halide bulbs are able to deliver high-dose therapy (60 mW/cm^2).[24] As a result of the higher energy and heat generated by the metal-halide lamps, they often require fans. Smaller units are meant to provide localized therapy (**Fig. 2**A), whereas standing UVA1 boxes are utilized for whole-body therapy (**Fig. 2**B).

Dosing

Dosing of UVA1 is divided into 3 categories. The low ranges span from 10 to 29 J/cm^2, medium ranges from 30 to 59 J/cm^2, and 60 to 120 J/cm^2 is considered to be high dose.[25] As mentioned previously, the lamp type will determine the feasibility of a given dose range capability (fluorescent lamp cubicles may require 45–60 minutes to

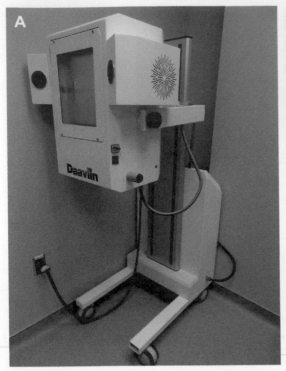
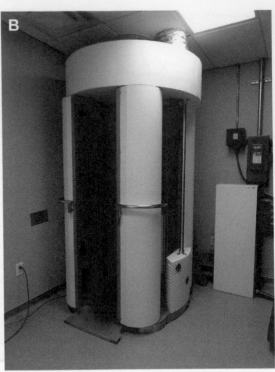

Fig. 2. UVA1 phototherapy equipment. Examples of equipment currently available in the United States includes(*A*) localized phototherapy units that utilize fluorescent lamp cubicles and emit low and medium doses and (*B*) whole-body units that produce high-output doses using metal halide sources.

deliver medium- to high-dose treatment, which most patients do not tolerate). Cumulative dose of radiation is another point of distinction for UVA1 therapy. Low is below 300 J/cm^2; medium is within the range of 300 to 975 J/cm^2, and high is from 975 J/cm^2 to 1840 J/cm^2.[26] Treatment dose, duration, and intervals per week may vary depending on the skin condition being treated; however, unlike UVB or PUVA, the dose is generally held constant during treatment rather than with incremental increases over time.

UVA1 FOR SPECIFIC DISORDERS
Sclerosing Skin Conditions

UVA1 has potential for therapeutic efficacy in sclerosing skin conditions via its effect on immune dysregulation and collagen metabolism, which may soften lesions, reduce inflammation, and decrease dermal thickness.[27] This has led to its use in morphea (localized scleroderma), systemic sclerosis (scleroderma), and lichen sclerosus. **Table 1** demonstrates the current level of evidence of different types of phototherapy for sclerosing skin conditions and various other skin conditions that will be discussed. A 2008 systematic review looked at the use of UVA1 for sclerotic skin conditions and found good results for all doses of UVA1

as an effective treatment for these conditions, although medium- to high-dose has proven consistently more efficacious.[28]

Morphea

Morphea characteristically has a high predominance of inflammatory CD4+ T cells and excessive collagen deposition. UVA1 phototherapy is considered to be one of the treatments of choice for morphea because of the level of evidence for its efficacy, which is similar to that of methotrexate.[29] The first study to look at high-dose UVA1 treatment was a 1997 study by Stege and colleagues.[30] This study demonstrated that high-dose UVA1 phototherapy was an effective therapeutic modality in reducing the thickness and increasing the elasticity of sclerotic plaques. Kroft and colleagues[28] found that UVA1 decreased the duration of active lesions for patients with morphea and prevented further disease progression. A 2010 retrospective and prospective study found good efficacy of UVA1 in treating 30 patients with morphea with a reduction in skin thickness (measured by ultrasound) and an increase in elasticity (measured by Cutometer).[19] A study comparing medium- versus low-dose UVA1 phototherapy with narrowband UVB (NBUVB) showed that medium-dose UVA1 therapy was superior to both low-dose UVA1 therapy and narrow band UVB therapy, with no significant difference between low-dose UVA1 and narrow band UVB.[31] Another 2006 study compared effectiveness of low-, medium-, and high-dose therapy on 32 patients with morphea.[32] Investigators noted better response to therapy among the medium- and high-dose groups, with a poorer response in the low-dose group. Su and colleagues[26] strengthened these findings in a study of 35 patients using medium-dose UVA1 therapy (30 J/cm2) over the course of 30 to 45 treatments. Clinical improvement was noted in 29 of 35 patients, and 13 MHz ultrasound examination demonstrated significantly reduced skin thickness.[26] Sator and colleagues[33] compared sonographic thickness of plaques after treatment with high- and low-dose UVA1 and found the medium dose to be more effective. A randomized control trial showed good efficacy from combined low-dose UVA1 and calcipotriol therapy.[31] At present, the best evidence for treating morphea is with medium- to high-dose regimens (60 J/cm^2, 3–5 times weekly) for a total of 40 sessions.[29] Importantly, an assessment of UVA1-treated patients with generalized, linear, plaque-type, and mixed morphea subtypes revealed a 46% recurrence rate within the first 2 years after treatment.[34] Recurrence did not appear to be associated with morphea subtype, skin phototype, cumulative dose, or duration of treatment, although it was associated with increased disease duration.[34] Thus, patients should continue to be monitored regularly following UVA1 phototherapy for new morphea lesions.

A key factor in treating patients with UVA1 phototherapy with morphea is appropriate patient selection. Although few studies have addressed this issue in a systematic manner, it is standard of care to avoid treating patients with soft tissue involvement of their morphea (subcutis or underlying fascia or muscle) with UVA1 phototherapy, because it does not reach the area of pathology and the high risk of long term functional sequalae in patients, who should be treated with systemic immunosuppressives. Further, it is important to choose patients with active, inflammatory morphea, as purely sclerotic or atrophic plaques do not respond to UVA1 phototherapy. Finally, patients must be counseled on the time course and expected outcomes of treatment. It is reasonable to expect lesions to stop enlarging and erythema to resolve during the 2- to 3-month course of treatment, but softening often continues for several months thereafter and may not reach maximum improvement for up to a year. Further, plaques with features of hyperpigmentation or atrophy will not respond at all to UVA1 phototherapy and may become more obvious because of increased hyperpigmentation. The use of photography is encouraged as an aid to assess improvement, as hyperpigmentation induced by UVA1 phototherapy makes clinical assessment challenging in some patients.

Systemic sclerosis

Systemic sclerosis (SSc) is a multisystem autoimmune connective tissue disease. Although there are various skin manifestations, cutaneous sclerosis, particularly acrosclerosis and sclerodactyly, is characteristic.[35] Acrosclerosis has combined features of Raynaud, phenomena with sclerosis of the distal digits, face, and neck. Studies investigating the effectiveness of UVA1 in the therapy of cutaneous sclerosis are mixed in terms of efficacy.[36,37] In a small study of 8 patients treated with medium-dose UVA1 4 times a week for 50 treatments of acrosclerosis, 7 patients experienced improvement in skin elasticity and joint range combined with a decreased number of digital ulcerations.[37] A later study with 18 patients treated with low-dose UVA1for acrosclerosis at varying frequencies (4 times a week for 8 weeks followed by 3 times a week for 6 weeks) observed softening of former stiffness reflected by a decrease in the hand score, reduction in skin thickness, and increase in overall skin distension.[38] Histopathological biopsies revealed a significant elevation of dermal collagenase on post-therapeutic MMP-1 immunolabeling when compared with pretherapeutic skin. Thus, low-dose UVA1 phototherapy was determined to be a viable treatment option that could help induce collagenases and reduce collagen deposition and cellular infiltration.[38] Sclerotic skin lesions were softened after 10 to 30 exposures of medium-dose UVA1 therapy, improving joint mobility and cutaneous elasticity in patients with systemic sclerosis.[39] However, in a randomized investigator-blinded study with comparison of a treated hand to untreated hand of the same patient in 9 patients receiving low-dose UVA1 phototherapy (40 J/cm2 3 times weekly over a period of 14 weeks), there was no significant improvement in joint flexion or extension despite an improved skin score and visual analog scale ($P<.05$).[40] Tewari and colleagues[41] reported successful reductions in microstomia in SSc patients treated with medium-dose UVA1. At this time, the data to support efficacy in SSc are mixed; therefore, it is not considered to be a first-line therapy, but remains a useful adjunct in cases in which patients do not tolerate or have contraindications to mycophenolate mofetil, methotrexate, or other immunosuppressive agents.

It is important to note that further study is needed before UVA1 phototherapy is considered without efficacy. The existing studies cited were limited in several important ways. Likely the largest obstacle was that they focused exclusively on treating patients' hands. From other studies in systemic sclerosis, it is known that the hands improve the least and much more slowly than other affected body surface sites, so it is not surprising that they would not show improvement with UVA1 phototherapy in the context of a controlled trial. Further, many of the patients enrolled in these studies had longstanding (multiyear) disease duration, which is also associated with less likelihood of improvement in other studies of systemic sclerosis skin disease. Finally, most of these studies were small and uncontrolled and lacked a validated outcome measure. Taken together, this makes it difficult to determine whether UVA1 phototherapy has efficacy in the treatment of systemic sclerosis skin disease. Additional controlled trials are needed of patients with early onset skin disease utilizing total-body treatment and validated outcome measures.

Lichen sclerosus

Lichen sclerosus (LS) is a chronic inflammatory disorder that results in atrophic, porcelain white plaques with palpable sclerosis. The condition can occur in genital or extragenital forms. Studies for treatment of LS with UVA1 therapy demonstrate efficacy.[42] A 2002 study of 10 patients with extragenital LS treated with low-dose UVA1 therapy for 10 weeks showed successful improvement in clinical symptoms and ultrasound findings.[43] In genital LS, topical corticosteroids remain the gold standard therapy, but UVA1 therapy is a promising second-line treatment. A 2-arm randomized clinical trial of 30 female patients with vulvar LS was performed, with 1 group receiving clobetasol proprionate (0.05%) ointment, applied once daily over 3 months, and the other group receiving medium-dose UVA1 (50 J cm^2) 4 times weekly over 12 weeks.[44] UVA1 demonstrated significant clinical improvement, but topical corticosteroid therapy was still superior, particularly for reduction in pruritus and improvement in overall quality of life. Based on the data available, UVA1 therapy is a second-line treatment option for LS when topical corticosteroid therapy is contraindicated or poorly tolerated, in cases of widespread disease, and/or if the disease is not well-managed on corticosteroid therapy alone. Of particular concern in the case of vulvar LS is the risk of photocarcinogenesis in a disorder that is already associated with increased risk of squamous cell carcinoma.

Chronic graft-versus-host disease

Graft-versus-host disease (GVHD) is a complication of allogenic stem cell transplant. Although cutaneous manifestations are varied, sclerodermoid or morpheaform lesions occur in up to 20% of patients with chronic GVHD.[45] UVA1 phototherapy can be used as an alternative or adjunct to immunosuppression for this condition, which can be refractory to conventional therapies. One case report of a patient who failed cyclosporine, prednisone, and mycophenolate mofetil exhibited clinical improvement with a combination of low-dose UVA1 therapy (single dose, 20 J/cm^2, 4 times a week over 6 weeks) and 2 g/d of mycophenolate mofetil. The results showed improvement of skin thickness to nearly normal levels when measured by ultrasound with a stable 9-month follow-up.[46] A subsequent study was conducted with 5 patients with chronic sclerodermoid GVHD who failed PUVA therapy and photophoresis and put on 5 J/cm^2 UVA1 phototherapy 5 times per week for 30 to 40 treatments. All patients had increased range of motion, improved ulcers, and skin softening with stable disease on follow-up.[47] Calzavara-Pinton and colleagues[48] also treated 5 patients with sclerodermoid GVHD successfully with medium-dose UVA1. A study in 2 pediatric patients with chronic GVHD revealed that high-dose UVA1 therapy followed by low-to-medium doses resulted in skin improvement that was sustained during follow-up 8 months later.[49] In 2010, Schlaak and colleagues[50] retroactively examined 70 patients with acute cutaneous GVHD. UVA1 treatment of these patients was effective in achieving complete or partial remission and allowed a more rapid taper of immunosuppression. Connolly and colleagues[51] found high-dose regimens to be more effective than low- and medium-dose regimens in retrospective analysis of 25 patients. Given that most of the evidence is limited to case studies or retrospective analyses, it is not possible. Also of note, bone marrow transplant patients are at increased risk of skin cancers because of immunosuppression and often use of voriconazole. Therefore, if considering UVA1 phototherapy in this situation, it is important to assess the patient's overall risk for skin cancer and initiate a conversation with the hematologist managing his or her care regarding minimizing exposure to immunosuppressive and voriconazole if possible.

ATOPIC DERMATITIS

Atopic dermatitis (AD) is a remitting and relapsing inflammatory disorder of the skin. The mechanisms by which UVA1 is thought to be effective in atopic dermatitis are through its immunoregulatory properties, specifically via inducing CD4+ T-cell apoptosis, killing Langerhans cells, and suppressing cytokine levels. In 1992, Krutmann and colleagues[52] first showed that UVA1 was useful for patients with AD. After several randomized control trials, UVA1 became a well-established therapeutic modality for AD patients.[53–55] A systematic review in 2007 established that phototherapy with medium-dose (50 J/cm^2) UVA1 can be used to control acute flares of AD.[56] This study found that treatment with UVA1 induced clinical improvement faster than conventional UVB, although UVB was still the recommended form of treatment for chronic AD. Initially, high-dose UVA1 was superior to UVB-UVA therapy.[54] However, later studies found that medium-dose UVA1 phototherapy was as effective as narrowband UVB in improving clinical scores and signs for patients with moderate-to-severe AD.[57] More recently, a large retrospective study found that UVA1 is an effective alternative for a diverse group of patients with severe AD.[58] The most frequent doses observed in this study were between 30 and 60 J/cm^2. Another recent study compared efficacy of UVA1 phototherapy in treating atopic dermatitis across different Fitzpatrick skin types. The authors found that there was no difference in efficacy in comparing lighter- or darker-skinned individuals and advocated for the use of high-dose UVA1 phototherapy in Fitzpatrick skin types IV or greater.[59]

Taken together, the current literature supports a role for UVA1 phototherapy of atopic dermatitis in patients who have failed standard topical treatments and appropriate emollient use. Because UVA1 phototherapy has not proven to be more efficacious than NBUVB phototherapy and there are more data on safety of NBUVB phototherapy, it is advisable to use UVA1 phototherapy for those patients who cannot tolerate or had poor response to NBUVB phototherapy. Because there are limited data on the safety of UVA-1 phototherapy in children in terms of photoaging and photocarcinogenesis, it should be undertaken with caution in the pediatric population.

DYSHIDROSIS

Dyshidrosis is an eczematous skin condition that results in a pruritic, vesicular eruption on the hands and feet. One of the first studies looking at the efficacy of UVA1 therapy in treating dyshidrosis examined 12 patients with an acute exacerbation of dyshidrotic hand eczema. Patients were treated on the palm and dorsum of the hand at 40 J/cm^2/d over 3 weeks. Of the 12 patients, 10 reported near resolution of their symptoms with no relapses at 3 months follow-up.[60] In a randomized, double-blind, placebo-controlled trial of UVA1 therapy for dyshidrotic hand eczema, 28 patients received either UVA1 irradiation at 30 J/cm^2 or placebo for 5 times a week for 3 weeks. Using a severity index (DASI) as an evaluation measure, UVA1 was shown to be significantly more effective after 2 to 3 weeks, and desquamation and area of affected skin also improved significantly more.[60] Polderman and colleagues[61] additionally reported efficacy for UVA1 in a double-blind placebo-controlled randomized controlled trial with 28 patients. Another study looking at high-dose UVA1 therapy with topical PUVA therapy found that UVA1 was as effective as PUVA in reducing the DASI score by 50%; no significant difference was found between the 2 therapies.[62] Therefore, at this time, UVA1 is an efficacious option for patients with dyshidrosis who have not had adequate response to first-line topical treatment and appropriate lifestyle modifications.

MYCOSIS FUNGOIDES/CUTANEOUS T-CELL LYMPHOMA

Mycosis fungoides, also known as cutaneous T-cell lymphoma (MF/CTCL) is an indolent non-Hodgkin T-cell lymphoma that primarily develops in the skin. The apoptosis promoting mechanisms of UVA1 provide a rational for use of this therapy in MF, and malignant T cells appear to be more sensitive than normal cells to UVA1 radiation-induced apoptosis.[11] In 1999, Plettenberg and colleagues[63] described the effects of UVA1 phototherapy in MF. They used daily whole-body UVA irradiations at either a high dose (130 J/cm^2 per exposure) or a medium dose (60 J/cm^2) for patients who had a biopsy-proven diagnosis of stages IA or IB CTCL. In all 3 patients, skin lesions began to resolve after a few UVA1 exposures, with complete clearance achieved between 16 to 20 exposures regardless of dose. In another studies, patients with CTCL stages ranging from IB to III received 100 J/cm^2 of UVA1 daily. Of the 13 patients observed, the 11 patients who had lesions accessible by UVA1 showed complete clinical and histologic responses.[64] Those who had lesions that could not be irradiated served as controls and did not experience any improvement in lesions. Immunocytologic studies of skin infiltrates determined that circulating CD4+/CD4RO+ and

CD4+/CD95+ lymphocytes were significantly reduced by therapy.[64] At follow-up 7 months later, 7 patients had stable remission, whereas 4 patients had relapsed within 4 months of ending phototherapy. In a study of the patients with MF, 13 of the 15 patients achieved complete remission, while 2 patients received partial remission, demonstrating that UVA1 phototherapy can be safe and effective in advanced stages of mycosis fungoides.[65] In 2013, these investigators treated 14 patients with low- (n = 3), medium- (n = 7), and high-dose (n = 4) UVA1. They noted complete (n = 11) or partial (n = 3) remission in all patients, concluding that UVA1 appears to be effective irrespective of dose.[66] In a study of 19 patients treated with 30 J/cm^2 for 5 days per week, 12 achieved a complete response, and 7 achieved a partial response by the end of 5 weeks of therapy.[67] The lack of a long and sustained response warrants additional optimization of dosing protocol and maintenance treatment. Of note, PUVA and NBUVB are also accepted treatments for mycosis fungoides, although these studies show UVA1 has good potential as an alternative to PUVA, especially when the side effects of oral psoralens are not suitable for the patient.

URTICARIA PIGMENTOSA

Urticaria pigmentosa (UP) is the most common manifestation of cutaneous mastocytosis in children and adults. Given the previously reported findings of UVA1 reducing the density of mast cells in the dermis, it has been effective in patients with UP. In 4 adult patients with urticaria pigmentosa treated initially with 60 J/cm^2 then subsequently increased to 130 J/cm^2 for 2 weeks, pruritus improved after 3 sessions, although the response of specific skin lesions to UVA1 was not reported.[68] One patient also had a reduced number of mast cells on bone marrow biopsy, and 2 patients also reported improvement of previous symptoms of diarrhea and migraine. This was complemented with the reduction of serum serotonin levels to normal after 10 exposures to UVA1. Follow-up at 10 months revealed that no patients experienced a relapse, which was sustained 2 years after cessation of therapy. In another study of patients with urticaria pigmentosa treated with medium- or high-dose UVA1, most patients did not experience reduction in the number of skin lesions, although there was a decrease in the number of mast cells in lesional skin and improvement in pruritus and quality of life by the completion of the treatment course and at 6 months follow-up.[69] For this study, no differences were noted between the high- and medium-dose UVA1.

LUPUS ERYTHEMATOSUS

Lupus erythematosus is a photosensitive T cell-driven autoinflammatory condition that can occur in systemic and/or skin-restricted variants. The first study to report UVA1 phototherapy in subacute cutaneous lupus (SCLE) was a 9-week series leading to a cumulative dose of almost 190 J/cm2 in 1993.[70] The authors reported improvement of lupus skin lesions for the patients observed. A later study treated 10 patients with systemic lupus erythematosus (SLE) with 6 J/cm^2 for 15 sessions for 3 weeks and observed marked clinical improvement and a reduction in serum antibody count.[71] A subsequent prospective, double-blind, placebo-controlled trial was performed, dividing patients into 2 groups. Group A received 60 kJ/m^2 of UVA1 irradiation 5 days a week for 3 weeks, and Group B (placebo) received an equal amount of visible light of greater than 430 nm.[72] The groups then crossed over for exposure to the other source for 3 weeks. Disease activity (SLAM) scores in Group A improved significantly after the first 3 weeks of UVA1 irradiation, while Group B exhibited negligible response during this time.[72] Anti-double stranded DNA antibodies also decreased significantly. Adverse effects were negligible. The authors concluded that low-dose UVA1 was effective in reducing signs and symptoms of SLE activity.[72] McGrath later reported a case of DLE that was exacerbated by UVA1 therapy.[73] Another double-blinded, placebo-controlled, cross-over study was used to examine the efficacy of low doses of UVA1 radiation (12 J/cm2 each day for 15 days) in 12 patients.[74] Polderman and colleagues also concluded that low-dose UVA1 therapy is a useful treatment for moderately active SLE. Clinical trials are currently in the recruiting phases to explore this treatment modality in patients with cutaneous lupus. Thus, low doses of UVA1 comprise a potential therapy for lupus; however, caution should be taken to avoid higher doses, which are shown to cause photoinduction of lesions.[75,76]

ADVERSE EFFECTS AND CONTRAINDICATIONS
Adverse Effects

Most studies report few to no serious adverse effects from UVA1. Common adverse effects include hyperpigmentation, erythema, xerosis, and pruritus.[77] Other uncommon adverse effects include polymorphous light eruption and recurrence of herpes simplex infection.[28,69,78] One study reported UVA1 as a potential trigger for bullous pemphigoid.[79] Severe acute adverse reactions to

UVA1 phototherapy have otherwise not been reported. UVA1, unlike UVB, is less erythemogenic; however, phototoxic episodes have occurred among light-skinned individuals.[80,81]

Photocarcinogenesis and photoaging in patients with UVA1 exposure are also concerns. Via its effects on collagen breakdown, there is a potential for UVA1 to promote photoaging.[82] The carcinogenic potential of UVA1 has not been assessed in people, but it is known to cause DNA damage via cyclobutene pyrimidine dimer formation.[83] UVA1 can also induce p53 and BRM mutations, which are associated with skin cancers.[84] There is 1 case report of a patient with mastocytosis who developed melanoma after intense UVA1 therapy.[85] However, because this patient had received PUVA bath therapy, the study was unable to determine a link between UVA1 and melanoma. Two cases of Merkel cell carcinoma were reported in immunocompromised patients who received high-dose UVA1 therapy, but the concomitant immunosuppression makes it difficult to draw a causal association.[86] Therefore, although the risk of photocarcinogenesis has not been formally established, it cannot be ignored at this time. Patients should be counseled on this prior to initiating UVA1 therapy, particularly in cases of immunosuppression or a longstanding history of phototherapy, particularly PUVA, or tanning bed use. Patients should also continue to receive regular skin checks during and after UVA1 therapy.

Contraindications

UVA1 is contraindicated in those with xeroderma pigmentosum, porphyria, skin cancer, photosensitivity disorders, or long-term immunosuppression.[87] It should not be used in patients taking photosensitizing drugs and should be used with caution in patients younger than 18 years.

FUTURE CONSIDERATIONS

Despite the fact that UVA1 phototherapy has been in use since the late 1990s, there are numerous unanswered questions regarding its use. To date, few studies have assessed the efficacy and safety of combination therapy with either topical or systemic treatments in combination with UVA1 phototherapy. Also largely unaddressed are the optimal total dose or duration of therapy for a given disorder. Finally, many of the conditions discussed herein are chronic, remitting relapsing disorders that will likely need ongoing treatment even after a course of successful UVA1 phototherapy. However, there is little information on the safety of either maintenance or recurrent courses of UVA1 phototherapy to inform therapeutic decision making in this patient population. It is important for future studies to examine these questions.

SUMMARY

Phototherapy is a viable form of treatment that can offer benefit to patients with many skin diseases with few systemic adverse effects. UVA1 is a newer form of phototherapy that produces long wavelengths of up to 340 to 400 nm, allowing it to penetrate deeper into the dermis and subcutis and target an array of cells, including lymphocytes, mast cells, fibroblasts, and dendritic cells. Dosage from UVA1 is described as low, ranging from 10 to 29 J/cm2; medium, ranging from 30 to 59 J/cm2; and high, for doses greater than 60 J/cm2. UVA1 can be sourced by either fluorescent lamps in the case of low-dose UVA1 therapy, or filtered metal-halide lamps for medium or high doses.

Through the use of UVA1 phototherapy, diseases with pathology or extracutaneous manifestations lying in the epidermal, dermal, and even subcutis layers of the skin can be targeted. Indications for UVA1 include sclerosing skin conditions, atopic dermatitis, urticaria pigmentosa, mycosis fungoides, and systemic lupus erythematosus. A 2017 study found benefit for these conditions in addition to others such as necrobiosis lipoidica, granuloma annulare, and keloids.[88] In some cases, UVA1 therapy has been shown to be superior to UVB therapy. Adverse effects are rare, and are most often limited to hyperpigmentation, erythema, xerosis, and pruritus. The long-term carcinogenic potential of UVA1 therapy has not been fully determined. UVA1 phototherapy should be considered an important tool in treating various skin conditions.

REFERENCES

1. York NR, Jacobe HT. UVA1 phototherapy: a review of mechanism and therapeutic application. Int J Dermatol 2010;49(6):623–30.
2. Parrish JA, Fitzpatrick TB, Shea C, et al. Photochemotherapy of vitiligo. Use of orally administered psoralens and a high-intensity long-wave ultraviolet light system. Arch Dermatol 1976;112(11):1531–4.
3. Ingram JT. The approach to psoriasis. Br Med J 1953;2(4836):591–4.
4. Goeckerman WH. The treatment of psoriasis. Northwest Med 1925;24:229–31.
5. Parrish JA, Fitzpatrick TB, Tanenbaum L, et al. Photochemotherapy of psoriasis with oral methoxsalen

and longwave ultraviolet light. N Engl J Med 1974; 291(23):1207–11.

6. Plewig G, Hofmann C, Braun-Falco O, et al. A new apparatus for the delivery of high intensity UVA and UVA+UVB irradiation, and some dermatological applications. Br J Dermatol 1978;98(1):15–24.

7. Grabbe J, Welker P, Humke S, et al. High-dose ultraviolet A1 (UVA1), but not UVA/UVB therapy, decreases IgE-binding cells in lesional skin of patients with atopic eczema. J Invest Dermatol 1996;107(3): 419–22.

8. Godar DE. UVA1 radiation triggers two different final apoptotic pathways. J Invest Dermatol 1999;112(1): 3–12.

9. Cai J, Yang J, Jones DP. Mitochondrial control of apoptosis: the role of cytochrome c. Biochim Biophys Acta 1998;1366(1–2):139–49.

10. Guhl S, Hartmann K, Tapkenhinrichs S, et al. Ultraviolet irradiation induces apoptosis in human immature, but not in skin mast cells. J Invest Dermatol 2003;121(4):837–44.

11. Yamauchi R, Morita A, Yasuda Y, et al. Different susceptibility of malignant versus nonmalignant human T cells toward ultraviolet A-1 radiation-induced apoptosis. J Invest Dermatol 2004; 122(2):477–83.

12. Bando N, Hayashi H, Wakamatsu S, et al. Participation of singlet oxygen in ultraviolet-a-induced lipid peroxidation in mouse skin and its inhibition by dietary beta-carotene: an ex vivo study. Free Radic Biol Med 2004;37(11):1854–63.

13. Gambichler T, Skrygan M, Tomi NS, et al. Significant downregulation of transforming growth factor-beta signal transducers in human skin following ultraviolet-A1 irradiation. Br J Dermatol 2007;156(5):951–6.

14. Skov L, Hansen H, Allen M, et al. Contrasting effects of ultraviolet A1 and ultraviolet B exposure on the induction of tumour necrosis factor-alpha in human skin. Br J Dermatol 1998;138(2):216–20.

15. Grewe M, Gyufko K, Schopf E, et al. Lesional expression of interferon-gamma in atopic eczema. Lancet 1994;343(8888):25–6.

16. Krutmann J, Honigsmann H, Elments CA, et al. Dermatological phototherapy and photodiagnostic methods. New York: Springer; 2001.

17. Gruss C, Reed JA, Altmeyer P, et al. Induction of interstitial collagenase (MMP-1) by UVA-1 phototherapy in morphea fibroblasts. Lancet 1997;350(9087): 1295–6.

18. Wang F, Garza LA, Cho S, et al. Effect of increased pigmentation on the antifibrotic response of human skin to UV-A1 phototherapy. Arch Dermatol 2008; 144(7):851–8.

19. Andres C, Kollmar A, Mempel M, et al. Successful ultraviolet A1 phototherapy in the treatment of localized scleroderma: a retrospective and prospective study. Br J Dermatol 2010;162(2):445–7.

20. Wlaschek M, Heinen G, Poswig A, et al. UVA-induced autocrine stimulation of fibroblast-derived collagenase/MMP-1 by interrelated loops of interleukin-1 and interleukin-6. Photochem Photobiol 1994;59(5): 550–6.

21. Hassani J, Feldman SR. Phototherapy in Scleroderma. Dermatol Ther (Heidelb) 2016;6(4): 519–53.

22. Gruss C, Stucker M, Kobyletzki G, et al. Low dose UVA1 phototherapy in disabling pansclerotic morphoea of childhood. Br J Dermatol 1997;136(2): 293–4.

23. Jacobe HT, Cayce R, Nguyen J. UVA1 phototherapy is effective in darker skin: a review of 101 patients of Fitzpatrick skin types I-V. Br J Dermatol 2008;159(3): 691–6.

24. Kerr AC, Ferguson J, Attili SK, et al. Ultraviolet A1 phototherapy: a British Photodermatology Group workshop report. Clin Exp Dermatol 2012;37(3):219–26.

25. Careta MF, Romiti R. Localized scleroderma: clinical spectrum and therapeutic update. An Bras Dermatol 2015;90(1):62–73.

26. Su O, Onsun N, Onay HK, et al. Effectiveness of medium-dose ultraviolet A1 phototherapy in localized scleroderma. Int J Dermatol 2011;50(8):1006–13.

27. Mutzhas MF, Holzle E, Hofmann C, et al. A new apparatus with high radiation energy between 320-460 nm: physical description and dermatological applications. J Invest Dermatol 1981;76(1):42–7.

28. Kroft EB, Berkhof NJ, van de Kerkhof PC, et al. Ultraviolet A phototherapy for sclerotic skin diseases: a systematic review. J Am Acad Dermatol 2008; 59(6):1017–30.

29. Gambichler T, Schmitz L. Ultraviolet A1 phototherapy for fibrosing conditions. Front Med (Lausanne) 2018;5:237.

30. Stege H, Berneburg M, Humke S, et al. High-dose UVA1 radiation therapy for localized scleroderma. J Am Acad Dermatol 1997;36(6 Pt 1):938–44.

31. Kreuter A, Hyun J, Stucker M, et al. A randomized controlled study of low-dose UVA1, medium-dose UVA1, and narrowband UVB phototherapy in the treatment of localized scleroderma. J Am Acad Dermatol 2006;54(3):440–7.

32. Tuchinda C, Kerr HA, Taylor CR, et al. UVA1 phototherapy for cutaneous diseases: an experience of 92 cases in the United States. Photodermatol Photoimmunol Photomed 2006;22(5):247–53.

33. Sator PG, Radakovic S, Schulmeister K, et al. Medium-dose is more effective than low-dose ultraviolet A1 phototherapy for localized scleroderma as shown by 20-MHz ultrasound assessment. J Am Acad Dermatol 2009;60(5):786–91.

34. Vasquez R, Jabbar A, Khan F, et al. Recurrence of morphea after successful ultraviolet A1 phototherapy: A cohort study. J Am Acad Dermatol 2014; 70(3):481–8.

35. Pearson DR, Werth VP, Pappas-Taffer L. Systemic sclerosis: current concepts of skin and systemic manifestations. Clin Dermatol 2018;36(4):459–74.

36. Pereira N, Santiago F, Oliveira H, et al. Low-dose UVA(1) phototherapy for scleroderma: what benefit can we expect? J Eur Acad Dermatol Venereol 2012;26(5):619–26.

37. von Kobyletzki G, Uhle A, Pieck C, et al. Acrosclerosis in patients with systemic sclerosis responds to low-dose UV-A1 phototherapy. Arch Dermatol 2000;136(2):275–6.

38. Kreuter A, Breuckmann F, Uhle A, et al. Low-dose UVA1 phototherapy in systemic sclerosis: effects on acrosclerosis. J Am Acad Dermatol 2004;50(5): 740–7.

39. Morita A, Kobayashi K, Isomura I, et al. Ultraviolet A1 (340-400 nm) phototherapy for scleroderma in systemic sclerosis. J Am Acad Dermatol 2000;43(4): 670–4.

40. Durand F, Staumont D, Bonnevalle A, et al. Ultraviolet A1 phototherapy for treatment of acrosclerosis in systemic sclerosis: controlled study with half-side comparison analysis. Photodermatol Photoimmunol Photomed 2007;23(6):215–21.

41. Tewari A, Garibaldinos T, Lai-Cheong J, et al. Successful treatment of microstomia with UVA1 phototherapy in systemic sclerosis. Photodermatol Photoimmunol Photomed 2011;27(2):113–4.

42. Rombold S, Lobisch K, Katzer K, et al. Efficacy of UVA1 phototherapy in 230 patients with various skin diseases. Photodermatol Photoimmunol Photomed 2008;24(1):19–23.

43. Kreuter A, Gambichler T, Avermaete A, et al. Low-dose ultraviolet A1 phototherapy for extragenital lichen sclerosus: results of a preliminary study. J Am Acad Dermatol 2002;46(2):251–5.

44. Terras S, Gambichler T, Moritz RK, et al. UV-A1 phototherapy vs clobetasol propionate, 0.05%, in the treatment of vulvar lichen sclerosus: a randomized clinical trial. JAMA Dermatol 2014;150(6): 621–7.

45. Inamoto Y, Storer BE, Petersdorf EW, et al. Incidence, risk factors, and outcomes of sclerosis in patients with chronic graft-versus-host disease. Blood 2013;121(25):5098–103.

46. Grundmann-Kollmann M, Behrens S, Gruss C, et al. Chronic sclerodermic graft-versus-host disease refractory to immunosuppressive treatment responds to UVA1 phototherapy. J Am Acad Dermatol 2000; 42(1 Pt 1):134–6.

47. Stander H, Schiller M, Schwarz T. UVA1 therapy for sclerodermic graft-versus-host disease of the skin. J Am Acad Dermatol 2002;46(5):799–800.

48. Calzavara Pinton P, Porta F, Izzi T, et al. Prospects for ultraviolet A1 phototherapy as a treatment for chronic cutaneous graft-versus-host disease. Haematologica 2003;88(10):1169–75.

49. Ziemer M, Thiele JJ, Gruhn B, et al. Chronic cutaneous graft-versus-host disease in two children responds to UVA1 therapy: improvement of skin lesions, joint mobility, and quality of life. J Am Acad Dermatol 2004;51(2):318–9.

50. Schlaak M, Schwind S, Wetzig T, et al. UVA (UVA-1) therapy for the treatment of acute GVHD of the skin. Bone Marrow Transplant 2010;45(12):1741–8.

51. Connolly KL, Griffith JL, McEvoy M, et al. Ultraviolet A1 phototherapy beyond morphea: experience in 83 patients. Photodermatol Photoimmunol Photomed 2015;31(6):289–95.

52. Krutmann J, Czech W, Diepgen T, et al. High-dose UVA1 therapy in the treatment of patients with atopic dermatitis. J Am Acad Dermatol 1992;26(2 Pt 1): 225–30.

53. Gambichler T, Othlinghaus N, Tomi NS, et al. Medium-dose ultraviolet (UV) A1 vs. narrowband UVB phototherapy in atopic eczema: a randomized crossover study. Br J Dermatol 2009;160(3): 652–8.

54. Krutmann J, Diepgen TL, Luger TA, et al. High-dose UVA1 therapy for atopic dermatitis: results of a multicenter trial. J Am Acad Dermatol 1998;38(4): 589–93.

55. von Kobyletzki G, Pieck C, Hoffmann K, et al. Medium-dose UVA1 cold-light phototherapy in the treatment of severe atopic dermatitis. J Am Acad Dermatol 1999;41(6):931–7.

56. Meduri NB, Vandergriff T, Rasmussen H, et al. Phototherapy in the management of atopic dermatitis: a systematic review. Photodermatol Photoimmunol Photomed 2007;23(4):106–12.

57. Garritsen FM, ter Haar NM, Spuls PI. House dust mite reduction in the management of atopic dermatitis. A critically appraised topic. Br J Dermatol 2013; 168(4):688–91.

58. Ordonez Rubiano MF, Arenas CM, Chalela JG. UVA-1 phototherapy for the management of atopic dermatitis: a large retrospective study conducted in a low-middle income country. Int J Dermatol 2018;57(7):799–803.

59. Pacifico A, Iacovelli P, Damiani G, et al. "High dose" versus "medium dose" UVA1 phototherapy in Italian patients with severe atopic dermatitis. J Eur Acad Dermatol Venereol 2019;33(4):718–24.

60. Schmidt T, Abeck D, Boeck K, et al. UVA1 irradiation is effective in treatment of chronic vesicular dyshidrotic hand eczema. Acta Derm Venereol 1998; 78(4):318–9.

61. Polderman MC, Govaert JC, le Cessie S, et al. A double-blind placebo-controlled trial of UVA-1 in the treatment of dyshidrotic eczema. Clin Exp Dermatol 2003;28(6):584–7.

62. Petering H, Breuer C, Herbst R, et al. Comparison of localized high-dose UVA1 irradiation versus topical cream psoralen-UVA for treatment of chronic

vesicular dyshidrotic eczema. J Am Acad Dermatol 2004;50(1):68–72.

63. Plettenberg H, Stege H, Megahed M, et al. Ultraviolet A1 (340-400 nm) phototherapy for cutaneous T-cell lymphoma. J Am Acad Dermatol 1999;41(1): 47–50.

64. Zane C, Leali C, Airo P, et al. "High-dose" UVA1 therapy of widespread plaque-type, nodular, and erythrodermic mycosis fungoides. J Am Acad Dermatol 2001;44(4):629–33.

65. Suh KS, Kang JS, Baek JW, et al. Efficacy of ultraviolet A1 phototherapy in recalcitrant skin diseases. Ann Dermatol 2010;22(1):1–8.

66. Jang MS, Kang DY, Jeon YS, et al. Ultraviolet A1 phototherapy of mycosis fungoides. Ann Dermatol 2013;25(1):104–7.

67. Adisen E, Tektas V, Erduran F, et al. Ultraviolet A1 phototherapy in the treatment of early mycosis fungoides. Dermatology 2017;233(2–3):192–8.

68. Stege H, Schopf E, Ruzicka T, et al. High-dose UVA1 for urticaria pigmentosa. Lancet 1996;347(8993):64.

69. Gobello T, Mazzanti C, Sordi D, et al. Medium-versus high-dose ultraviolet A1 therapy for urticaria pigmentosa: a pilot study. J Am Acad Dermatol 2003;49(4):679–84.

70. Sonnichsen N, Meffert H, Kunzelmann V, et al. [UV-A-1 therapy of subacute cutaneous lupus erythematosus]. Hautarzt 1993;44(11):723–5.

71. McGrath H Jr. Ultraviolet-A1 irradiation decreases clinical disease activity and autoantibodies in patients with systemic lupus erythematosus. Clin Exp Rheumatol 1994;12(2):129–35.

72. McGrath H, Martinez-Osuna P, Lee FA. Ultraviolet-A1 (340-400 nm) irradiation therapy in systemic lupus erythematosus. Lupus 1996;5(4):269–74.

73. McGrath H Jr. Ultraviolet A1 (340-400 nm) irradiation and systemic lupus erythematosus. J Investig Dermatol Symp Proc 1999;4(1):79–84.

74. Polderman MC, le Cessie S, Huizinga TW, et al. Efficacy of UVA-1 cold light as an adjuvant therapy for systemic lupus erythematosus. Rheumatology (Oxford) 2004;43(11):1402–4.

75. Klein LR, Elmets CA, Callen JP. Photoexacerbation of cutaneous lupus erythematosus due to ultraviolet A emissions from a photocopier. Arthritis Rheum 1995;38(8):1152–6.

76. Lehmann P, Holzle E, Kind P, et al. Experimental reproduction of skin lesions in lupus erythematosus by UVA and UVB radiation. J Am Acad Dermatol 1990;22(2 Pt 1):181–7.

77. Richer V, Lui H. Cross-sectional evaluation of acute adverse reactions during ultraviolet A1 phototherapy. Br J Dermatol 2017;177(1):258–9.

78. Gambichler T, Al-Muhammadi R, Boms S. Immunologically mediated photodermatoses: diagnosis and treatment. Am J Clin Dermatol 2009;10(3): 169–80.

79. Sacher C, Konig C, Scharffetter-Kochanek K, et al. Bullous pemphigoid in a patient treated with UVA-1 phototherapy for disseminated morphea. Dermatology 2001;202(1):54–7.

80. Gambichler T, Terras S, Kampilafkos P, et al. T regulatory cells and related immunoregulatory factors in polymorphic light eruption following ultraviolet A1 challenge. Br J Dermatol 2013;169(6):1288–94.

81. Beattie PE, Dawe RS, Ferguson J, et al. Dose-response and time-course characteristics of UV-A1 erythema. Arch Dermatol 2005;141(12):1549–55.

82. Wang F, Smith NR, Tran BA, et al. Dermal damage promoted by repeated low-level UV-A1 exposure despite tanning response in human skin. JAMA Dermatol 2014;150(4):401–6.

83. Tewari A, Sarkany RP, Young AR. UVA1 induces cyclobutane pyrimidine dimers but not 6-4 photoproducts in human skin in vivo. J Invest Dermatol 2012; 132(2):394–400.

84. Halliday GM, Byrne SN, Damian DL. Ultraviolet A radiation: its role in immunosuppression and carcinogenesis. Semin Cutan Med Surg 2011;30(4):214–21.

85. Wallenfang K, Stadler R. Association between UVA1 and PUVA bath therapy and development of malignant melanoma. Hautarzt 2001;52(8):705–7 [in German].

86. Calzavara-Pinton P, Monari P, Manganoni AM, et al. Merkel cell carcinoma arising in immunosuppressed patients treated with high-dose ultraviolet A1 (320-400 nm) phototherapy: a report of two cases. Photodermatol Photoimmunol Photomed 2010;26(5): 263–5.

87. Totonchy MB, Chiu MW. UV-based therapy. Dermatol Clin 2014;32(3):399–413. ix-x.

88. Attili SK, Dawe RS, Ibbotson SH. Ultraviolet A1 phototherapy: one center's experience. Indian J Dermatol Venereol Leprol 2017;83(1):60–5.

Phototherapy in the Pediatric Population

Michelle C. Juarez, BS[a], Anna L. Grossberg, MD[b],*

KEYWORDS

- Phototherapy • Pediatric • Children • Narrowband • NBUVB • PUVA • Excimer • Atopic dermatitis

KEY POINTS

- Evidence to support the use of phototherapy has been demonstrated in a wide range of pediatric skin conditions, including vitiligo, atopic dermatitis, psoriasis, alopecia areata, pityriasis lichenoides, and mycosis fungoides.
- Special considerations must be taken before starting phototherapy in children, including optimal dosage and frequency, scheduling demands, safe delivery, and long-term safety.
- Future studies are needed to assess the long-term safety of phototherapy in children and its utility in other pediatric skin conditions.

INTRODUCTION

Phototherapy has been used successfully to treat a wide range of dermatologic conditions in adults. Given the growing body of evidence demonstrating its efficacy and safety in this population, the use of phototherapy as a treatment modality for pediatric skin conditions has become more widely accepted. Some of the childhood dermatoses in which phototherapy has been used successfully include vitiligo, atopic dermatitis (AD), psoriasis, alopecia areata (AA), pityriasis lichenoides (PL), and mycosis fungoides (MF), among others. The mechanism of action varies with disease and treatment modality used, but it is thought that UV light may aid in the modulation of the immune response underlying various inflammatory and autoimmune dermatologic conditions.[1] Treatment modalities include broadband UVB (BBUVB, 280–315 nm), narrowband UVB (NBUVB, 311–313 nm), UVA (315–400 nm) alone or in combination with psoralen (psoralen + UVA; PUVA), combination UVA and UVB (UVAB, 280–400 nm), and the excimer laser (308 nm). Indications for the use of these modalities differ depending on the disease, age of the child, and desired outcome.

Despite the growing body of literature on the use of phototherapy in children, there are no randomized controlled trials, and data are primarily limited to retrospective studies. As a result, treatment parameters and dosing remain largely empirical and have not been specifically regulated. Furthermore, special considerations must be taken when using phototherapy in the pediatric population, such as safe delivery, scheduling, and long-term safety. In this review, the authors highlight the most compelling evidence supporting the efficacy and safety of phototherapy in children. They also discuss the potential challenges of using phototherapy in children, provide recommendations for the use of phototherapy in pediatric skin disease, and emphasize the need for further research to assess for long-term safety and utility of phototherapy in other pediatric skin conditions.

Disclosure Statement: The authors have no conflicts of interest or disclosures.
a The Johns Hopkins School of Medicine, 733 North Broadway, Baltimore, MD 21205, USA; b Department of Dermatology, Division of Pediatric Dermatology, The Johns Hopkins University School of Medicine, 200 North Wolfe Street, Unit 2107, Baltimore, MD 21287, USA
* Corresponding author.
E-mail address: agrossb2@jhmi.edu

Dermatol Clin 38 (2020) 91–108
https://doi.org/10.1016/j.det.2019.08.012
0733-8635/20/

APPROACH TO PHOTOTHERAPY IN CHILDREN

The approach to phototherapy in children begins with a careful history and physical examination to determine if the patient is an ideal candidate for treatment. Various factors need to be taken into consideration and are outlined in **Table 1**. Absolute contraindications to phototherapy include photosensitive and skin cancer–predisposing disorders, such as xeroderma pigmentosum, systemic lupus erythematosus, and Gorlin syndrome.[2] During this time it is also important to discuss expectations and potential barriers to treatment with the patient and family. An orientation to the clinic and treatment unit may aid in helping patients and families understand and familiarize themselves with the treatment process.[3]

Once phototherapy is deemed appropriate, the next step is determining the optimal treatment modality and protocol, which is dependent on a multitude of factors. The evidence-based efficacy for each of the different modalities in the most common pediatric skin conditions is discussed in subsequent sections of this review. Dosing and frequency protocols vary, because there are no set guidelines for treatment parameters in children, but are primarily based on initial calculation of the minimal erythema dose (MED). The starting dose for children is typically 70% MED or lower and may be increased by 20% per treatment. However, some studies in children propose a more gradual increase in dose by 10% rather than 20% per session to help ameliorate acute side effects, such as erythema and burning, and to improve overall tolerability.[4,5] Frequency and duration of treatment vary depending on disease type and severity

and other patient characteristics, but most regimens range from delivering treatments 2 to 3 times per week for several months.

CHALLENGES OF PHOTOTHERAPY IN CHILDREN
Safe Delivery

Safe delivery is of utmost importance for all patients treated with phototherapy, but safe treatment in children may pose additional challenges. For young children, particularly those less than 5 years of age, there may be poor compliance with wearing protective eyewear. Poor compliance with eyewear may especially be an issue in those undergoing PUVA, in which prolonged eye protection is necessary even following the session, which may be challenging even for older children. In addition, children may have difficulty holding still for treatment, which is critical for providing targeted therapy to affected areas and reducing potential side effects. Children may also experience anxiety when faced with entering the light box alone, and as a result of this anxiety, urinary incontinence has been reported.[5,6] In 1 study, urinary incontinence in the light box resulted in a short circuit in a base fan unit, highlighting the extent to which anxiety may significantly impact the safe delivery of phototherapy.[6] To help ameliorate anxiety, the authors suggest allowing a parent (wearing proper covering) to go into the light box with the child or to consider partially opening the door of the light box so that the child can easily see outside. Other suggestions to help reduce anxiety include playing music during treatment, hanging drawings or decorations, and arranging for a pretreatment tour of the phototherapy unit.[3] Use of a parent's phone or tablet may also aid in

Table 1
Approach to evaluating a child for treatment with phototherapy

History	Physical Examination
• Age • Dermatologic condition • Severity of disease • Duration of disease (acute or chronic) • Impact on quality of life • Previous treatments • Comorbidities • Contraindications, including history of photosensitive skin condition, (eg, lupus erythematosus) or skin cancer-predisposing condition, (eg, xeroderma pigmentosa, Gorlin syndrome) • Potential scheduling difficulties • Current medications • Family history of skin cancers	• Fitzpatrick skin type • Examination findings consistent with a light-sensitive dermatologie disease process • Location and distribution • Body surface area involvement • Other indicators of severity

distraction so long as it does not block the areas needing to be treated on the child's skin.

Scheduling

Most skin conditions treated with phototherapy require treatment sessions 2 to 3 times per week, making scheduling treatments difficult not only for the child but also for the parent or guardian as well. Scheduling is particularly challenging in school-aged children, in whom it may result in a significant amount of missed time from school. This may be a deterrent for some families to even consider light therapy, and in others may greatly limit compliance with sessions. In children, the authors strongly recommended a trial of in-office therapy to demonstrate efficacy and tolerability for each child. However, in many cases, obtaining home units may be preferable for convenience. Home units may also help in alleviating anxiety because children can be treated in their own homes with a parent close by. In addition, many home units have open designs, which are less intimidating than office units. These benefits may be outweighed by the fact that home units often require longer sessions and may be cost-prohibitive, because obtaining insurance coverage can be challenging.

Adverse Effects

Phototherapy is generally well tolerated in children, with the most common acute side effects being erythema, burning, xerosis, pruritus, and peeling. There have been some reports of varicella and herpes simplex virus reactivation as well as rare occurrences of blistering.[4,5,7–9] The most concerning long-term risk of phototherapy in children is the potential for cutaneous malignancy development with repeat UV exposure. This risk warrants special consideration in children compared with adults, because of longer life expectancy in children and the assumption that there may be increased carcinogenicity risks that may manifest later in life. However, data are scarce, particularly long-term follow-up studies, supporting a link between the use of phototherapy in children and skin carcinogenicity.

Much of what can be inferred regarding the risk of cutaneous malignancy with phototherapy comes from data on another form of phototherapy that is often used in children: neonatal blue light phototherapy (NBLP). This treatment modality has been used since the 1970s to treat neonatal jaundice. Blue light (400–520 nm), a wavelength of visible light, is adjacent to UV on the light spectrum and may have similar biologic effects because it can stimulate immature melanocytes in the newborn skin. There have been several studies examining whether there is an increased risk of NBLP in the development of acquired melanocytic nevi, which may then be associated with an increased risk of melanoma. Data have been conflicting across studies. In a twin study of 59 pairs of monozygotic and dizygotic twins, a significantly higher prevalence of melanocytic nevi was seen in the twin with a history of NBLP exposure compared with the unexposed twin sibling.[10] However, a 2016 metaanalysis found no evidence to conclude an increased risk for melanocytic nevi in children who had been treated with NBLP.[11]

A link between the use of PUVA and carcinogenicity has been proposed in a patient who had received long-term PUVA between ages 1 and 8, who developed 2 basal cell carcinomas before age 21.[12] In 1978, the American Academy of Pediatrics issued an advisory recommending against PUVA in children less than 12 years of age, because of increased rates of nonmelanoma skin cancer development. Although studies in children may not directly demonstrate this risk, they are limited by having very short follow-up periods, and it is important to consider a lag phase between when treatments were administered and when skin cancers may develop many years later. It is also important when considering the carcinogenicity of phototherapy and PUVA not to generalize results taken from studies examining the risks in adults, because adults may be more likely to have been treated with multiple treatment modalities, including immunosuppressants, which may have confounding effects in terms of promotion of carcinogenicity.

In addition, studies have suggested an increased risk of nevus development with phototherapy. One study that included both adults and children treated with NBUVB showed that many benign changes occurred in nevi present at the start of treatment; however, none were concerning for malignancy.[13] In nevi with globular pigment networks before phototherapy, 63% increased in color intensity, size, and number of dots or globules. Of those that enlarged, all were noted to return to baseline upon cessation of therapy. Taken together, the evidence does point to a possibility of changing melanocytic nevi and new melanocytic nevus development in children treated with phototherapy, but the significance of these changes remains unclear.

USE IN PEDIATRIC SKIN CONDITIONS
Vitiligo

Vitiligo is a common disease characterized by loss of functioning melanocytes and resultant depigmentation of the skin. It affects approximately 0.06% to 2.28% of the population worldwide,[14] with about half of these cases beginning before the age of 20.[15] Vitiligo in childhood can be associated with significant psychosocial impairment, and the cause remains largely unknown, making treatment challenging. Topical therapies are first-line treatment in children, but phototherapy may be considered after failure of topical treatment modalities or in extensive or rapidly progressive disease. A variety of phototherapy modalities has been used in children with vitiligo, including NBUVB, PUVA, combined UVA1 and UVB, and the 308-nm excimer laser. However, there are no randomized controlled trials, and most of the data are limited to retrospective studies and a few small prospective trials.

Historically, PUVA was commonly used in the treatment of vitiligo, but it has now largely been replaced by NBUVB because of excellent repigmentation outcomes with NBUVB and because of the potential risks associated with PUVA in children, including increased malignancy risk.[16] The mechanism of NBUVB repigmentation remains incompletely understood, although it is thought to be a 2-fold process with an initial stabilization of the depigmentation process followed by stimulation of residual follicular melanocytes.[17] The first study on NBUVB use in childhood vitiligo was by Njoo and colleagues[18] in which disease stabilization occurred in about 80% of pediatric patients with generalized vitiligo treated with NBUVB twice weekly, and more than half of the patients experienced greater than 75% repigmentation. The investigators also found significant improvement in quality of life (QOL) and concluded that NBUVB was safe and effective for vitiligo in children.[18] Several other prospective and retrospective studies have demonstrated similar findings, with significant repigmentation rates ranging from 40% to 75% and overall mild adverse effects (**Table 2**).[5,7,19–23] In many of these studies, response to therapy was positively correlated with location of the lesions, with greater improvement noted for face and neck lesions and less on acral lesions, which is attributed to the lower density of hair follicles in these areas and therefore decreased ability of UV light to stimulate residual follicular melanocytes.[22] Several studies note correlations between an earlier response to treatment and higher overall rates of repigmentation. There were no associations between response to treatment and patients' sex, age, or family history of vitiligo.

Data on long-term effects of NBUVB therapy in childhood vitiligo are limited. To date, there has only been 1 long-term study performed by Lommerts and colleagues,[24] in which the investigators collected follow-up data from 18 of the 51 patients in the initial study by Njoo and colleagues, who were treated for their childhood vitiligo 20 years before. They found that 22% of patients did not receive any additional treatment after the NBUVB course, and this inversely correlated with the extent of body surface area involvement, suggesting that in a small subset of patients vitiligo was not reactivated or slowly progressed after the initial treatment. In this study, none of the patients reported occurrence of melanoma or nonmelanoma skin cancers.[24]

Treatment of childhood vitiligo with other modalities, such as combined UVA1 and UVB, as well as with the monochromatic 308-nm excimer laser has also been reported.[7] The excimer laser, in particular, may be an attractive option when treating smaller surface areas because it provides targeted phototherapy while sparing normal surrounding skin from exposure. In addition, excimer light therapy often requires less frequent sessions that may improve patient compliance. Overall, these studies demonstrate a similar side-effect profile and response pattern as in NBUVB phototherapy for pediatric vitiligo (see **Table 2**). As for NBUVB, response rates for vitiligo treated with excimer laser are better in facial and neck lesions compared with acral lesions, and improved response also correlates positively with initiation of treatment earlier in the disease course.[7,25] Importantly, there is no evidence in any reviewed studies of any light or laser modality for increased improvement in pediatric vitiligo with higher cumulative doses of phototherapy, and therefore, it is recommended to discontinue therapy if there is no improvement noted by 6 months to reduce the potential adverse effects and mitigate hypothetical long-term risks.[26]

In pediatric patients with treatment-resistant vitiligo, combination therapy with topical immunomodulatory agents and phototherapy may be more beneficial than phototherapy alone. One open-label study looked at combination therapy for NBUVB with 0.03% tacrolimus ointment in children with symmetric vitiligo lesions and found a significant increase in the percentage of repigmentation at 4 to 6 months with combination therapy compared with phototherapy alone, and lower

Table 2
Summary of studies using phototherapy in children with vitiligo

Author, y	Light Modality	Study Type	No. Patients; Age Range Vitiligo Type Disease Duration	Mean Treatment (tx) No. Mean Cumulative Dose (MCD; J/cm^2)	Main Findings	Adverse Effects
Njoo et al,[18] 2000	NBUVB	Prospective	16; ages: 4–16 Generalized vitiligo Mean disease duration: 4 y	• Mean 78 tx • MCD: 91.3	53% of patients experienced >75% repigmentation; best response noted on face, neck > trunk, extremities > acral	Itching, xerosis
Kanwar et al,[19] 2005	NBUVB	Prospective	20; ages: 5–14 Generalized vitiligo Mean disease duration: 1.63 y	• Mean 34 tx • MCD: 39.7	75% of patients had >75% repigmentation; response better for face/neck > trunk/ proximal extremities > acral	Burning/itching, xerosis
Brazzelli et al,[20] 2005	NBUVB	Prospective	10; ages: 6–14 8 localized, 2 generalized Mean disease duration: 3.15 y	• Mean 48 tx • MCD: 47.7	50% of patients had >75% repigmentation	Erythema
Ersoy-Evans et al,[21] 2008	NBUVB	Retrospective	9; ages 7–13 11 generalized, 7 localized Mean disease duration: unknown	• Mean 24 tx • MCD: 70	>50% repigmentation achieved in 50% of patients	Erythema
	PUVA	Retrospective	8; ages 14–16 11 generalized, 7 localized Mean disease duration: unknown	• Mean 14 tx • MCD dose: 303	57% of patients achieved >50% repigmentation	Erythema

(continued on next page)

Table 2
(continued)

Author, y	Light Modality	Study Type	No. Patients; Age Range Vitiligo Type Disease Duration	Mean Treatment (tx) No. Mean Cumulative Dose (MCD; J/cm²)	Main Findings	Adverse Effects
Cho et al,[26] 2011	Excimer laser	Retrospective	30; ages 5–17 Vitiligo types: unknown Disease duration: 1 mo to 10 y	• Mean tx number unknown • MCD: 18.58	56.7% of patients achieved >50% repigmentation at end of the treatment. Best responses on face, neck, and trunk. Treatment response did not correlate with the cumulative dose or duration of treatment	First- and second-degree burns, folliculitis, perilesional hyperpigmentation
Percivalle et al,[22] 2012	NBUVB	Prospective	28; ages: 3–15 17 generalized, 5 focal, 5 segmental, 3 acrofacial Mean disease duration: 2.96 y	• Mean 62 tx • MCD: 156	14.3% of patients had >75% repigmentation; 43% had >50% repigmentation; 66.7% had sustained improvement at 11 mo follow-up; best response achieved on face and trunk	Mild erythema
Sen et al,[5] 2014	NBUVB	Retrospective	36; ages: 6–16 Vitiligo types: unknown Disease duration: unknown	• Mean 125 tx • MCD: 232	44.5% had >75% repigmentation (16% with complete repigmentation)	Erythema in 12%, blistering, VZV reactivation, urinary incontinence in booth

Koh et al,[7] 2015	NBUVB, combined UVA1 and UVB, excimer laser, PUVA	Retrospective	71; ages: 5–15 >1/2 with generalized, >1/3 segmental vitiligo Disease duration: 2 mo to 12 y	• Range: 20–209 tx • MCD: unknown	Patients with generalized vitiligo had a better response than those with segmental vitiligo. Response rates were highest with NBUVB followed by combined UVA1 and UVB, 308-nm excimer laser, phototherapy, and lowest for PUVA	Itching, scaling, erythema, pain, sunburn, blistering, phototoxicity
Yazici et al,[23] 2017	NBUVB	Retrospective	26; ages 2–18 16 generalized, 4 focal, 6 acrofacial Disease duration: 6 mo to 12 y	• Mean 83 tx • MCD: 34.66	45.4% had >75% repigmentation; 21% had >25% repigmentation	Mild erythema

Abbreviation: VZV, varicella zoster virus.

mean cumulative doses and number of phototherapy sessions were required for clinically visible response with combination therapy.[27] Similarly, combination therapy for 308-nm excimer laser with either 1% pimecrolimus cream or halometasone topically has resulted in higher rates of repigmentation compared with those receiving laser alone.[28,29]

Atopic Dermatitis

AD is an inflammatory skin disorder with a relapsing and remitting course that commonly presents in childhood, with approximately 85% of cases beginning by age 5.[30] In children, it often presents as pruritic, eczematous plaques on the face, neck, and extensor surfaces and can significantly affect QOL, to a similar extent as those with other pediatric chronic illnesses such as cystic fibrosis.[31] Topical therapy with emollients, steroids, and/or calcineurin inhibitors is the first-line treatment in children. Phototherapy is recommended as a second-line treatment in patients with moderate to severe AD, and several studies have demonstrated its efficacy in pediatric patients.

NBUVB is the most studied light modality for pediatric AD, with numerous studies supporting its safety and efficacy in children. In one of the largest retrospective studies by Clayton and colleagues,[9] 40% of children with AD treated with NBUVB demonstrated complete clearance or minimal residual disease following therapy, whereas 23% showed good disease improvement with a median time to remission of approximately 3 months. Several other studies have also validated the efficacy and tolerability of NBUVB in children with AD and have shown overall good response with NBUVB, with clearance rates ranging from 40% to 90% in addition to improvement in QOL indices (**Table 3**).[4,6,8,9,32–41] Most of these studies were performed over an average of 3 months; however, dosing and treatment regimens varied considerably by study. A recent consensus statement the American Academy of Dermatology (AAD) provides dosing guidelines for various phototherapy modalities that may be useful for providers in treating their patients with AD.[42] In addition, in all of these studies, most children with AD who cleared after treatment with NBUVB were able to achieve long periods of remission. One study found that more than half of their pediatric patients remained clear at 1-year follow-up after completion of NBUVB therapy.[4] Long-term studies on NBUVB treatment in childhood AD, to better address maintenance regimens and assess long-term adverse effects, are lacking.

Other modalities used to treat pediatric AD include PUVA, combination UVA/UVB, the 308-nm excimer laser, and BBUVB (see **Table 3**). Use of PUVA for the treatment of AD in children has largely been replaced by NBUVB for reasons similar to those previously discussed in this review. Overall, studies in children using the various modalities are limited, and there are no trials or comprehensive comparative studies to support 1 modality as being more efficacious than another. Given the limited evidence, the AAD currently endorses NBUVB therapy over these other modalities.[42]

Psoriasis

Psoriasis is one of the most common chronic inflammatory skin conditions, affecting approximately 2% to 3% of adults, with an estimated 30% of patients presenting with their first symptoms during childhood and adolescence.[43] Psoriasis in children can present differently than in adults, with more frequent reports of pruritus and lesions that are thinner, softer, and less scaly.[44] In a recent consensus statement, the AAD endorsed phototherapy as a second-line treatment of psoriasis in children who fail initial topical therapy or in extensive psoriatic disease.[45] Phototherapy has been used to treat various forms of psoriasis but has been more effective in thin plaque and guttate forms. Reported modalities include BBUVB, NBUVB, Goeckerman treatment (coal tar + UVB), and UVA with topical or systemic psoralen (PUVA).

NBUVB is the preferred treatment modality owing to strong evidence documenting its efficacy, safety, and ease of administration in children with psoriasis. In the largest study, Pavlovsky and colleagues[38] reported 88 pediatric patients with psoriasis treated with NBUVB and observed greater than 75% improvement in disease in 92% of children treated. More recently, Eustace and colleagues[4] reported 15 pediatric patients who underwent NBUVB treatment with an initial clearance of 86%, and at 1-year follow-up 43% of patients remained clear. Numerous other studies have also documented significant reductions in extent of disease with clearance rates ranging between 50% and 90%, sustained remissions, and minimal adverse effects over an average of 25 to 34 treatments (**Table 4**).[4–6,21,35,37,38,40,46–53] One study found that pediatric patients with psoriasis responded better to phototherapy than children with AD and required fewer treatments.[37] As in AD, combination therapy for NBUVB with topical agents may increase the efficacy of phototherapy in childhood

Table 3
Summary of studies using phototherapy in children with atopic dermatitis

Author, y	Light Modality	Study Type	No. Patients; Age Range Disease Severity	Mean or Median tx No.; MCD (J/cm²)	Main Findings	Adverse Effects
Atherton et al,[33] 1988	PUVA	Prospective	15; ages: 10–14 "Long-standing severe eczema"	• Median 16 wk tx • Median cumulative dose: 155	Clearance in 93% of patients; 60% of patients maintained remission	HSV reactivation, photoonycholysis, freckle development
Sheehan et al,[34] 1993	PUVA	Prospective	53; ages: 6–16 Severity: unknown	• Mean 19 tx • MCD: 280	74% of patients achieved clearance or near clearance (>90% BSA reduction); 69% of patients remained in remission at 1-y follow-up	HSV reactivation, erythema, pruritus, blistering, freckling, acute exacerbations of asthma
Collins et al,[41] 1995	NBUVB	Retrospective	40; ages <16 y "Moderate to severe AD"	• Mean 25 tx • MCD: 17.8	28% with excellent response, 23% with good response	Erythema, xerosis, herpes labialis, burning
Tay et al,[40] 1996	BBUVB	Prospective	5; ages: 16 mo to 11 y Severity >50% BSA	• Mean 41 tx • MCD: 5.6	No patients cleared completely, but all were moderately improved with reduction of extent of eczema and decrease in pruritus	Erythema, burning
Pasic et al,[35] 2003	Combined UVA/UVB	Retrospective	21; ages: 4–15 >40% BSA	• Mean 18 tx • MCD: 6.14 for UVB and 69.7 for UVA	45.5% with >90% improvement in SCORAD; 68.2% with >70% reduction in SCORAD	Erythema
Clayton et al,[9] 2006	NBUVB	Retrospective	60; ages: 4–16 "Severe AD"	• Median 30 tx • MCD: 29.3	40% of patients with complete clearance; 100% sustained clearance at 3 mo, 65% at 6 mo	Erythema, HSV reactivation

(continued on next page)

Table 3
(continued)

Author, y	Light Modality	Study Type	No. Patients; Age Range Disease Severity	Mean or Median tx No.; MCD (J/cm²)	Main Findings	Adverse Effects
Jury et al,[6] 2006	NBUVB	Retrospective	25; ages: 4–16 Severity: unknown	• Median 24 tx • MCD: unknown	68% showed minimal residual disease at the end of treatment	HSV reactivation, anxiety, erythema, blistering, VZV reactivation
Nistico et al,[36] 2008	Excimer laser	Prospective	6; ages: 6–16 Moderate to severe AD by SCORAD	• Range 6–12 tx • MCD: 21.89	66.7% obtained complete remission and significant improvement in SCORAD; 44% maintained remission at 16 wk follow-up	Erythema, pruritus, vesicle formation, edema, hyperpigmentation
Tan et al,[37] 2010	NBUVB	Prospective	61; ages: 2–15 Severity: unknown	• Mean 33 tx • MCD: 29.7	71% achieved >75% improvement	Erythema
Pavlovsky et al,[38] 2011	NBUVB	Retrospective	41; ages: 2–18 Severity: unknown	• Mean tx duration: 3.3 mo • MCD: 51.6	25% of patients cleared; 69% with >75% improvement; mean duration of remission 5 mo	Erythema, first-degree burn, pruritus
Darne et al,[32] 2014	NBUVB	Prospective	29; ages: 3–16 Mean 48% BSA	• Mean 24 tx • MCD: 28.6	61% mean improvement in SASSAD score in treated group vs 6% worsening in controls; 41% of treated patients cleared; 29% sustained response at 6 mo	Erythema

Study	Modality	Type	Patients	Treatment	Outcomes	Adverse effects
Mok et al,[39] 2014	NBUVB	Retrospective	15; ages: 7–15 Severity >70% BSA	• Mean 60 tx • MCD: 1.175	66% of patients achieved >70% improvement in BSA; 90% sustained improvement at 1-y follow-up	Pruritus, peeling, erythema, eczema herpeticum
	Combined UVA and NBUVB	Retrospective	9; ages: 7–15 Severity >70% BSA	• Mean 22 tx • MCD: 1.3 for UVA and 0.01 for NBUVB	44% had >70% improvement in BSA	Pruritus, erythema, eczema herpeticum
	Combined UVA and BBUVB	Retrospective	2; ages: 7–15 Severity >70% BSA	MCD: 1.5 for UVA and 0.0125 for BBUVB	Both patients had worsening of symptoms requiring cessation of treatment after 2–4 mo	Unknown
Dayal et al,[8] 2017	NBUVB	Prospective	30; ages: 4–14 Mean 34% BSA Moderate to severe eczema by SCORAD	• Mean 24 tx • MCD: 2.1	90% of patients with clearance by week 24 and sustained at 2-y follow-up; improved pruritus and sleep	Erythema, HSV reactivation, VZV reactivation
Eustace et al,[4] 2017	NBUVB	Retrospective	44; ages: 3–17 "Severe disease" in 79% of patients	• Mean 29 tx • MCD: 53	76% response rate; 52% sustained response at 12-mo follow-up	Erythema, HSV reactivation
	PUVA	Retrospective	4; ages: 3–17 "Severe hand eczema"	• Mean 17 tx • MCD: 15.1	1 patient cleared after treatment, 2 with continued moderate disease, 1 failed to complete course	None

Abbreviations: BSA, body surface area; HSV, herpes simplex virus; SASSAD, six area, six sign atopic dermatitis severity score; SCORAD, SCORing Atopic Dermatitis index.

Table 4
Summary of studies using phototherapy in children with psoriasis

Author, y	Light Modality	Study Type	No. Patients; Age Range; Disease Severity	Mean or Median tx No.; MCD (J/cm²)	Main Findings	Adverse Effects
Menter et al,[46] 1984	Goeckerman treatment	Retrospective	31; ages: 0–16 >60% BSA involvement in half of the patients	• Mean 12 tx • MCD: 1.92	64% of patients with >90% clearance	Unknown
al-Fouzan & Nanda,[47] 1995	BBUVB	Prospective	20; ages: 5–12 Mean 61% BSA	• Mean 25 tx • MCD: 3.31	88% of patients with >80% clearance	None
Tay et al,[40] 1996	BBUVB	Prospective	10; ages: 14 mo to 12 y 30%–60% BSA	• Mean 36 tx • MCD: 7.8	All patients cleared with therapy (defined as >90% reduction in BSA)	Erythema, swelling, pain
Pasic et al,[35] 2003	NBUVB	Retrospective	20; ages: 6–14 30%–60% BSA	• Mean 19 tx • MCD: 6.61	45% of patients with >90% reduction; 65% showed >70% improvement in PASI	None
Pahlajani et al,[48] 2005	Excimer laser	Prospective	4; mean age: 11 y Severity: unknown	• Mean 12.5 tx • MCD: unknown	91.3% reduction in PSS	Hyperpigmentation, blisters
Jury et al,[6] 2006	NBUVB	Retrospective	35; ages: 4–16 Severity: unknown	• Median 17.5 tx • MCD: unknown	63% of patients achieved clearance or had minimal disease by the end of treatment	Erythema (30%); HSV reactivation; anxiety; urinary incontinence resulting in short circuit in a base fan unit
Jain et al,[49] 2007	NBUVB	Prospective	20; ages: 5–14 24%–60% BSA	• Mean 24 tx • MCD: 4	60% of patients with >90% reduction; 15% with >70% reduction	Erythema, erythroderma, burning, itching
Borska et al,[50] 2007	Goeckerman treatment	Prospective	26; ages: 8–17 Severity: unknown	• Mean 19 d tx • MCD: unknown	PASI decreased significantly	Unknown

Study	Treatment	Study type	Population	Parameters	Results	Side effects
Ersoy-Evans et al,[21] 2009	NBUVB	Retrospective	65; mean age 12 Severity: unknown	• Mean 4 mo tx • MCD: 20	92.9% of patients with >75% reduction using NBUVB	Erythema, pruritus
	BBUVB	Retrospective		• Mean 3 mo tx • MCD: 21	93.3% of patients with >75% reduction using BBUVB	Erythema, pruritus
	PUVA	Retrospective		• Mean 27 mo tx • MCD: 498	83.3% of patients with >75% reduction using PUVA	Erythema, pruritus
Zamberk et al,[51] 2010	NBUVB	Retrospective	20; ages: 5–17 Median PASI 8.25	• Median 28 tx • MCD: 40.8	52% of patients with >90% improvement in PASI score; 70% with >75% improvement in PASI; maintained improvement for mean of 8 mo	Erythema
Tan et al,[37] 2010	NBUVB	Prospective	38; ages: 8–15 Severity: unknown	• Mean 28 tx • MCD: 20.4	90% of patients achieved >75% improvement.	Erythema
Kortuem et al,[52] 2010	Goeckerman treatment	Retrospective	65; ages: 3 mo to 18 y 25 to >75% BSA affected	• Mean 20 d • MCD: unknown	62% of patients with >90% clearance; 23% with 80%–89% clearance; Mean duration of remission: 2.61 y	Folliculitis
Pavlovsky et al,[38] 2011	NBUVB	Retrospective	88; ages: 2–18 Severity: unknown	• Mean 3 mo • MCD: 46.5	51% of patients cleared; 92% achieved 75% or more improvement; mean duration of remission 20 mo	Erythema, first-degree burn, pruritus

(continued on next page)

Table 4
(continued)

Author, y	Light Modality	Study Type	No. Patients; Age Range; Disease Severity	Mean or Median tx No.; MCD (J/cm²)	Main Findings	Adverse Effects
Sen et al,[5] 2014	NBUVB	Retrospective	30; ages: 5–16 Severity: unknown	• Mean 32 tx • MCD: 30.9	60% of patients showed complete clearance; 73% showed at least 75% improvement	Erythema, blistering, VZV reactivation, urinary incontinence in light box
Wong et al,[53] 2015	NBUVB	Retrospective	12; ages: 6–13 2%–70% BSA affected	• Mean 57.3 tx • MCD: unknown	50% of patients achieved >90% improvement; 40% achieved 70%–90% improvement	Burning, pain, erythema, itching
Eustace et al,[4] 2017	NBUVB	Retrospective	21; ages: 3–17 Moderate to severe psoriasis by PASI or PGA	• Mean 30 tx • MCD: 52.4	86% of patients showed 90% improvement in PASI score; at 12-mo follow-up, 43% of patients sustained improvement, 28% started on systemics	Erythema, HSV reactivation

Abbreviations: PASI, psoriasis area and severity index; PGA, physician global assessment; PSS, psoriatic severity score.

psoriasis while decreasing overall exposure to UV light.[54]

BBUVB and Goeckerman treatment have also been reported to be safe and effective in childhood psoriasis (see **Table 4**).[21,46,50,52,55] PUVA has also been used with excellent efficacy; however, as previously noted, PUVA is used with extreme caution in children given its carcinogenic risks and other adverse effects.[21] There are no large studies examining excimer laser therapy in childhood psoriasis; however, 1 pilot study in which 4 children were treated with excimer laser reported a significant reduction of 91.3% in the mean psoriasis severity score after an average of 12 treatments.[48]

Alopecia Areata

AA is an autoimmune disease causing nonscarring hair loss. It most commonly manifests as patchy hair loss on the scalp, although other parts of the body may be affected, and its presentation can vary in severity. AA is common in the pediatric population and is associated with a significant psychosocial burden and impaired QOL in childhood.[56] Several treatments are available for AA, with topical therapy encouraged as first-line treatment in children. Although there are several studies demonstrating the efficacy of phototherapy in AA for adults, studies in children are limited. Reported modalities in the literature include the 308-nm excimer laser, NBUVB, and PUVA.

In a retrospective review, Ersoy-Evans and colleagues[21] reported 10 children, ages 14 to 16, with varying severities of AA who were treated with PUVA. Of these 10 patients, only 2 (30%) responded with complete hair regrowth. Similarly, another study reported the use of NBUVB in treating 6 children with AA and found poor response rates, with 83% of patients reporting no improvement.[6] Based on the lack of evidence demonstrating its efficacy, phototherapy is not currently recommended as standard therapy for the treatment of AA in the pediatric population.

In contrast, some studies have shown the 308-nm excimer laser as being an effective treatment option for AA in children. In an open study including 11 children with AA treated with excimer laser twice weekly for a period of 12 weeks, 60% reported regrowth of hair in treated areas of the scalp compared with no growth on control areas not treated with excimer laser. In addition, 1 recent case report observed significant hair regrowth in a 5-year-old patient with extensive, refractory AA, treated with khellin and excimer laser.[57] Khellin is similar to psoralens with regard to phototherapeutic properties but incurs less phototoxic and carcinogenic effects. More studies are needed to verify its safety and efficacy in children.

Pityriasis Lichenoides

PL is a chronic inflammatory disorder spanning the clinical spectrum from pityriasis lichenoides et varioliformis acute to pityriasis lichenoides chronica (PLC). PL is predominantly a pediatric disease and often presents with a relapsing-remitting course, making management difficult. First-line therapy consists of corticosteroids or oral antibiotics, but because of frequent failure of these modalities, systemic medications or phototherapy is often required.[58] Evidence supporting the efficacy of phototherapy in pediatric PL is well documented in the literature and includes treatment with NBUVB, BBUVB, and PUVA.

NBUVB is the most studied modality in the treatment of pediatric PL, with strong evidence supporting its efficacy. Most recently, Eustace and colleagues[4] reported 3 patients with PLC who underwent treatment with NBUVB and experienced significant improvement in their disease, with clear to almost clear skin in all patients and minimal side effects. At 1-year follow-up, all patients were able to be managed on topical treatment alone. Other studies have also supported the use of NBUVB in the management of refractory PL.[59,60] In a recent systematic review analyzing 9 studies on a total of 29 children treated with NBUVB, complete clearance occurred in 74% of the cases, partial clearance in 13%, and no clearance in 13%, with an average of 19 sessions to achieve response.[1] BBUVB and PUVA have also demonstrated efficacy in the management of PL.[1,21,61] NBUVB has been the preferred treatment modality given its favorable adverse effect profile and strong track record for efficacy and remission induction in PL.

Mycosis Fungoides

MF is the most common form of cutaneous T-cell lymphoma in both children and adults. MF is rare in the pediatric population, with an estimated incidence of 0.5% to 5% before the age of 20, and it tends to present in earlier stages than in adults.[62] Given the rare nature of the disease in children, there is currently no established consensus regarding the treatment of MF in this population. Importantly, MF in young patients is a disease in which phototherapy may be considered a first-line therapy, with studies supporting the efficacy of both NBUVB and PUVA. NBUVB has demonstrated particularly favorable outcomes in pediatric patients with the hypopigmented variant of MF.[63]

Evidence is lacking comparing the efficacy of NBUVB with PUVA, but some studies have suggested more frequent recurrence of lesions with the use of NBUVB than with PUVA. Most recently in 2019, Brazzelli and colleagues[62] found that the effectiveness of NBUVB was better when used as a first-line therapy for younger children and when used in early-stage MF. In this study, the mean remission in patients in the 15- to 19-year age group was 11 months following NBUVB, and 30 months following PUVA. In those less than 15, complete remission for a mean of 59 months was seen following NBUVB only. These findings are in concordance with previous studies on the efficacy of phototherapy in children with MF, highlighting higher rates of remission with PUVA but an overall safer therapeutic index with NBUVB. In an earlier study by Laws and colleagues,[64] 26 pediatric patients with MF were treated with light as a first-line agent, with 18 receiving NBUVB and 8 receiving PUVA. Eighty percent of the patients treated with NBUVB achieved either complete or partial remission, whereas all patients treated with PUVA achieved complete or partial remission. After NBUVB, 58% of patients who responded required a further course of phototherapy after a median of 4 months, compared with the PUVA group, in which 50% of patients who initially responded required a further course of treatment after a median of 45.5 months. Taken together, NBUVB is recommended as a first-line therapy for early stage MF, especially in younger patients with hypopigmented disease, and consideration should be taken for the use of PUVA in refractory cases, weighing the hypothetical long-term risks of PUVA against its potential benefits in the management of this cutaneous malignancy on a case-by-case basis.

Other Skin Conditions

Although evidence for the use of phototherapy in children is most abundant in the aforementioned diseases, it is also commonly used in several other pediatric dermatoses, including morphea, graft-versus-host disease, urticaria pigmentosa, and pruritic dermatoses. Evidence regarding the efficacy of phototherapy in these conditions is limited to a few studies and case reports, however, and further research is needed to provide recommendations on its use in these conditions.

SUMMARY

There is strong evidence supporting the efficacy and safety of phototherapy in the pediatric population. Indications for the use of various light modalities differ depending on the skin condition, age of the child, and desired outcome. NBUVB has become the preferred modality for many pediatric skin conditions because of the rarity of severe adverse effects and more favorable long-term side-effect profile. Short-term risks and benefits of phototherapy are similar in children and adults, although treatments may be more challenging in children and require ongoing support of parents and supervision by trained staff to safely administer treatments and provide comfort for the child. Because of the dearth of studies reporting long-term follow-up of children treated with phototherapy, it should be used with caution in children, particularly PUVA. It is always prudent to prescribe phototherapy conscientiously when it comes to treating children and maintain close follow-up so that the shortest course needed can be used, in order to mitigate potential long-term effects. The use of adjunctive therapies for many skin conditions may help enhance clearance and minimize phototherapy needs and should be considered when appropriate. Finally, avoidance of PUVA in favor of NBUVB for management of the most common light-sensitive dermatoses discussed herein is reasonable, with special consideration for the use of PUVA in children with more refractory cases or severe diseases, such as pediatric MF, after risks and benefits have been thoroughly reviewed with the patient and family.

REFERENCES

1. Maranda EL, Smith M, Nguyen AH, et al. Phototherapy for pityriasis lichenoides in the pediatric population: a review of the published literature. Am J Clin Dermatol 2016;17(6):583–91.
2. Lara-Corrales I, Ramnarine S, Lansang P. Treatment of childhood psoriasis with phototherapy and photochemotherapy. Clin Med Insights Pediatr 2013;7:25–33.
3. Song E, Reja D, Silverberg N, et al. Phototherapy: kids are not just little people. Clin Dermatol 2015;33(6):672–80.
4. Eustace K, Dolman S, Alsharqi A, et al. Use of phototherapy in children. Pediatr Dermatol 2017;34(2):150–5.
5. Sen BB, Rifaioglu EN, Ekiz O, et al. Narrow-band ultraviolet B phototherapy in childhood. Cutan Ocul Toxicol 2014;33(3):189–91.
6. Jury CS, McHenry P, Burden AD, et al. Narrowband ultraviolet B (UVB) phototherapy in children. Clin Exp Dermatol 2006;31(2):196–9.
7. Koh MJ, Mok ZR, Chong WS. Phototherapy for the treatment of vitiligo in Asian children. Pediatr Dermatol 2015;32(2):192–7.
8. Dayal S, Pathak K, Sahu P, et al. Narrowband UV-B phototherapy in childhood atopic dermatitis:

efficacy and safety. An Bras Dermatol 2017;92(6): 801–6.

9. Clayton TH, Clark SM, Turner D, et al. The treatment of severe atopic dermatitis in childhood with narrowband ultraviolet B phototherapy. Clin Exp Dermatol 2007;32(1):28–33.

10. Csoma Z, Tóth-Molnár E, Balogh K, et al. Neonatal blue light phototherapy and melanocytic nevi: a twin study. Pediatrics 2011;128(4):e856–64.

11. Lai YC, Yew YW. Neonatal blue light phototherapy and melanocytic nevus count in children: a systematic review and meta-analysis of observational studies. Pediatr Dermatol 2016;33(1):62–8.

12. Stern RS, Nichols KT, Bauer E, et al. Therapy with orally administered methoxsalen and ultraviolet A radiation during childhood increases the risk of basal cell carcinoma. J Pediatr 1996;129(6):915–7.

13. Lin CY, Oakley A, Rademaker M, et al. Effect of narrowband ultraviolet B phototherapy on melanocytic naevi. Br J Dermatol 2013;168(4):815–9.

14. Kruger C, Schallreuter KU. A review of the worldwide prevalence of vitiligo in children/adolescents and adults. Int J Dermatol 2012;51(10):1206–12.

15. Halder RM. Childhood vitiligo. Clin Dermatol 1997; 15(6):899–906.

16. Veith W, Deleo V, Silverberg N. Medical phototherapy in childhood skin diseases. Minerva Pediatr 2011;63(4):327–33.

17. Fitzpatrick TB. Mechanisms of phototherapy of vitiligo. Arch Dermatol 1997;133(12):1591–2.

18. Njoo MD, Bos JD, Westerhof W. Treatment of generalized vitiligo in children with narrow-band (TL-01) UVB radiation therapy. J Am Acad Dermatol 2000; 42(2 Pt 1):245–53.

19. Kanwar AJ, Dogra S. Narrow-band UVB for the treatment of generalized vitiligo in children. Clin Exp Dermatol 2005;30(4):332–6.

20. Brazzelli V, Prestinari F, Castello M, et al. Useful treatment of vitiligo in 10 children with UV-B narrowband (311 nm). Pediatr Dermatol 2005;22(3):257–61.

21. Ersoy-Evans S, Altaykan A, Sahin S, et al. Phototherapy in childhood. Pediatr Dermatol 2008;25(6): 599–605.

22. Percivalle S, Piccinno R, Caccialanza M, et al. Narrowband ultraviolet B phototherapy in childhood vitiligo: evaluation of results in 28 patients. Pediatr Dermatol 2012;29(2):160–5.

23. Yazici S, Gunay B, Baskan EB, et al. The efficacy of narrowband UVB treatment in pediatric vitiligo: a retrospective analysis of 26 cases. Turk J Med Sci 2017;47(2):381–4.

24. Lommerts JE, Njoo MD, de Rie MA, et al. Twenty-year follow-up using a postal survey of childhood vitiligo treated with narrowband ultraviolet B phototherapy. Br J Dermatol 2017;177(3):e60–1.

25. Do JE, Shin JY, Kim DY, et al. The effect of 308nm excimer laser on segmental vitiligo: a retrospective study of 80 patients with segmental vitiligo. Photodermatol Photoimmunol Photomed 2011;27(3): 147–51.

26. Cho S, Zheng Z, Park YK, et al. The 308-nm excimer laser: a promising device for the treatment of childhood vitiligo. Photodermatol Photoimmunol Photomed 2011;27(1):24–9.

27. Dayal S, Sahu P, Gupta N. Treatment of childhood vitiligo using tacrolimus ointment with narrowband ultraviolet B phototherapy. Pediatr Dermatol 2016; 33(6):646–51.

28. Hui-Lan Y, Xiao-Yan H, Jian-Yong F, et al. Combination of 308-nm excimer laser with topical pimecrolimus for the treatment of childhood vitiligo. Pediatr Dermatol 2009;26(3):354–6.

29. Li L, Liang Y, Hong J, et al. The effectiveness of topical therapy combined with 308-nm excimer laser on vitiligo compared to excimer laser monotherapy in pediatric patients. Pediatr Dermatol 2019;36(1): e53–5.

30. Kay J, Gawkrodger DJ, Mortimer MJ, et al. The prevalence of childhood atopic eczema in a general population. J Am Acad Dermatol 1994;30(1): 35–9.

31. Beattie PE, Lewis-Jones MS. A comparative study of impairment of quality of life in children with skin disease and children with other chronic childhood diseases. Br J Dermatol 2006;155(1):145–51.

32. Darne S, Leech SN, Taylor AE. Narrowband ultraviolet B phototherapy in children with moderate-to-severe eczema: a comparative cohort study. Br J Dermatol 2014;170(1):150–6.

33. Atherton DJ, Carabott F, Glover MT, et al. The role of psoralen photochemotherapy (PUVA) in the treatment of severe atopic eczema in adolescents. Br J Dermatol 1988;118(6):791–5.

34. Sheehan MP, Atherton DJ, Norris P, et al. Oral psoralen photochemotherapy in severe childhood atopic eczema: an update. Br J Dermatol 1993;129(4):431–6.

35. Pasic A, Ceovic R, Lipozencic J, et al. Phototherapy in pediatric patients. Pediatr Dermatol 2003;20(1): 71–7.

36. Nistico SP, Saraceno R, Capriotti E, et al. Efficacy of monochromatic excimer light (308 nm) in the treatment of atopic dermatitis in adults and children. Photomed Laser Surg 2008;26(1):14–8.

37. Tan E, Lim D, Rademaker M. Narrowband UVB phototherapy in children: a New Zealand experience. Australas J Dermatol 2010;51(4):268–73.

38. Pavlovsky M, Baum S, Shpiro D, et al. Narrow band UVB: is it effective and safe for paediatric psoriasis and atopic dermatitis? J Eur Acad Dermatol Venereol 2011;25(6):727–9.

39. Mok ZR, Koh MJ, Chong WS. Is phototherapy useful in the treatment of atopic dermatitis in Asian children? A 5-year report from Singapore. Pediatr Dermatol 2014;31(6):698–702.

40. Tay YK, Morelli JG, Weston WL. Experience with UVB phototherapy in children. Pediatr Dermatol 1996;13(5):406–9.

41. Collins P, Ferguson J. Narrowband (TL-01) UVB air-conditioned phototherapy for atopic eczema in children. Br J Dermatol 1995;133(4):653–5.

42. Sidbury R, Davis DM, Cohen DE, et al. Guidelines of care for the management of atopic dermatitis: section 3. Management and treatment with phototherapy and systemic agents. J Am Acad Dermatol 2014;71(2):327–49.

43. Paller AS, Singh R, Cloutier M, et al. Prevalence of psoriasis in children and adolescents in the United States: a claims-based analysis. J Drugs Dermatol 2018;17(2):187–94.

44. Benoit S, Hamm H. Childhood psoriasis. Clin Dermatol 2007;25(6):555–62.

45. Menter A, Korman NJ, Elmets CA, et al. Guidelines of care for the management of psoriasis and psoriatic arthritis: section 5. Guidelines of care for the treatment of psoriasis with phototherapy and photochemotherapy. J Am Acad Dermatol 2010;62(1): 114–35.

46. Menter MA, Whiting DA, McWilliams J. Resistant childhood psoriasis: an analysis of patients seen in a day-care center. Pediatr Dermatol 1984;2(1):8–12.

47. al-Fouzan AS, Nanda A. UVB phototherapy in childhood psoriasis. Pediatr Dermatol 1995;12(1):66.

48. Pahlajani N, Katz BJ, Lozano AM, et al. Comparison of the efficacy and safety of the 308 nm excimer laser for the treatment of localized psoriasis in adults and in children: a pilot study. Pediatr Dermatol 2005; 22(2):161–5.

49. Jain VK, Aggarwal K, Jain K, et al. Narrow-band UV-B phototherapy in childhood psoriasis. Int J Dermatol 2007;46(3):320–2.

50. Borska L, Fiala Z, Krejsek J, et al. Immunologic changes in TNF-alpha, sE-selectin, sP-selectin, sI-CAM-1, and IL-8 in pediatric patients treated for psoriasis with the Goeckerman regimen. Pediatr Dermatol 2007;24(6):607–12.

51. Zamberk P, Velazquez D, Campos M, et al. Paediatric psoriasis–narrowband UVB treatment. J Eur Acad Dermatol Venereol 2010;24(4):415–9.

52. Kortuem KR, Davis MD, Witman PM, et al. Results of Goeckerman treatment for psoriasis in children: a 21-year retrospective review. Pediatr Dermatol 2010;27(5):518–24.

53. Wong Y, Koh MJ, Chong WS. Role of narrowband ultraviolet B phototherapy in the treatment of childhood psoriasis in Asian children. Pediatr Dermatol 2015;32(5):e221–3.

54. Marqueling AL, Cordoro KM. Systemic treatments for severe pediatric psoriasis: a practical approach. Dermatol Clin 2013;31(2):267–88.

55. Yones SS, Palmer RA, Garibaldinos TT, et al. Randomized double-blind trial of the treatment of chronic plaque psoriasis: efficacy of psoralen-UV-A therapy vs narrowband UV-B therapy. Arch Dermatol 2006;142(7):836–42.

56. Bilgic O, Bilgic A, Bahali K, et al. Psychiatric symptomatology and health-related quality of life in children and adolescents with alopecia areata. J Eur Acad Dermatol Venereol 2014;28(11): 1463–8.

57. Fenniche S, Hammami H, Zaouak A. Association of khellin and 308-nm excimer lamp in the treatment of severe alopecia areata in a child. J Cosmet Laser Ther 2018;20(3):156–8.

58. Zang JB, Coates SJ, Huang J, et al. Pityriasis lichenoides: long-term follow-up study. Pediatr Dermatol 2018;35(2):213–9.

59. Farnaghi F, Seirafi H, Ehsani AH, et al. Comparison of the therapeutic effects of narrow band UVB vs. PUVA in patients with pityriasis lichenoides. J Eur Acad Dermatol Venereol 2011;25(8):913–6.

60. Koh WL, Koh MJ, Tay YK. Pityriasis lichenoides in an Asian population. Int J Dermatol 2013;52(12): 1495–9.

61. Romani J, Puig L, Fernandez-Figueras MT, et al. Pityriasis lichenoides in children: clinicopathologic review of 22 patients. Pediatr Dermatol 1998; 15(1):1–6.

62. Brazzelli V, Bernacca C, Segal A, et al. Photo-photochemotherapy in juvenile-onset mycosis fungoides: a retrospective study on 9 patients. J Pediatr Hematol Oncol 2019;41(1):34–7.

63. Boulos S, Vaid R, Aladily TN, et al. Clinical presentation, immunopathology, and treatment of juvenile-onset mycosis fungoides: a case series of 34 patients. J Am Acad Dermatol 2014;71(6): 1117–26.

64. Laws PM, Shear NH, Pope E. Childhood mycosis fungoides: experience of 28 patients and response to phototherapy. Pediatr Dermatol 2014;31(4): 459–64.

Home UV Phototherapy

Jason Jacob, MD[a,b,*], Adrian Pona, MD[c,1], Abigail Cline, MD, PhD[c,1],
Steven Feldman, MD, PhD[d,e,f,1]

KEYWORDS

- Home-based phototherapy • Narrowband ultraviolet B • Psoriasis • Eczema • Vitiligo
- Tanning beds

KEY POINTS

- Home phototherapy has similar efficacy to office-based phototherapy.
- Home phototherapy is associated with lower cost over the duration of treatment, and increased adherence.
- In the right setting, home phototherapy should be considered for its economic value, tolerance, adherence, and efficacy in patients with psoriasis, vitiligo, and atopic dermatitis.

INTRODUCTION

Phototherapy is a first-line treatment for extensive psoriasis, vitiligo, atopic dermatitis, and other photosensitive dermatoses. Anecdotal accounts report that the ancient Egyptians used sunlight for its therapeutic properties.[1] The earliest reports of phototherapy use for skin disorders are from India around 1400 BC where patients with depigmentation disorders were given plant extracts thought to contain psoralens, and then exposed to the sun.[2,3] Starting in 1903, phototherapy was used for managing lupus vulgaris, tuberculosis, leg ulcers, skin diseases, and smallpox.[1] In the mid-1900s, oral psoralens with total body UVA was found to be more effective than previously used phototherapy modalities[4]; subsequently, other wavelengths of ultraviolet light were introduced including broadband UVB (BB-UVB) and narrowband UVB (NB-UVB).[5–7]

In 1925 at the Mayo clinic, Goeckerman developed the use of BB-UVB in combination with day and night applications of crude coal tar for the successful treatment of psoriasis, which entailed a multiweek inpatient admission stay.[8,9] Several modifications and simplifications were made, the most well-known being the Ingram regimen developed in the 1950s, which replaced crude coal tar with anthralin.[9] In 1981, investigators found that, for psoriasis, phototherapy was most efficacious in the 308 to 312 nm range, optimizing therapeutic response while minimizing erythemogenic response to nontherapeutic light wavelengths.[2,7,10]

Phototherapy does have limitations. For example, the scalp, genitals, and nails are difficult areas to treat that may not be responsive to light therapy.[11–14] Office-based phototherapy can be time-consuming, expensive, and inconvenient. Patients must have access to frequent office sessions, pay direct costs including copayments, and incur lost wages from attending treatment sessions.[11–14] Patients have reported inconvenience and inability to afford treatment as common reasons to stop NB-UVB.[12,14]

[a] Department of Medicine, Hartford Hospital, 80 Seymour Street, Hartford, CT 06102, USA; [b] University of Connecticut School of Medicine and Internal Medicine Residency, Farmington, CT, USA; [c] Center for Dermatology Research, Wake Forest School of Medicine, Winston-Salem, NC, USA; [d] Department of Dermatology, Wake Forest School of Medicine, Winston-Salem, NC, USA; [e] Department of Pathology, Wake Forest School of Medicine, Winston-Salem, NC, USA; [f] Department of Social Sciences & Health Policy, Wake Forest School of Medicine, Winston-Salem, NC, USA
[1] Present address: 1 Medical Center Blvd, Winston-Salem, NC 27157.
* Corresponding author. Department of Medicine, Hartford Hospital, 80 Seymour Street, Hartford, CT 06102.
E-mail address: jasonjac@gmail.com

Dermatol Clin 38 (2020) 109–126
https://doi.org/10.1016/j.det.2019.09.001
0733-8635/20/© 2019 Elsevier Inc. All rights reserved.

Home phototherapy devices may overcome many of the logistical and financial barriers associated with outpatient phototherapy treatment. Use of home treatment for psoriasis was published in 1979.[15] Since then, additional home phototherapy studies have been performed in early plaque stage mycosis fungoides, vitiligo, photosensitive dermatoses, and hand eczema.[15–28]

The aim of this article is to explore the history of home phototherapy and discuss the devices currently available on the market, including their cost, efficacy, and patient adherence. The current evidence on tanning beds is also reported.

The History of Home Phototherapy

Although home NB-UVB equipment has been commercially available since the 1980s, the lack of well-controlled clinical trials and standardized guidelines along with the need for close monitoring, extensive patient education, and appropriate screening delayed the incorporation of NB-UVB as a routinely used therapeutic modality in dermatology.[11,29,30] Although home NB-UVB is now widely accepted, it is unclear just when this paradigm shift occurred. Randomized control trials and other studies showing safety and efficacy may have helped encourage acceptance of home-based phototherapy.

In 2009, a multicenter, single-blind, randomized clinical trial of 196 subjects with psoriasis reported that home NB-UVB is as effective as office-based NB-UVB.[17] About 70% of subjects treated with home phototherapy reached a 50% decrease in Psoriasis Area and Severity Index (PASI 50) compared with 73% of subjects managed with office-based phototherapy ($P<.001$).[10,17] Although quality of life improved in both groups, 42% of subjects treated at home rated their experience as "excellent" compared with 23% of subjects managed in the office setting ($P = .001$).[17] Based on these findings, the authors concluded that patients with psoriasis who are compliant, motivated, and adherent to instructions and follow-up visits could, under the supervision of a dermatologist, be considered appropriate candidates for home UVB phototherapy.[17]

Subsequent guidelines began to reflect the evidence for safety and efficacy of home phototherapy. In 2010, the American Academy of Dermatology Guidelines of Care for the Management of Psoriasis and Psoriatic Arthritis contended that home-based UVB phototherapy is a safe and effective treatment, although care must be taken to inform and educate the patient on potential long-term side effects including increased risk of skin cancer, cataracts, and premature aging.[9]

Current Home Phototherapy Devices

The National Psoriasis Foundation currently recommends 6 home phototherapy equipment vendors—Clarify Medical, National Biological Corporation, Daavlin, Luma Therapeutics, Solarc Systems, Inc, and UVBioTek Phototherapy.[30] Web site review and correspondence with the vendors were used to obtain information on devices and available associated costs. There are many home phototherapy devices and we discuss some of these; please note that the following is not an exhaustive list of available devices.

LIMITED CUTANEOUS DISEASE

For small-to-medium areas of cutaneous disease, the Daavlin line of home phototherapy devices includes the DermaPal (retail value $1000) and Levia (retail value $1400) as scalp and spot devices (Fig. 1), as well as small panels including the 1-series which can be used for localized treatment. The National Biological Corporation

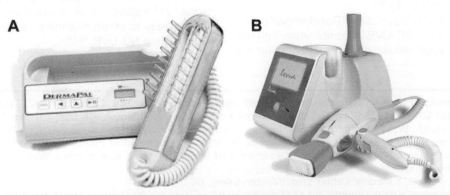

Fig. 1. (*A*) DermaPal. Light-weight and portable, the DermaPal wand is used for spot treatments and hard to reach areas. (*B*) Levia. This powerful and unique device offers both a fiber-optic brush for scalp treatment and a targeted spot light for small areas. (*Courtesy of* Daavlin Company, Bryan, OH; with permission.)

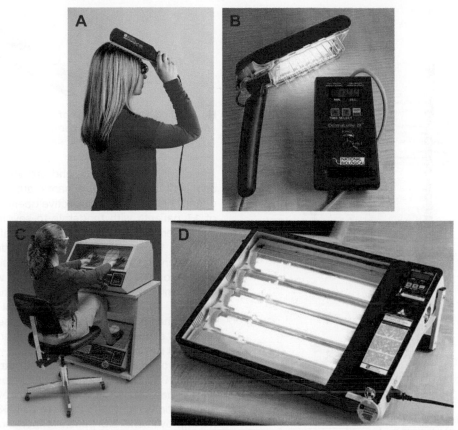

Fig. 2. (*A*) Dermalight-90 scalp treatment. (*B*) The DermaLume 2x Phototherapy Wand. (*C*) HandFoot II. (*D*) D Handisol II. (*Courtesy of* National Biological Corp., Beachwood, OH; with permission.)

line includes the Dermalight-90 scalp treatment (retail value $849), Dermalume 2X Handheld (retail value $1095), Hand/Foot II (retail value $2195), and Handisol II (retail value $1,995, **Fig. 2**). Other brands include Clarify Medical, with a home light therapy system featuring scheduling and dosing algorithm managed on a smartphone (**Fig. 3**). Luma Therapeutics also offers a smartphone dosing algorithm (Illuvinate system), along with an occlusive hydrogel with coal tar. UVBioTek Phototherapy offers the Versa Lite small panel for localized treatments (**Fig. 4**), the more portable Mobile Lite for flat surfaces, such as hands and feet (**Fig. 5**), and the Handwand for the scalp, bottom of feet, and back of arms (**Fig. 6**).

EXTENSIVE CUTANEOUS DISEASE

For extensive disease, the Daavlin line includes the 7 series and UV series (retail value $5000; **Fig. 7**). Solarc Systems, Inc, offers the SolRx 1000-Series (retail value $1995–2895; **Fig. 8A**) and the SolRx E-series (retail value $1195–4895;

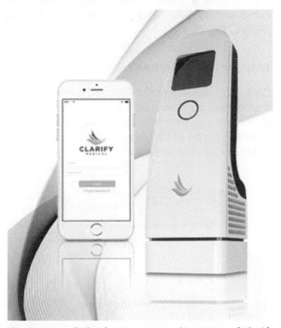

Fig. 3. Home light therapy system. (*Courtesy of* Clarify Medical, San Diego, CA; with permission.)

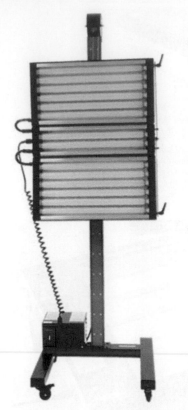

Fig. 4. Versa Lite system. (*Courtesy of* UV BioTek Phototherapy, Hudson Falls, NY; with permission.)

Fig. 8B). National Biological Corporation offers the Panosol II panel ($1995–2595), Panasol 3D Full-Body ($4980) and Foldalite III Full-Body ($6995; **Fig. 9**).

TANNING BED THERAPY

Carlin and colleagues[31] performed a retrospective medical record review of 26 patients who had used a commercial bed in conjunction with acitretin, examining type of tanning bed used, dose of acitretin, duration of combination treatment, severity

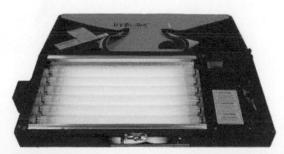

Fig. 5. Mobile Lite system. (*Courtesy of* UV BioTek Phototherapy, Hudson Falls, NY; with permission.)

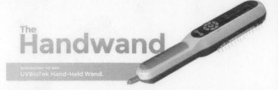

Fig. 6. Hand wand. (*Courtesy of* UV BioTek Phototherapy, Hudson Falls, NY; with permission.)

and duration of psoriasis, and previous systemic and light therapies. The same authors subsequently performed a prospective open-label study of 17 patients with moderate-to-severe plaque-type psoriasis. In the prospective trial, patients received 12 weeks of daily oral acitretin (25 mg) and commercial tanning bed UV exposure (mean UVB output 4.7%) for 4 to 5 days per week. The Wolff tanning beds used had a manufacturer-reported UVB output close to 5% of the total output, the rest being UVA. Acitretin use and tanning bed exposure was reduced if clearance was achieved before 12 weeks.

In the outcomes reported on the retrospective review, 19 of 23 (83%) of patients achieved clearance or near clearance, 2 of 23 (9%) showed moderate improvement, and 2 out of 23 (2%) showed no improvement. No patient experienced worsening of psoriasis, and patients reported a high degree of satisfaction. In the outcomes reported on the prospective trial, the PASI score decreased an average mean of 78.6% from baseline. Patients who began with moderate psoriasis showed a 72.2% reduction in PASI scores, whereas those with severe psoriasis showed an average reduction of 85.9% in PASI scores. The authors conclude that acitretin in combination with commercial tanning bed exposure is effective and useful for those patients in areas with limited access to physician-administered phototherapy. An earlier study also supported the efficacy of tanning beds for psoriasis, demonstrating greater clearing with more exposure.[32] Long-term safety data were not collected in these studies.[31,32]

Barriers to Home Phototherapy

The landmark PLUTO study, discussed below in detail, reviewed the economics of average cost of phototherapy between home-based phototherapy and office-based phototherapy in the Netherlands. In the PLUTO study, home phototherapy cost slightly more on average than in-office phototherapy, potentially because of upfront costs incurred by home phototherapy as opposed to in-office phototherapy, which incurs costs

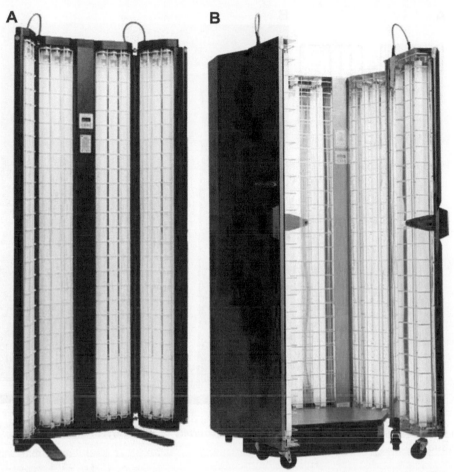

Fig. 7. (*A*) 7 series. A 6-foot-tall panel with optional doors, the 7 series is highly efficient and offers full-body treatment in a space-saving design. (*B*) UV series. A full-body cabinet with a unique elliptical shape and interior platform that ensures an even treatment every time. (*Courtesy of* Daavlin Company, Bryan, OH; with permission.)

spread over the entire treatment schedule.[33] The upfront cost of home phototherapy can be significant and may be a deterrent for many patients. In 1 study, 72% of patients failed to fill their home phototherapy prescription because of high out-of-pocket costs up to $2000.[27]

An unfortunate additional limitation is the amount of training needed to manage a panel of patients who opt for home-based phototherapy; in 1 study, only 35% of dermatology residents received any formal training on home phototherapy.[28] Inadequate insurance reimbursements have also been cited as an additional reason for the decrease in prescriptions and why the trend is toward more expensive biologics.[28] As an example, less than 1100 prescriptions have been written for home phototherapy in 1 year, suggesting provider preference and additional training gaps in the dermatology curriculum may be implicated.[28]

Efficacy of Home Phototherapy

Table 1

Psoriasis

The landmark PLUTO study for home-based phototherapy was a single-blinded randomized control trial that compared home-based phototherapy with office-based phototherapy in 196 patients with psoriasis. The primary outcome was greater than 50% reduction of baseline PASI or SAPASI (Self-Administered Psoriasis Area and Severity Index) scores (termed PASI 50 or SAPASI 50), reduction in median scores, and proportion of patients reaching PASI 75 and SAPASI 90.[10,17] Secondary outcomes were quality of life using the psoriasis disability index score and SF-36, burden of treatment (questionnaire), patients' preferences, satisfaction (questionnaire), dosimetry, and short-term side effects (diary).[10,17] Of the

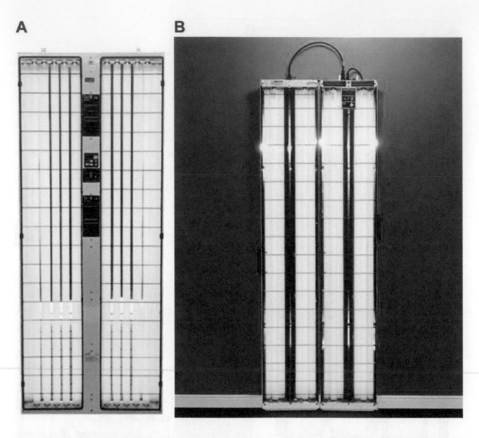

Fig. 8. (*A*) SolRx 1000-Series. (*B*) SolRx E-Series, 2 panels. (*Courtesy of* SolarC Systems Inc., Minesing, ON, Canada; with permission.)

patients receiving at home phototherapy, 82% reached SAPASI 50 compared with 79% of patients receiving office-based phototherapy (95% CI, −8.6 to 14.2), and 70% compared with 73% reached PASI 50 (95% CI, −15.7 to 11.1). For patients treated at home, the median SAPASI score decreased 82% and the median PASI score decreased 74% compared with 79% and 70%, respectively, for patients treated in the office setting. End of therapy was defined and included up to 46 irradiations. Treatment effect and side effects were similar between the 2 arms. Although the quality of life increased regardless of treatment setting, 42% of patients receiving home phototherapy more often rated their experiences as "excellent" compared with 23% of patients receiving office-based phototherapy (*P* = .001).[17]

The perceived burden of treatment was measured using a 4-item questionnaire assessed after 23 irradiations and at end of therapy. The overall average burden associated with phototherapy was lower for patients in the home phototherapy group compared with the office-based group. No specific values or CIs were reported. The

difference in mean scores, however, for the 4 domains were 1.23 to 3.01 (*P*<.0001).[17] The Psoriasis Disability Index (PDI) (max of 45, higher scores indicating more impairment) decreased from 32.8 at inclusion (n = 98) to 20.9 at the end of therapy (n = 93) for the home UVB group. The PDI decreased from 34.3 in the outpatient UVB group (n = 98) at inclusion to 22 at the end of therapy (n = 91).[17] The 8 SF-36 domains and its 2 component scores were similar across the groups.[17] Patients treated at home evaluated their treatment more positively than patients treated in the outpatient setting (*P* = .001); 92% (83/90) of patients treated at home and 60% (53/88) of those treated in the office reported they would prefer home phototherapy in the future (difference 32%; 95% CI, 19.5–44.5).[17]

Patient waiting time before start of phototherapy was also studied. Of the patients treated at home and in the office, 26% (22/86) and 45% (26/58), respectively, thought waiting time was not a problem; 48% (41/86) and 35% (20/58) thought the waiting time was acceptable. Waiting time was considered too long in 17% of home group arm

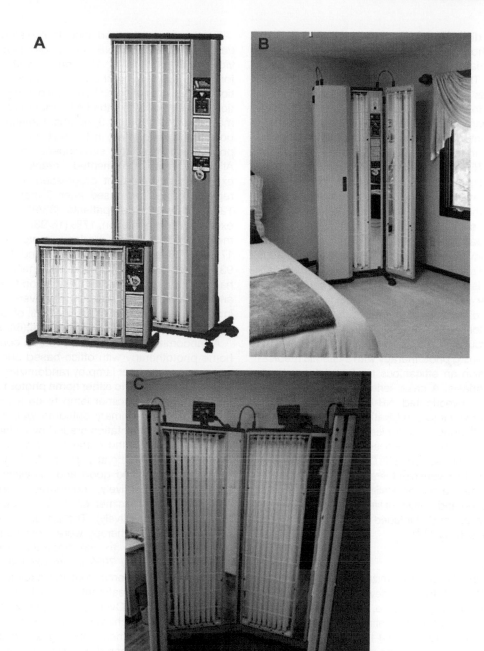

Fig. 9. (*A*) Panosol II panel. (*B*) Panasol 3D Full-Body. (*C*) Foldalite III Full-Body. (*Courtesy of* National Biological Corp., Beachwood, OH; with permission.)

versus 16% in the outpatient group arm. It was considered far too long by 9% in the home arm versus 5% in the outpatient arm (*P* = .038).[17]

Patients (n = 98 for both arms) treated at home had a higher mean total number of irradiations than patients in the outpatient group (34.4 versus 28.6; difference of 5.8; 95% CI, 2.7–9.0). The

mean cumulative dose (J/cm^2) at 23 irradiations was 21.2 for the home arm (n = 85) and 26.9 for outpatient arm (n = 68). At end of therapy, the mean cumulative dose (J/cm^2) was 51.5 for the home arm (n = 91) and 46.1 for the outpatient arm (n = 93), a difference of 5.4 J/cm^2 (95% CI, −5.2 to 16.0). The final cumulative dose of UVB did not differ significantly between the 2 groups. The authors concluded that the risk of skin cancer from treatment would be similar across the groups. The possible difference of 5.4 J/cm^2 corresponds to a difference of about 9 minimal erythema doses (MEDs) (95% CI, −9 to 26), which they deem insignificant and insufficient to favor outpatient therapy over home treatment. For comparison, in the Netherlands, the mean solar exposure is 75 MEDs annually for indoor workers and 170 MEDs annually for outdoor workers.[17]

There was no significant difference in side effects between home and office phototherapy. A burning sensation occurred in 7.1% of home-treated patients versus 10.0% of office-treated patients; severe erythema occurred in 5.5% versus 3.6%, blistering in 0.3% versus 0.6%, and mild erythema is 29.8% versus 28.6%. The mean probability per irradiation of experiencing a side effect did not differ between the groups. The patients' perception of safety also did not differ between the 2 groups.[17]

Combining phototherapy with systemic medication is also an efficacious treatment for patients with psoriasis. A case series of 27 patients with psoriasis investigated NB-UVB phototherapy 3 times per week in combination with daily oral acitretin.[10,34] Concurrent topical regimens and emollients were permitted. Efficacy was assessed with PASI and Dermatology Life Quality Index scores at 2, 4, 8, and 12 weeks of therapy.[10,34] Most patients (22/27) had a lower PASI score with greater satisfaction and quality of life.[10,34] Adverse effects were mild, and included mild alopecia and photosensitivity.[10,34]

Vitiligo

In a double-blind, randomized trial of 2 handheld NB-UVB phototherapy devices or placebo for treatment of vitiligo at home, 86% (25/29) of participants were adherent, defined as administering home phototherapy 3 to 4 times a week. Participants in the active groups were more likely to be satisfied with their treatment than participants in the placebo group (31.5% versus 20%); 68% of participants said they would use the handheld device again and 64% would recommend it to others. In the active groups, 75% of all lesions had some repigmentation compared with 39% of lesions in the placebo group at week 16. The face and neck responded best to treatment. Adverse effects included erythema grade 1 and 2 reported in 27% and 13% of active group participants, compared with 6% in the placebo group. Other reported adverse effects in the active group included pruritus (7%), hyperpigmentation around the lesions (10%), and dry skin (10%).[20]

Another open-label and uncontrolled study evaluated a home-based NB-UVB phototherapy device in 93 patients for 12 months, with clinical follow-up every 3 months to assess repigmentation and adverse effects.[21] The rate of repigmentation was fastest within the first 3 months and was maintained for the next 3 months. Patients with a poor therapeutic effect in the first 3 months had poor response to subsequent treatments. Although the repigmented areas gradually expanded as treatment progressed, the rate of repigmentation decreased after 6 months. After 12 months, 38% of patients (35/93) achieved excellent repigmentation, 17% (16/93) good repigmentation, 16% (15/93) moderate repigmentation, 17% (16/93) poor repigmentation, and 12% (11/93) no repigmentation. Face and neck lesions had the best response, with lesions on the hands and feet being most resistant.[21] Adverse effects included burning or pruritus in 12% of patients (11/93) and dry skin in 6% of patients (6/93).[21]

A randomized, parallel group study compared home phototherapy with office-based phototherapy using an excimer lamp by randomizing 44 patients with psoriasis to either home phototherapy 3 times a week or excimer lamp twice a week for 6 months.[22] The primary outcome was the percentage of repigmentation graded by an independent dermatologist and worsening of vitiligo. In the home-based phototherapy group, 72% and 50% of subjects achieved good and excellent repigmentation, respectively, compared with 54% and 36% in the excimer group ($P = .3066$ and $P = .0971$, respectively). The patients receiving home-based phototherapy were more compliant, with 92% sticking to the treatment regimen, compared with only 70% in the excimer group. Furthermore, 3 patients from the excimer group discontinued the treatment completely because of time constraints. Overall, the home-based phototherapy group achieved a higher mean total number of the treatments and higher average cumulative dose compared with the excimer group. The only adverse effect reported was a single case of phototherapy burn caused by overuse.[22]

Eczema and acne

A case series compared the efficacy of a home phototherapy unit to office-based phototherapy in 26 patients with chronic hand eczema. Eleven patients were treated at home and 15 were treated at an outpatient clinic.[35] Patients received UVB irradiation 4 to 5 times a week for 10 weeks. Although none of the patients cleared during the study, 69% of all patients (18/26) were much improved. In the home treatment group, 63% (7/11) were much improved and 37% (4/11) were

Table 1
Trials of home phototherapy

Study	Methodology	Significant Results	Conclusions
Larko & Swanbeck,[15] 1979	Patients with psoriasis (n = 28)—daily high-dose BB-UVB with induction of slight erythema as home phototherapy	*Efficacy:* 20/28 patients achieved complete remission studied over 6.5 wk. 2/28 patients with no improvement *Adverse effects:* in 25/28 patients' phototoxicity warranted a change in dosing.	
Jordan et al,[16] 1981	Patients with recalcitrant psoriasis (n = 56); home phototherapy with broad-spectrum UVB and concurrent topical tar	*Efficacy:* Psoriatic lesion clearance achieved in 55/56 patients after 8 wk of UVB treatment *Adverse effects:* Nothing significant reported	
Milstein et al,[25] 1982	Early mycosis fungoides (N = 31) and parapsoriasis en plaques (N = 3) treated with UV phototherapy (280–350 nm) at home using a light source containing 4 Westinghouse FS40 lamps	*Efficacy:* Complete clinical and histologic remission of disease (N = 19) was achieved on average in 18 mo	Although higher complete response rates generally are achieved with other therapeutic modalities, UV phototherapy with its minimal adverse effects may be indicated for selected patients. Controlled studies are encouraged.
Resnik & Vonderheid,[26] 1993	Early patch and plaque stage mycosis fungoides (n = 31); home phototherapy UVB with Westinghouse FS 40 lamps delivering erythmogenic doses	*Efficacy:* Complete clearance both clinically and histologically with sustained remission in 28/31 patients. Phototherapy was well tolerated *Adverse effects:* Minor phototoxic episodes occurred as dose vwas increased but was not great enough to warrant cessation of treatment	Home UVB phototherapy may be an appropriate therapeutic option for the treatment of patients with early mycosis fungoides

(continued on next page)

Table 1
(continued)

Study	Methodology	Significant Results	Conclusions
Sjovall & Christenson,[35] 1994	Patients with chronic hand eczema (n = 26) given high output UVB irradiation delivered by a Handylux device 4–5 times a wk for approximately 10 wk at home or at outpatient clinics	*Efficacy:* 15 patients treated as outpatients and 11 at home. No patient demonstrated complete clearance. Overall, 18/24 patients felt much improved and 6/24 were improved, after 2 dropped out of study. In the home treatment group, 7/11 were much improved and 4/11 were improved. In the outpatient group, 11/13 were much improved and 2/13 were improved *Adverse effects:* Burning and stinging were dose dependent. This also correlated with topical corticosteroid use	High-dose UVB is effective and offers opportunity to treat patients with chronic, recalcitrant hand eczema
Cameron et al,[19] 2002	Patients with photosensitive dermatoses (n = 23) received home NB-UVB phototherapy using TL-01 unit with accurate dosimetry	*Efficacy:* Complete clearance was achieved in 18/23 patients with psoriasis and moderate improvement in 3/23 patients with psoriasis. Clearance was achieved in a guttate psoriasis patients subset. Atopic dermatitis (n = 4), 1 with minimal residual activity and 3 showed marked/moderate improvement. Granuloma annulare (n = 2), 1 demonstrated minimal residual activity and the other had moderate clearance. One patient with lichen planopilaris had marked improvement and 1 patient with psoriasiform dermatitis had moderate improvement *Adverse effects:* grade 1 erythema, 62%; grade 2 erythema, 42%; grade 3 erythema, 26%; grade 4 erythema, 0%	UVB TL-01 is a useful practical development that is similar to outpatient treatment. It is safe and cost-effective

Yelverton et al,[34] 2008	Patients with moderate-to-severe psoriasis (PASI [Psoriasis Area Severity Index] > 12). N = 27 received narrowband UVB phototherapy 3 times per wk (with exposure time based on skin type and response) in combination with oral acitretin daily (25 mg dose as needed). Concurrent topical regimens and emollients were permitted. Efficacy assessed with PASI and DLQI (Dermatology Life Quality Index) scores at 2, 4, 8, and 12 wk of therapy	*Efficacy:* 22/27 patients completed the study. Mean baseline PASI decreased from 18.6 to 13.9 after 12 wk of combined therapy. DLQI responses revealed increased quality of life and high level of satisfaction with treatment *Adverse effects:* Mild alopecia and photosensitivity were reported in all subjects. Four patients required dosage change in acitretin because of increased triglycerides	Home phototherapy with narrowband UVB and oral acitretin is effective and well tolerated in patients with psoriasis Subjects were interested in continuing therapy after completion of study
Van Coevorden et al,[23] 2004	Patients (n = 158) with moderate-to-severe chronic hand eczema of more than 1 y randomized to oral PUVA (psoralens with UVA light) with portable tanning unit at home or hospital-administered bath PUVA *Primary outcome* was clinical assessment by a hand eczema score (evaluated desquamation, erythema, vesiculation, infiltration, fissures, itch, and pain on a 4-point scale) after 10 wk of treatment *Secondary outcome* was hand eczema score at 8 wk follow-up after treatment completion *Tertiary outcome* was travel cost and time off work	*Efficacy:* Both groups showed a comparable and substantial decrease in hand eczema score (equating to clinical improvement). The decrease was maintained during the follow-up period. Patients treated with oral PUVA at home had lower travel costs and less time off work	Authors concluded oral PUVA at home had a clinically relevant efficacy similar to that of hospital-administered bath PUVA. This effect was maintained during the 8 wk follow-up period and resulted in lower travel costs and less time off work

(continued on next page)

Table 1
(continued)

Study	Methodology	Significant Results	Conclusions
Koek et al,[17] 2009 PLUTO study	Patients (n = 196) with psoriasis eligible for NB-UVB phototherapy. Pragmatic single-blind RCT (randomized clinical trial) comparing NB-UVB home phototherapy using a TL-01 unit and standard NB-UVB outpatient phototherapy *Primary outcomes* was >50% reduction of baseline PASI or SAPASI (Self-administered Psoriasis Area and Severity Index), reduction in median scores, and proportion reaching PASI 75 and SAPASI 90 *Secondary outcomes* were quality of life, burden of treatment, patients' preferences and satisfaction, dosimetry, and short-term side effects.	*Efficacy:* Patients treated at home, 82% reached SAPASI 50 and 70% reached PASI 50. In the home phototherapy arm, SAPASI decreased by 82% and PASI decreased by 74%. Treatment effect, side effects, and increase in quality of life were similar between the 2 arms. Burden associated with treatment was significantly lower for patients in the home phototherapy group *Adverse effects:* Similar in the 2 groups and included burning sensation, mild and severe erythema, and blistering	Home UVB phototherapy is equally safe and effective (in terms of clinical resolution and improvement in quality of life) compared with standard outpatient UVB phototherapy. In addition, home UVB phototherapy demonstrated a lower burden of treatment and associated greater patient satisfaction
Kwon et al,[24] 2013	Patients (n = 35) with mild-to-moderate acne were randomized to either a home-use irradiation group using an LED device, or a control group using a sham device. The treatment group was instructed to serially irradiate their forehead and cheeks with 420-nm blue light and 660-nm red light for 2–5 min twice daily for 4 wk	*Efficacy:* At the final visit at 12 wk, both inflammatory and noninflammatory acne lesions had decreased significantly by 77% and 54%, respectively, in the treatment group. No significant difference was observed in the control group. In the treatment group, sebum output reduction, attenuated inflammatory cell infiltrations, and a decreased size of the sebaceous gland were found. The immunostaining intensities for interleukin-8 (IL-8), IL-1α, matrix metalloproteinase-9, toll-like receptor-2, nuclear factor-κB, insulin-like growth factor-1 receptor and sterol response element binding protein (SREBP-1 [sterol regulatory element binding protein-1]) were reduced concomitantly. Messenger RNA expression of SREBP-1c was also decreased *Adverse effects:* No severe adverse reactions were reported	

Eleftheriadou et al,[20] 2014 HI-Light Trial	A feasibility, double-blind, multicenter, parallel group randomized placebo-controlled trial of handheld NB-UVB phototherapy for the treatment of vitiligo at home. Patients (N = 29) with vitiligo were followed for 7 mo (3 mo recruitment and 4 mo treatment) and randomized to active (N = 19) and placebo (N = 10) groups in 2:1 ratio *Primary outcome* was the proportion of eligible participants who were willing to be randomized *Secondary outcomes* included proportion of participants expressing interest in the trial and fulfilling eligibility criteria, withdrawal rates and missing data, proportion of participants adhering to and satisfied with the treatment, and incidence of NB-UVB short-term adverse events	*Efficacy:* 83% (45/54) of vitiligo patients who expressed interest in the trial were willing to be randomized. Because of time and financial constraints, only 29/45 potential participants were booked to attend a baseline hospital visit. All 29 (100%) potential participants were confirmed as being eligible and were subsequently randomized; 86% (25/29) of patients adhered to the treatment and 65% (7/11) in the active group had some degree of repigmentation. Both devices used (Dermfix 1000 NB-UVB [N = 10] and Waldmann NB-UVB 109 [N = 9]) were acceptable to participants *Adverse effects:* Only 1 patient in the active group reported erythema grade 3 (3%)	Hand-held NB-UVB devices need evaluation in a large, pragmatic RCT. A pilot trial has explored many of the uncertainties that need to be overcome before embarking on a full-scale trial, including the development of a comprehensive training package and treatment protocol. The study has shown strong willingness of participants to be randomized, very good treatment adherence and repigmentation rates, and provided evidence of feasibility for a definitive trial

(continued on next page)

Table 1
(continued)

Study	Methodology	Significant Results	Conclusions
Shan et al,[21] 2014	Open and uncontrolled study of (N = 93) patients with vitiligo; 46 males and 47 females were treated with home phototherapy using the SS-01 UV phototherapy instrument which bears 2 Philips TL-9W/01 lamps	*Efficacy:* Patients were examined at baseline and reviewed every 3 mo for up to 1 y, to assess repigmentation and any side effects. At the end of 1 y, 35 patients achieved excellent repigmentation, 16 achieved good repigmentation, 15 showed moderate repigmentation, 16 had poor repigmentation, and 11 had no repigmentation. The best response (excellent repigmentation) after 1 y was seen in 27/36 cases with face and neck lesions followed by 16/43 cases with truncal vitiligo and 9/34 with limb lesions. Lesions on the hands and feet were resistant to treatment and excellent repigmentation was achieved in only 2/29 such cases *Adverse effects:* Were reported as minimal and did not necessitate treatment discontinuation. Eleven patients complained of burning or pruritus in the lesions and 6 reported dryness of skin. These minor problems were addressed by adjusting the irradiation dose or by application of emollients	The effectiveness of home phototherapy appears to be similar to that of hospital-based phototherapy and appears to be safe and cost-effective. Repigmentation was usually observed after 1 mo and some patients with localized lesions achieved complete repigmentation within 3 mo. They indicated that excellent results can be achieved when a positive response is seen in the early stages of treatment. They recommend consideration of discontinuation of treatment if no response within 3 mo. Patients with extensive vitiligo lesions need longer to complete each treatment as the portable device used could only irradiate a small area. However, the slightly greater time taken for each session of home phototherapy is trivial compared with the total time and cost of frequent visits to a hospital phototherapy unit. The advantage of this portable device is that lesions on different body sites can be given different doses of radiation. Long-term side effects: most patients received phototherapy for longer than 1 y and no cutaneous malignancy was found, although a significantly longer follow-up is required to document the frequency of this complication

| Guan et al,[22] 2015 | Randomized parallel group trial comparing home-based phototherapy with institution-based phototherapy using an excimer lamp; 44 patients were recruited based on literature review to show a difference in effectiveness of 10% or more. These patients had stable focal vitiligo and were randomized into 2 groups: 1 using home-based phototherapy (Daavlin DermaPal system, three times a wk, and 1 using institution-based excimer lamp treatment twice a wk for 6 mo. Images were taken at 0 (baseline), 3, and 6 mo. At the end of the study, the percentage repigmentation was graded by an independent dermatologist as: worsening of vitiligo, no change, slight repigmentation (<50%), good repigmentation (>50% but <75%), excellent repigmentation (>75% but less than complete), and complete repigmentation | *Efficacy:* There was no statistical difference in baseline variables between the 2 groups in terms of demographics and clinical characteristics. The home-based phototherapy group seemed to have better efficacy, with 72% and 50% in the group achieving good and excellent repigmentation, respectively, in contrast to only 54% and 36% in the excimer group. However, this difference in response was not statistically significant. *Adverse effects:* There was only 1 case of phototherapy burn caused by overenthusiastic application of home phototherapy but the patient subsequently recovered completely | The authors concluded that the observed difference in efficacy could be explained because of difference in compliance. The patients using home-based phototherapy were more compliant, with 92% sticking to the treatment regimen, whereas this figure was only 70% in the excimer group. In addition, 3 patients from the excimer group discontinued the treatment completely because of a lack of time. Overall, the patients from the home-based phototherapy group achieved a much higher mean total number of treatments and higher average cumulative dose as opposed to the excimer group. Compliance in the home-based therapy group was better probably because patients can perform phototherapy sessions as per their convenience. This study demonstrated that, with careful selection of the patients, home-based phototherapy can be as effective as institution-based treatment options |

Data from Refs.[10,15–26,34,35]

improved.[35] In the office-based group, 85% (11/13) were much improved and 15% (2/13) were improved after 2 dropped out of study. Burning and stinging were dose-dependent adverse effects.[35]

An open-label trial randomized 158 patients with moderate-to-severe chronic hand eczema to oral PUVA with a home phototherapy unit or hospital-administered bath PUVA. During the treatment period, 33 subjects (21%) dropped out: 15 in the home group and 18 in the hospital group (P = .66; 95% CI, −0.17 to 0.11). At week 10, the mean reduction in hand eczema score in the home group was 41% (95% CI, 2.4–4.1) and 31% in the hospital group (95% CI, 1.7–3.2). Although both groups had reductions from their baseline (P<.001), there was no statistical difference between them (P = .15; 95% CI, −0.31 to 2.0). The authors concluded that oral PUVA at home and hospital-administered bath PUVA had similar clinical improvement. Patients treated with oral PUVA at home had lower travel costs and less time off work. Adverse effects occurred in both groups, such as temporary nausea in the home group and mild stinging in the hospital group. Only side effects that were a reason to discontinue were analyzed: 3 in the home group (all temporary nausea) and 1 in the hospital group (burn).[23]

A double-blind controlled trial randomized 35 patients with mild-to-moderate acne to either a home phototherapy device or a control group with a sham device. Participants were instructed to use their device twice daily for 4 weeks.[24] After 12 weeks, both inflammatory and noninflammatory acne were reduced by 77% and 54%, respectively, in the home-based group, with significant improvement noted in control group.[24] Patients in the treatment group were also more satisfied than the control group from weeks 2 to 12 (P<.05). Patient adherence to treatment was measured based on their submitted usage diaries. Except for 1 patient who skipped their daily uses once, both the treatment and control groups consistently used their devices during the study period. Adverse effects included mild dryness, erythema, and desquamation.[24]

Mycosis fungoides

In a case series, 31 patients with early mycosis fungoides and 3 patients with parapsoriasis en plaques were treated with home phototherapy. Nineteen patients (61%) achieved complete clinical and histologic remission of disease, lasting for a median duration in excess of 18 months.[25] Fifteen years later, researchers presented follow-up data on those original 31 patients. Twenty-

three patients (74%) achieved a complete clinical and histologic response to home phototherapy. The maximum duration of the response ranged from 5 months to more than 15 years, with a median of 15 months. After discontinuing maintenance phototherapy, 7 patients (23%) had a sustained disease-free interval lasting more than 58 months (median >90 months).[25] Home phototherapy was well tolerated without evidence of significant photodamage or photocarcinogenicity.[26]

FUTURE TRENDS AND CURRENT PERSPECTIVES

Although there are numerous clinical trials in home phototherapy, each trial has used different protocols; including treatment schedules, units, patient selection criteria, UVB instruments, and different outcome measures to assess treatment response. This makes it difficult to analyze and compare efficacy outcomes from the established studies to achieve population-based generalization.[36] However, 1 common theme seen in these trials is that patients have higher satisfaction and adherence with their home unit.[10,15–26,34,35]

Other limitations include identifying the appropriate patient population, providing treatment education, having an increase in time between visits, and ensuring the home phototherapy unit is periodically checked, calibrated, and replaced.[36] In addition, concern for an "open prescription" by health care providers and lack of controls for the UV irradiation dose makes the decision to place someone on home phototherapy challenging.[27,28] Fortunately, many home phototherapy devices are programmed to require patients to seek follow-up from their physician after a designated number of treatments. Moreover, home phototherapy (and even tanning beds) give physicians and patients more control over dosimetry than can be achieved with sun exposure.

Additional trials may be helpful for assuring physicians of the benefits of home UV. A large, randomized, pragmatic trial—the LITE study (https://www.pcori.org/research-results/2017/comparing-home-versus-clinic-based-phototherapy-treatment-psoriasis-lite-study)—will compare the effectiveness and safety of 12 weeks of home-based versus office-based phototherapy in 1050 patients with psoriasis aged 6 years and older among 20 to 40 clinical sites around the country.[36] An additional burden that needs to be addressed, however, is the high upfront costs many patients face; removing disincentives to home phototherapy could help reduce the overall cost of psoriasis management if patients can be managed with home phototherapy instead of far more costly biologic alternatives.

A home phototherapy system (and perhaps commercial tanning[37]) is a good option for convenient treatment of photoresponsive dermatologic conditions. Studies consistently demonstrate home phototherapy can be safe, effective, and appealing to patients. An at home phototherapy system can reduce the obstacles of time, expense, and travel, which may lead to better patient adherence and improved clinical outcomes.

DISCLOSURE

S. Feldman received research, speaking and/or consulting support from a variety of companies including Galderma, GSK/Stiefel, Almirall, Leo Pharma, Boehringer Ingelheim, Mylan, Celgene, Pfizer, Valeant, Abbvie, Samsung, Janssen, Lilly, Menlo, Merck, Novartis, Regeneron, Sanofi, Novan, Ourient, National Biological Corporation, Caremark, Advance Medical, Sun Pharma, Suncare Research, Informa, UpToDate, and National Psoriasis Foundation. He is founder and majority owner of www.DrScore.com and part owner of Causa Research, a company dedicated to enhancing patients' adherence to treatment. A. Cline, A. Pona, and J. Jacob have no conflicts of interest to disclose.

REFERENCES

1. Roelandts R. The history of phototherapy: something new under the sun? J Am Acad Dermatol 2002; 46(6):926–30.
2. Dogra S, Kanwar AJ. Narrow band UVB phototherapy in dermatology. Indian J Dermatol Venereol Leprol 2004;70(4):205–9.
3. Fitzpatrick TB, Pathak MA. Historical aspects of methoxsalen and other furocoumarins. J Invest Dermatol 1959;32(2, Part 2):229–31.
4. Parrish JA, Fitzpatrick TB, Tanenbaum L, et al. Photochemotherapy of psoriasis with oral methoxsalen and longwave ultraviolet light. N Engl J Med 1974; 291(23):1207–11.
5. Wiskemann A. UVB-phototherapy of psoriasis using a standing box developed for PUVA-therapy. Z Hautkr 1978;53(18):633–6 [in German].
6. van Weelden H, De La Faille HB, Young E, et al. A new development in UVB phototherapy of psoriasis. Br J Dermatol 1988;119(1):11–9.
7. Green C, Ferguson J, Lakshmipathi T, et al. 311 nm UVB phototherapy—an effective treatment for psoriasis. Br J Dermatol 1988;119(6):691–6.
8. Gupta R, Debbaneh M, Butler D, et al. The Goeckerman regimen for the treatment of moderate to severe psoriasis. J Vis Exp 2013;77:e50509.
9. Menter A, Korman NJ, Elmets CA, et al. Guidelines of care for the management of psoriasis and psoriatic arthritis: stion 5. Guidelines of care for the treatment of psoriasis with phototherapy and photochemotherapy. J Am Acad Dermatol 2010;62(1): 114–35.
10. Nolan BV, Yentzer BA, Feldman SR. A review of home phototherapy for psoriasis. Dermatol Online J 2010;16(2):1.
11. Foundation NP. Pros and cons of phototherapy. Available at: https://www.psoriasis.org/advance/pros-and-cons-phototherapy. Accessed December 2, 2018.
12. Yeung H, Wan J, Van Voorhees AS, et al. Patient-reported reasons for the discontinuation of commonly used treatments for moderate-to-severe psoriasis. J Am Acad Dermatol 2013;68(1):64–72.
13. Yelverton CB, Kulkarni AS, Balkrishnan R, et al. Home ultraviolet B phototherapy cost-effective option for severe psoriasis. Manag Care Interface 2006;19(1):33–6, 39.
14. Dothard EH, Sandoval LF, Yentzer BA, et al. Home ultraviolet light therapy for psoriasis: why patients choose other options. Dermatol Online J 2014; 21(2) [pii:13030/qt7943r72j].
15. Larko O, Swanbeck G. Home solarium treatment of psoriasis. Br J Dermatol 1979;101(1):13–6.
16. Jordan WP, Clarke AM, Hale RK. Long-term modified Goeckerman regimen for psoriasis using an ultraviolet B light source in the home. J Am Acad Dermatol 1981;4:584–91.
17. Koek MB, Buskens E, van Weelden H, et al. Home versus outpatient ultraviolet B phototherapy for mild to severe psoriasis: pragmatic multicentre randomised controlled non-inferiority trial (PLUTO study). BMJ 2009;338:b1542.
18. Lowe NJ. Home ultraviolet phototherapy. Semin Dermatol 1992;11(4):284–6.
19. Cameron H, Yule S, Moseley H, et al. Taking treatment to the patient: development of a home TL-01 ultraviolet B phototherapy service. Br J Dermatol 2002;147(5):957–65.
20. Eleftheriadou V, Thomas K, Ravenscroft J, et al. Feasibility, double-blind, randomized, placebo controlled, multi-center trial of hand held NB-UVB phototherapy for the treatment of vitiligo at home (HI-Light trial: Home Intervention of Light therapy). Trials 2014;15:51. Available at: https://www.ncbi.nlm.nih.gov/pmc/articles/PMC3923442/pdf/1745-6215-15-51.pdf.
21. Shan X, Wang C, Tian H, et al. Narrow-band ultraviolet B home phototherapy in vitiligo. Indian J Dermatol Venereol Leprol 2014;80(4):336–8.
22. Guan STT, Theng C, Chang A. Randomized, parallel group trial comparing home-based phototherapy with institution-based 308 excimer lamp for the treatment of focal vitiligo vulgaris. J Am

Acad Dermatol 2015;72(4):733–5. Available at: https://www.jaad.org/article/S0190-9622(14)02311-1/fulltext.

23. Van Coevorden AM, Kamphof WG, van Sonderen E, et al. Comparison of oral psoralen UV-A with a portable tanning unit at home vs hospital administered bath psoralen UV-A in patients with chronic hand eczema: an open label randomized controlled trial of efficacy. Arch Dermatol 2004;140(12):1463–6.

24. Kwon HH, Lee JB, Yoon JY, et al. The clinical and histological effect of home-use, combination blue-red LED phototherapy for mild to moderate acne vulgaris in Korean patients: a double-blind randomized controlled trial. Br J Dermatol 2013;68(5):1088–94.

25. Milstein HJ, Vonderheid EC, Van Scott EJ, et al. Home ultraviolet phototherapy of early mycosis fungoides: preliminary observations. J Am Acad Dermatol 1982;6:355–62.

26. Resnik KS, Vonderheid EC. Home UV phototherapy of early mycosis fungoides: long-term follow-up observations in thirty-one patients. J Am Acad Dermatol 1993;29:73–7.

27. Feldman SR, Clark A, Reboussin DM, et al. An assessment of potential problems of home phototherapy treatment of psoriasis. Cutis 1996;58(1):71–3.

28. Yentzer BA, Feldman SR. Trends in home phototherapy adoption in the US: monetary disincentives are only the tip of the iceberg. J Dermatolog Treat 2011;22(1):27–30.

29. Bhutani T, Liao W. A practical approach to home UVB phototherapy for the treatment of generalized psoriasis. Pract Dermatol 2010;7(2):31–5.

30. Foundation NP. Moderate to severe psoriasis. Home UVB equipment. Available at: https://www.psoriasis.org/about-psoriasis/treatments/phototherapy/uvb/home-equipment. Accessed December 3, 2018.

31. Carlin CS, Callis KP, Krueger G. Efficacy of Aciretin and commercial tanning bed therapy for psoriasis. Arch Dermatol 2003;139:436–42.

32. Fleischer AB, Clark AR, Rapp SR, et al. Commercial tanning bed treatment is an effective psoriasis treatment: results from an uncontrolled clinical trial. J Invest Dermatol 1997;109(2):170–4.

33. Koek MB, Sigurdsson V, van Weelden H, et al. Cost effectiveness of home ultraviolet B phototherapy for psoriasis: economic evaluation of a randomised controlled trial (PLUTO study). BMJ 2010;340:c1490.

34. Yelverton CB, Yentzer BA, Clark A, et al. Home narrowband UV-B phototherapy in combination with low-dose acitretin in patients with moderate to severe psoriasis. Arch Dermatol 2008;144(9):1224–5.

35. Sjovall P, Christensen OB. Treatment of chronic hand eczema with UV-B Handylux in the clinic and at home. Contact Dermatitis 1994;31(1):5–8.

36. Franken SM, Vierstra CL, Rustemeyer T. Improving access to home phototherapy for patients with psoriasis: current challenges and future prospects. Psoriasis (Auckl) 2016;6:55–64.

37. Su J, Pearce DJ, Feldman SR. The role of commercial tanning beds and ultraviolet A light in the treatment of psoriasis. J Dermatolog Treat 2009;16(5–6):324–6.

Phototherapy for Cutaneous T-Cell Lymphoma

Arthur Marka, BS[a], Joi B. Carter, MD[b,c],*

KEYWORDS

- Mycosis fungoides • Cutaneous T- cell lymphoma • Ultraviolet • Phototherapy • Narrowband UVB
- Psoralen and ultraviolet A • Psoralen

KEY POINTS

- Narrowband ultraviolet B radiation (NBUVB) and psoralen with ultraviolet A radiation (PUVA) are first-line treatments for mycosis fungoides (MF) stages IA, IB, and IIB.
- A phototherapy protocol for early stage MF includes an induction phase, a consolidation phase, and a maintenance phase with dosing based on skin phototype or minimal erythema dosing.
- Most studies comparing PUVA and NBUVB report a small but statistically significant difference in efficacy favoring PUVA; however, PUVA is associated with long-term photocarcinogenicity risk.
- PUVA is more effective than NBUVB for plaque disease and folliculotropic MF, although its advantage in skin of color remains theoretic.

INTRODUCTION

Cutaneous T-cell lymphoma (CTCL) encompasses a rare and clinicopathologically heterogenous group of neoplasms of skin-homing T-cells, which account for approximately 75% of all primary cutaneous lymphomas.[1] Several subtypes of CTCL have been described, but mycosis fungoides (MF) is the most common, representing more than half of all CTCL cases.[1] In general, the natural history of MF follows an indolent course, with an overall 5-year survival rate of 88%.[1] Classically, MF presents as erythematous scaly patches that gradually progress to plaques, tumors, and erythroderma over the course of months to decades, with the potential for extracutaneous progression. Given the protracted course of MF and the ease of access to the lymphoma in the skin, the initial treatment recommendations for early-stage disease include skin-directed therapies such as topical steroids, nitrogen mustard, and phototherapy.

Phototherapy, with psoralen and ultraviolet A radiation (PUVA) or narrowband ultraviolet B radiation (NBUVB), is considered among the first-line treatments for the early stages of MF. Initially developed as a treatment for psoriasis, PUVA was first used for MF in 1976 by Gilchrest and colleagues,[2] who demonstrated a treatment response in 9 patients, 4 of whom showed complete clearance. Broadband ultraviolet B (BB-UVB) was later reported as a treatment for MF in 1982 by Milstein and colleagues,[3] who demonstrated complete remission in 19 of 31 patients. The first report of NBUVB for MF followed in 1999 when Hofer and colleagues[4]

Disclosure Statement: The authors have nothing to disclose.
[a] Geisel School of Medicine at Dartmouth College, Box 163, Kellogg Building, 45 Dewey Field Road, Hanover, NH 03755, USA; [b] Geisel School of Medicine at Dartmouth College, Hanover, NH, USA; [c] Section of Dermatology, Department of Surgery, Dartmouth-Hitchcock Medical Center, Dartmouth-Hitchcock Heater Road, 18 Old Etna Road, Lebanon, NH 03766, USA
* Corresponding author. Dartmouth-Hitchcock Heater Road, 18 Old Etna Road, Lebanon, NH 03766.
E-mail address: Joi.B.Carter@Hitchcock.org

Dermatol Clin 38 (2020) 127–135
https://doi.org/10.1016/j.det.2019.08.013

showed complete remission in 19 of 21 patients, and NBUVB has now all but completely replaced BB-UVB.[5] Today, subtypes of cutaneous lymphoma remain the only malignant conditions for which UV-phototherapy is indicated.[6] This article provides an overview of the most recent, evolving research in UV-phototherapy for CTCL, with a focus on practical guidelines for the design and implementation of a phototherapy protocol for early stage MF.

PHOTOTHERAPY USE IN CUTANEOUS T-CELL LYMPHOMAS
Amenability by Cutaneous T-Cell Lymphoma Subtype

CTCL subtyping is currently based on the joint classification scheme defined by the World Health Organization (WHO) and the European Organization for Research and Treatment of Cancer (EORTC).[7] The latest WHO-EORTC scheme defines over 12 discrete forms of CTCL; however, UV-phototherapy is predominately used for MF, Sézary Syndrome (SS), and lymphomatoid papulosis (LyP). Its use is limited to adjuvant therapy in SS, where systemic modalities are considered the mainstays of treatment given the aggressive nature of the malignancy. In contrast, LyP, while displaying histologic features suggestive of malignancy and associated with the development of secondary lymphomas, is not clinically malignant in and of itself. However, given the itching, tenderness, and possible scarring associated with LyP, phototherapy is an option for symptomatic relief.[8] There are 2 MF subtypes, pagetoid reticulosis (PR) and granulomatous slack skin (GSS), which are exceedingly rare but have reported success with PUVA in case reports.[9–11] Given that most phototherapy use in cutaneous lymphomas is specific to MF, this article will focus on UV-phototherapy as it pertains to conventional MF and folliculotropic MF.

Amenability by Mycosis Fungoides Stage

Accurate staging of MF is critical, as it informs both clinical management and prognosis. Staging of MF is based on the TNMB (tumor-node-metastasis-blood) classification scheme, developed in 2007 as a consensus recommendation of the joint task force formed by the EORTC and the International Society for Cutaneous Lymphomas (ISCL).[12] Staging should include a total body skin examination with skin biopsy, complete blood count with quantification of peripheral blood involvement via flow cytometry or Sézary count, clinical lymph node examination with potential biopsy if lymphadenopathy is detected, and imaging studies if visceral involvement is suspected. Treatment selection for MF varies by stage of disease and is largely based on consensus recommendations.[13] These guidelines recommend phototherapy with PUVA and NBUVB as a first-line therapy only for stages IA, IB, and IIA, which feature variable body surface area affected by patches and plaques but no tumors or erythroderma. Given that most available data on UV-phototherapy for MF pertain to stage IA, IB, and IIA disease,[14] the remainder of this article will focus on these stages, hereinafter referred to as early stage MF.

PLANNING A PHOTOTHERAPY PROTOCOL FOR MYCOSIS FUNGOIDES
Treatment Phases and Response Criteria

Currently, the only possible cure for MF involves hematopoietic stem cell transplantation. Thus, the goal of all other MF treatments, including UV-phototherapy, is palliation and improvement in quality of life. A standard phototherapy protocol for MF can be broadly divided into 3 phases of treatment: induction, consolidation, and maintenance. The induction phase includes initial treatment and dose escalation, which is continued until there is complete clinical resolution of disease. The United States Cutaneous Lymphoma Consortium (USCLC) has made recommendations for the initial phototherapy dose and dose titration based on Fitzpatrick skin type (**Table 1**), as well as recommendations for dose adjustments after missed treatments (**Table 2**) during the induction phase.[14] Alternatively, some dermatologists may choose to use minimal erythema dose (MED) testing to guide phototherapy dosing, typically starting at 70% of MED and increasing by 20% with each subsequent treatment, or decreasing by 10% if a photoreaction occurs. Of note, MED-directed phototherapy is associated with a greater cumulative UVL dose for clearance compared with dosing based on skin phototype.[14] PUVA treatments for early stage MF are typically administered twice weekly, at least 48 hours apart, using a recommended dose of 0.6 mg/kg of 8-methoxypsoralen (8-MOP) administered 2 hours prior to UVA, or 0.5 mg/kg of Oxsoralen-Ultra (Valeant Pharmaceuticals, Bridgewater, New Jersey) administered 1 to 1.5 hours prior to UVA.[14] For NBUVB, the standard induction treatment frequency is 3 treatments per week; however, twice weekly treatments may be sufficiently effective, albeit slower, if cost and

Table 1
Recommendations for induction phase phototherapy dosing in early stage mycosis fungoides based on skin phototype

Skin Phototype	NBUVB		PUVA	
	Initial dose (mJ/cm²)	Increments (mJ/cm²)	Initial dose (J/cm²)	Increments (J/cm²)
I	130	15	0.5	0.5
II	220	25	1.0	0.5
III	260	40	1.5	1.0
IV	330	45	2.0	1.0
V	350	60	2.5	1.5
VI	400	65	3.0	1.5

If no response is seen after 20 treatments, exposure may be increased relative to the prior increment by an additional 50 to 100 J/cm² for NBUVB or by 0.5 to 1.0 J/cm² for PUVA, if tolerated.
Data from Refs.[14,50,51]

transportation are prohibitive. The induction phase continues until the patient has a complete response (CR). It is important to note that there has been significant variation in the definitions of treatment response and relapse in the literature on UV-phototherapy for MF. To address this, a joint task force published a statement in 2011, which provided consensus definitions for these clinical endpoints.[15] Whereas many prior studies had defined CR as greater than 90% to 95% clearance, the consensus group presented a more stringent definition of 100% clearance of skin lesions persisting for a minimum of 4 weeks (**Fig. 1**). In addition, partial response was defined as 50% to 99% clearance over the same minimum duration, and relapse was defined as any disease recurrence following complete resolution. Of note, these consensus guidelines state that biopsy of normal-appearing skin is

unnecessary for the assessment of CR but may be useful if there is a question of residual disease in a patient otherwise displaying CR.

After induction, the consolidation phase that follows is a period in which the dose and frequency of phototherapy are held constant, typically lasting from 1 to 3 months. The maintenance phase then involves a gradual decrease in the frequency of treatments before eventual discontinuation of UV-phototherapy, with the intention of extending the relapse-free interval (RFI). As will be discussed in a later section, the utility of the maintenance phase is debated, and regimens are highly variable, with some opting for no maintenance, while others continue for years. The dose of UVL during maintenance is initially held constant from the preceding consolidation phase, and treatment frequency is decreased in a stepwise fashion, typically once every 1 to 2 months. A widely used tapering schedule involves the reduction of treatment frequency from 3 times per week, to twice weekly, to weekly, to every 10 days, to twice monthly, and finally to every 3 weeks if tolerated. For patients treated with PUVA, maintenance treatment frequency may be further decreased to as low as once monthly. For NBUVB, the USCLC recommends decreasing the phototherapy dose by 25% relative to the end of the consolidation phase when twice-monthly treatments are initiated and then by 50% when the treatment frequency is reduced to every 3 weeks, if tolerated (**Table 3**).[14]

Light Source Selection

The selection of light source in MF is based predominately on primary lesions (patch vs plaque), follicular involvement, and availability. Although EORTC-CLTF guidelines recommend either NBUVB or PUVA as first-line therapy for early

Table 2
Recommendations for resumption of induction phase phototherapy in early-stage mycosis fungoides after missing a scheduled treatment session

Time Between Treatments	NBUVB	PUVA
4–7 d	Dose the same	Dose the same
8–14 d	Decrease by 25%	Decrease by 25%
15–21 d	Decrease by 50%	Decrease by 50%
22–28 d	Start over	Decrease by 75%
>4 wk	Start over	Start over

Data from Refs.[14,50,51]

A   B

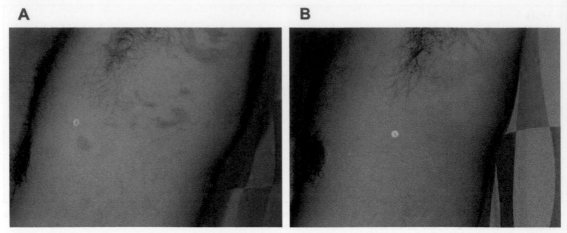

Fig. 1. Axillary mycosis fungoides patches before (*A*) and after (*B*) narrowband-UVB phototherapy in a man with early stage disease who achieved a complete response.

stage MF, they also note that NBUVB is favored in patients with T1a and T2a disease, which is limited to patches, whereas PUVA is preferred for patients with plaque disease (T1b, T2b),[13] in whom the relatively deeper dermal penetration of UVA is advantageous. In general, PUVA is also preferred in the folliculotropic variant of MF for this same reason, and evidence for its superiority relative to NBUVB in this context has been demonstrated.[16] It has also been shown that dermatologists have a clear preference for PUVA for the treatment of MF in skin of color.[17] However, there have thus far been no definitive data showing an effect of Fitzpatrick skin type on the efficacy of phototherapy modality.[14] To assess the relative efficacy of UV-phototherapy modalities, Phan and colleagues[18] conducted a meta-analysis of studies that directly compared PUVA versus NBUVB for early stage MF that included 778 patients. The results showed that 90.9% (479/527) of PUVA-treated patients

showed any response to treatment, compared with 87.6% (220/251) of patients who were treated with NBUVB, a difference that was not statistically significant (odds ratio [OR], 1.40; 95% confidence interval [CI], 0.84–2.34; *P*=.20). However, the rate of CR was found to be significantly greater in patients who received PUVA, of whom 73.8% (389/527) achieved CR, versus those who received NBUVB, of whom 62.2% (156/251) achieved CR (OR, 1.68; 95% CI, 1.02–2.76; *P*=.04). With respect to the relative cost of treatment, PUVA is nearly twice as expensive as NBUVB ($10,582 vs $5604); however, patients may be reassured that, in general, UV-phototherapy has been shown to be the most cost-effective option for generalized disease.[19]

Efficacy of Narrowband Ultraviolet B

Over 95% of patients in studies of NBUVB monotherapy for the treatment of MF have had stage IA

Table 3
Recommendations for maintenance phase phototherapy dosing in early stage mycosis fungoides

Treatment Frequency	NBUVB		PUVA	
	Weeks	Dose relative to end consolidation	Weeks	Dose relative to end consolidation
Twice weekly	4–8	Same	4–8	Same
Weekly	4–8	Same	4–8	Same
Every 10 d	4–8	Same	4–8	Same
Every 2 weeks	4–8	Decrease by 25%	4–8	Same
Every 3 weeks	NA	Decrease by 50%	4–8	Same
Every 4 weeks	NA	NA	4–8	Same

Abbreviation: NA, not applicable.
Data from Refs.[14,50,51]

or IB disease, with the remainder having primarily stage IIA disease. Among these studies, treatment was generally continued until the observation of a plateau in response or CR, which has ranged from 1.5 months to 14 months.[14] CR in these studies has generally been defined as greater than 90% to 95% clearance, which is in contradistinction to the aforementioned consensus recommendation of 100% clearance. The overall response rates for NBUVB range from 54% to 91%, with a mean rate of 77%.[14] Early stage MF stage is associated with excellent CR rates, which have ranged from 42% to 82% among stage IA patients and between 67% to 84% in those with stage IB disease.[14] Among patients with patch disease receiving NBUVB, CR rates tend to be higher (92%–100%) when compared with CR rates in plaque disease (60% to 83%).[14]

Efficacy of Psoralen and Ultraviolet A

There is greater variability in reported CR rates between studies of PUVA for the treatment of MF than there is between NBUVB studies. Although the literature for both modalities is marked by a wide degree of heterogeneity in quality, sample size, patient selection, and the definition of outcome measures, summative interpretation of the PUVA literature is further complicated by substantial differences between treatment protocols, inconsistency of weight-based psoralen dosage adjustment, and the use of 5-methoxypsoralen in some European studies. As such, clinical responses in studies of PUVA-treated early stage MF have ranged from no complete remission to 100% CR rate.[14] The effect of stage on response to PUVA varies by study. In a large series on PUVA for early stage MF, in which 49 of 68 patients achieved clinical and histopathologic CR, Herrmann and colleagues[20] showed that the time to response is typically 2 to 3 months, independent of stage; however, the CR rates were higher in stage IA compared with stage IB (79% vs 59%). Nikolaou and colleagues[21] found both stage of disease (89.9% CR IA vs 63.9% CR IB, $P<.001$) and clinical presentation (91.3% CR patch vs 70.6% CR plaque, $P<.003$) to be predictive of a CR to PUVA. It is clear that a subset of patients with early stage MF requires extended treatment with PUVA to achieve CR, likely attributable to the presence of thicker, more infiltrated plaques.[21]

Efficacy of Bath Psoralen and Ultraviolet A

If locally available, bath PUVA is another option for phototherapy that avoids the systemic adverse effects of psoralen. A recent study demonstrated excellent clearance rates for early stage MF in 158 patients treated with bath PUVA.[22] Their protocol included bath PUVA twice per week until remission, followed by a taper over 7 months. Their CR rate was 88.6%, with an RFI of 43.3 months.

Role of Maintenance Therapy

The role of maintenance therapy after the consolidation phase of UV-phototherapy is debated, and this is complicated by the relative scarcity of available data.[14] Moreover, the duration of follow-up and definition of RFI are not consistent across studies, and most studies do not explicitly use the strict definition of relapse that was established by expert consensus for clinical trials.

In studies of NBUVB for early-stage MF, relapse rates among patients who did not receive maintenance therapy have ranged from 29% to 100%, with mean RFI ranging from 5.9 to 14.5 months, whereas relapse rates among those who did receive maintenance therapy ranged from 4% to 83%, with mean RFI ranging from 3 to 26 months.[14] Conflicting evidence was presented by Elcin and colleagues,[23] who examined the effect of maintenance therapy duration on relapse rate and RFI in early stage MF patients treated with NBUVB. The study compared 15 patients who underwent a short maintenance phase of less than 12 months with 16 patients who underwent maintenance for more than 12 months, although the mean maintenance phase duration for each group was not provided. The results showed that the short maintenance group had a lower rate of relapse (33% vs 37%) and a greater median RFI (42 months vs 39 months); however, these results were not statistically significant. Moreover, this study defined CR as greater than 95% clearing of skin lesions, whereas among the studies of NBUVB that have defined CR as 100% clearance, maintenance phototherapy is associated with decreased relapse rate and increased RFI.[14] A follow-up study by Pavlotsky and colleagues[24] demonstrated 80% CR to NBUVB in stage I MF, and 60% of patients remained disease-free for 5 years without prolonged maintenance therapy. It was recommended that all patients proceed with maintenance taper from twice weekly for 4 weeks, to once weekly for 4 weeks, and then every other week for a duration of 3 to 6 months. The authors did not comment on the number of patients able to complete this taper, and as such it remains uncertain if this was a factor in their long-term remission.

The research on maintenance after PUVA is similarly conflicting. In a study of 24 patients with stage IA or IIA MF who did not receive maintenance phototherapy after achieving CR with PUVA, Ahmad and colleagues[25] found that 100% patients relapsed after a median RFI of 15 months. On the other hand, Hönigsmann and colleagues[26] showed that, among 35 patients with stage IA or IB disease, 42% achieved a mean RFI of 4 years after only a 2-month maintenance phase, suggesting that sustained remission is possible without prolonged maintenance. However, Wackernagel and colleagues[27] found that in early stage MF, both relapse rate and time to relapse did not differ significantly between 25 patients without maintenance therapy after CR and 9 patients who received 15 maintenance-phase treatments. Although the utility of short-term PUVA maintenance is uncertain, the evidence for prolonged RFI with more long-term maintenance treatment is more robust. For example, in a study of 66 patients with early stage MF who achieved CR with PUVA and were on continuous maintenance therapy, Querfeld and colleagues[28] showed that half relapsed after a median RFI of 39 months, while the other half had sustained remission for a median duration of 7 years. A recent prospective, randomized clinical trial by Vieyra-Garcia and colleagues[29] randomized 19 early stage MF patients who had achieved CR to either no maintenance or a 9-month PUVA maintenance phase. They demonstrated a significant prolongation of the median RFI from 4 months to 15 months ($P=.02$) with the use of maintenance therapy.

Although maintenance phototherapy may extend remission in early stage MF, this must be weighed against the risk of adverse effects from chronic phototherapy and the psychological, financial, and time cost to the patient. On the other hand, all of these risks and expenses would be amplified in the event of a relapse, which would require restarting therapy at induction-phase frequency. It is important to note that the prolongation of the RFI seen with long-term maintenance is not correlated with an increase in overall survival, but it is reassuring that patients with stage IA disease are highly likely to achieve CR even after relapse.[30]

PHOTOCARCINOGENICITY

It is well-established that high cumulative doses of PUVA are associated with the development of nonmelanoma skin cancer (NMSC), especially cutaneous squamous cell carcinoma (cSCC).[31–33] One meta-analysis of PUVA for psoriasis found a 14-fold increase in incidence of cSCC in patients who had received high-dose PUVA (>200 treatments or >2000 J/cm^2) relative to those who had received low-dose PUVA (<100 treatments or

<1000 J/cm^2).[34] Moreover, studies of psoriasis patients treated with PUVA have also demonstrated that the male genitalia is particularly susceptible to the development of cSCC in this context.[34] Thus it is recommended that this area be covered during PUVA treatment unless it has an MF lesion that is recalcitrant to alternative therapy. Similarly, it is generally acceptable to shield the face during phototherapy for early stage disease if it is uninvolved.[14] Whether there is an increased risk of developing melanoma with PUVA exposure remains a topic of controversy. Although many studies in the psoriasis literature have failed to show an increased risk of melanoma after PUVA,[35–37] 1 study did demonstrate a nearly tenfold increase in the incidence of invasive melanoma after a 15-year latency period in a cohort of psoriasis patients receiving high-dose PUVA (>250 treatments).[38]

In contrast to PUVA, there does not appear to be an increased risk of developing NMSC after NBUVB.[39,40] It has been shown that there is an increase in p53 mutations exhibiting a UVB signature in tumor-stage MF relative to plaque MF, suggesting that UVB-induced DNA damage may contribute to disease progression in MF.[41] However, in a retrospective study of 43 patients with stage IA or IB MF who progressed to tumor stage, Hoot and colleagues[42] showed that the 30 patients who received UV-phototherapy had a significantly longer median time to tumor progression than the 13 patients who had not received treatment (3.5 years vs 1.2 years; $P=.001$), as well as greater median overall survival (6.9 years vs 3.8 years; $P=.001$). It is important to note that this study included all forms of UV-phototherapy (PUVA, NBUVB, and sunlight). Thus, based on these limited data, it appears that the therapeutic benefit of UV-phototherapy in early stage MF outweighs the theoretic concern for UVB-induced p53 mutagenesis; however, further studies are indicated to explore this concern.

UNIQUE USES OF PHOTOTHERAPY IN MYCOSIS FUNGOIDES
Maintenance Therapy After Total Skin Electron Beam Therapy

Total skin electron beam therapy (TSEBT) is currently recommended as a second-line treatment for early stage MF (mainly stage T2b) and as first-line therapy for patients with stage IIB, IIIA, and IIIB MF.[13] Quirós and colleagues[43] investigated the use of PUVA as a maintenance phase therapy in 114 patients with T1 or T2 disease who had achieved CR after being treated with TSEBT at a total dose of 36 Gy. A slow, tapering course of adjuvant PUVA was initiated by 14 of these patients, while the other 100 patients received alternative adjuvant therapy or no further treatment. The 5-year overall survival rates were 100% for the PUVA group and 82% for the non-PUVA group, but this difference did not reach statistical significance (*P*<.10). However, there was a significant difference in disease-free interval at 5 years, which was observed in 85% for those who received PUVA after TSEBT, versus just 50% for those who had received alternative therapy or no additional treatment (*P*<.02). There were several important limitations in this study, including incomplete staging information, lack of randomization, and the fact that not all patients had achieved CR at the time of initiation of adjuvant therapy.

Combination Therapies

Combination treatments are often used to improve efficacy and potentially prolong remission in early stage MF cases wherein an inadequate response to PUVA has been demonstrated or is expected, such as in patients with thick, infiltrated plaques or those with folliculotropic disease. Combining PUVA with systemic therapy may allow for a reduction in cumulative PUVA dose and may therefore reduce PUVA-associated adverse effects. The agents most commonly used in combination with PUVA for MF are retinoids and interferon-alfa,[14] which may provide a degree of intrinsic suppression of NMSC beyond what is conferred by the relative reduction in PUVA dose needed to achieve CR.[44–46] A multimodality approach combining PUVA with extracorporeal photophoresis (ECP) and various biologic agents has also been reported for the treatment of erythrodermic disease, but the literature on this is sparse.[14] In contrast to PUVA, the available data on the combination of NBUVB with other modalities are minimal, although case reports have demonstrated an enhanced effect of NBUVB in combination with bexarotene, a retinoid X receptor-selective retinoid.[47,48] Methotrexate has also been used with both NBUVB and PUVA, but this combination is not recommended given the possibility of a rare radiation recall reaction, and, more importantly, the increased photocarcinogenesis that has been associated with this combination.[49] Finally, an important use of combination therapy in MF is for the treatment of sanctuary sites, which may be treated with localized radiation, topical nitrogen mustard, or topical steroids.

SUMMARY

In summary, phototherapy with NBUVB or PUVA for treatment of MF has been in use for over 40 years and is a first-line treatment option for early-stage MF. Patients with plaque MF or folliculotropic MF benefit from PUVA therapy over NBUVB. Although not curative, phototherapy with either modality results in CR in most patients, and sustained remission is possible with maintenance therapy. However, the most effective maintenance therapy protocol remains unknown. Several factors should be considered when designing a phototherapy protocol, including treatment availability, MF subtype, stage of disease, adverse effects, and patient preference, including impact of treatment on quality of life.

REFERENCES

1. Willemze R. Cutaneous T-Cell lymphoma. In: Bolognia JL, Schaffer JV, Cerroni L, editors. Dermatology. 4th edition. Philadelphia, PA: Elsevier Limited; 2018. p. 2127–47.
2. Gilchrest BA, Parrish JA, Tanenbaum L, et al. Oral methoxsalen photochemotherapy of mycosis fungoides. Cancer 1976;38:683–9.
3. Milstein HJ, Vonderheid EC, Van Scott EJ, et al. Home ultraviolet phototherapy of early mycosis fungoides: preliminary observations. J Am Acad Dermatol 1982;6:355–62.
4. Hofer A, Cerroni L, Kerl H, et al. Narrowband (311-nm) UV-B therapy for small plaque parapsoriasis and early-stage mycosis fungoides. Arch Dermatol 1999;135:1377–80.
5. Hönigsmann H. Phototherapy. In: Milestones in investigative dermatology: photobiology/photomedicine. J Invest Dermato 2013;133(1):18–20.
6. Herzinger T, Berneburg M, Ghoreschi K, et al. S1-Guidelines on UV phototherapy and photochemotherapy. J Dtsch Dermatol Ges 2016;14(8):853–76.
7. Willemze R, Cerroni L, Kempf W, et al. The 2018 update of the WHO-EORTC classification for primary cutaneous lymphomas. Blood 2019;133(16):1703–14.
8. Fernández-de-Misa R, Hernández-Machín B, Servitje O, et al. First-line treatment in lymphomatoid papulosis: a retrospective multicentre study. Clin Exp Dermatol 2018;43(2):137–43.
9. Puno MIBL, Dimagiba MTE, Jamora MJJ, et al. Granulomatous slack skin presenting as diffuse poikiloderma and necrotic ulcers, with features of granulomatous vasculitis and response to oral prednisone, acitretin, and oral psoralen plus ultraviolet light therapy-a case report. JAAD Case Rep 2017;3(4):294–300.
10. Lichte V, Ghoreschi K, Metzler G, et al. Pagetoid reticulosis (Woringer-Kolopp disease). J Dtsch Dermatol Ges 2009;7(4):353–4.
11. Lee J, Viakhireva N, Cesca C, et al. Clinicopathologic features and treatment outcomes in Woringer-

Kolopp disease. J Am Acad Dermatol 2008;59(4):
706–12.

12. Olsen E, Vonderheid E, Pimpinelli N, et al. Revisions
to the staging and classification of mycosis fungoides and Sézary syndrome: a proposal of the International Society for Cutaneous Lymphomas
(ISCL) and the cutaneous lymphoma task force of
the European Organization of Research and Treatment of Cancer (EORTC). Blood 2007;110(6):
1713–22.

13. National Comprehensive Cancer Network. Guidelines
for primary cutaneous lymphomas (Version 1.2019).
Available at: https://www.nccn.org/professionals/
physician_gls/pdf/primary_cutaneous.pdf. Accessed
April 29, 2019.

14. Olsen EA, Hodak E, Anderson T, et al. Guidelines for
phototherapy of mycosis fungoides and Sézary syndrome: A consensus statement of the United States
Cutaneous Lymphoma Consortium. J Am Acad Dermatol 2016;74(1):27–58.

15. Olsen EA, Whittaker S, Kim YH, et al. Clinical end
points and response criteria in mycosis fungoides
and Sézary syndrome: a consensus statement of
the International Society for Cutaneous Lymphomas,
the United States Cutaneous Lymphoma Consortium, and the Cutaneous Lymphoma Task Force
of the European Organisation for Research and
Treatment of Cancer. J Clin Oncol 2011;29(18):
2598–607.

16. Gerami P, Rosen S, Kuzel T, et al. Folliculotropic
mycosis fungoides: an aggressive variant of cutaneous T-cell lymphoma. Arch Dermatol 2008;
144(6):738–46.

17. Carter J, Zug KA. Phototherapy for cutaneous T-cell
lymphoma: online survey and literature review. J Am
Acad Dermatol 2009;60(1):39–50.

18. Phan K, Ramachandran V, Fassihi H, et al. Comparison of narrowband UV-B with psoralen-UV-A phototherapy for patients with early-stage mycosis
fungoides: a systematic review and meta-analysis.
JAMA Dermatol 2019;155(3):335–41.

19. Xia FD, Ferket BS, Huang V, et al. Local radiation
and phototherapy are the most cost-effective treatments for stage IA mycosis fungoides: a comparative decision analysis model in the United States.
J Am Acad Dermatol 2019;80(2):485–92.

20. Herrmann JJ, Roenigk HH Jr, Hurria A, et al. Treatment of mycosis fungoides with photochemotherapy
(PUVA): longterm follow-up. J Am Acad Dermatol
1995;33(2):234–42.

21. Nikolaou V, Sachlas A, Papadavid E, et al. Phototherapy as a first-line treatment for early-stage mycosis
fungoides: the results of a large retrospective analysis. Photodermatol Photoimmunol Photomed
2018;34(5):307–13.

22. Archier E, Devaux S, Castela E, et al. Carcinogenic
risks of psoralen UV-A therapy and narrowband

UV-B therapy in chronic plaque psoriasis: a systematic literature review. J Eur Acad Dermatol Venereol
2012;26(3):22–31.

23. Elcin G, Duman N, Karahan S, et al. Long-term
follow-up of early mycosis fungoides patients
treated with narrowband ultraviolet B phototherapy.
J Dermatolog Treat 2014;25(3):268–73.

24. Pavlotsky F, Dawood M, Barzilai A. The potential of
narrow band UVB to induce sustained durable complete remission off-therapy in stage I mycosis fungoides. J Am Acad Dermatol 2019;80(6):1550–5.

25. Ahmad K, Rogers S, McNicholas PD, et al.
Narrowband UVB and PUVA in the treatment of
mycosis fungoides: a retrospective study. Acta
Derm Venereol 2007;87:413–7.

26. Hönigsmann H, Brenner W, Rauschmeier W, et al.
Photochemotherapy for cutaneous T cell lymphoma. A follow-up study. J Am Acad Dermatol 1984;
10(2):238–45.

27. Wackernagel A, Hofer A, Legat F, et al. Efficacy of 8-
methoxypsoralen vs. 5-methoxypsoralen plus ultraviolet A therapy in patients with mycosis fungoides.
Br J Dermatol 2006;154:519–23.

28. Querfeld C, Rosen ST, Kuzel TM, et al. Long-term
follow-up of patients with early-stage cutaneous
T-cell lymphoma who achieved complete remission
with psoralen plus UV-A monotherapy. Arch Dermatol 2005;141:305–11.

29. Vieyra-Garcia P, Fink-Puches R, Porkert S, et al. Evaluation of low-dose, low-frequency oral psoralen-UV-A
treatment with or without maintenance on early-stage
mycosis fungoides: a randomized clinical trial. JAMA
Dermatol 2019;155(5):538–47.

30. Quaglino P, Pimpinelli N, Berti E, et al. Time course,
clinical pathways, and long-term hazards risk trends
of disease progression in patients with classic
mycosis fungoides. Cancer 2012;118(23):5830–9.

31. Stern RS, Thibodeau LA, Kleinerman RA, et al. Risk
of cutaneous carcinoma in patients treated with oral
methoxsalen photochemotherapy for psoriasis.
N Engl J Med 1979;300:809–13.

32. Stern RS, Laird N, Melski J, et al. Cutaneous
squamous-cell carcinoma in patients treated with
PUVA. N Engl J Med 1984;310:1156–61.

33. Nijsten TE, Stern RS. The increased risk of skin cancer is
persistent after discontinuation of psoralen1ultraviolet
A: a cohort study. J Invest Dermatol 2003;121:252–8.

34. Stern RS, Lunder EJ. Risk of squamous cell carcinoma and methoxsalen (psoralen) and UV-A radiation (PUVA). A meta-analysis. Arch Dermatol 1998;
134:1582–5.

35. Morison WL, Baughman RD, Day RM, et al.
Consensus workshop on the toxic effects of long-
term PUVA therapy. Arch Dermatol 1998;134:595–8.

36. Lindelof B. Risk of melanoma with psoralen/ultravio-
let A therapy for psoriasis. Do the known risks now
outweigh the benefits? Drug Saf 1999;20:289–97.

37. Chuang TY, Heinrich LA, Schultz MD, et al. PUVA and skin cancer. A historical cohort study on 492 patients. J Am Acad Dermatol 1992;26(2):173–7.

38. Stern RS, Nichols KT, Vakeva LH. Malignant melanoma inpatients treated for psoriasis with methoxsalen (psoralen) and ultraviolet A radiation (PUVA). The PUVA follow-up study. N Engl J Med 1997;336: 1041–5.

39. Lee E, Koo J, Berger T. UVB phototherapy and skin cancer risk: a review of the literature. Int J Dermatol 2005;44:355–60.

40. Hearn RM, Kerr AC, Rahim KF, et al. Incidence of skin cancers in 3867 patients treated with narrowband ultraviolet B phototherapy. Br J Dermatol 2008;159:931–5.

41. McGregor JM, Crook T, Fraser-Andrews EA, et al. Spectrum of p53 gene mutations suggests a possible role for ultraviolet radiation in the pathogenesis of advanced cutaneous lymphomas. J Invest Dermatol 1999;112:317–21.

42. Hoot JW, Wang L, Kho T, et al. The effect of phototherapy on progression to tumors in patients with patch and plaque stage of mycosis fungoides. J Dermatolog Treat 2018;29(3):272–6.

43. Quirós PA, Jones GW, Kacinski BM, et al. Total skin electron beam therapy followed by adjuvant psoralen/ultraviolet-A light in the management of patients with T1 and T2 cutaneous T-cell lymphoma (mycosis fungoides). Int J Radiat Oncol Biol Phys 1997;38:1027–35.

44. Bavinck JN, Tieben LM, Van der Woude FJ, et al. Prevention of skin cancer and reduction of keratotic skin lesions during acitretin therapy in renal transplant recipients: a double-blind, placebo-controlled study. J Clin Oncol 1995;13: 1933–8.

45. Stern RS. Oral retinoid use reduces cutaneous squamous cell carcinoma risk in patients with psoriasis treated with psoralen-UVA: a nested cohort study. J Am Acad Dermatol 2003;49:644–50.

46. Rodríguez-Villanueva J, McDonnell TJ. Induction of apoptotic cell death in non-melanoma skin cancer by interferon-alpha. Int J Cancer 1995;61(1):110–4.

47. Lokitz ML, Wong HK. Bexarotene and narrowband ultraviolet B phototherapy combination treatment for mycosis fungoides. Photodermatol Photoimmunol Photomed 2007;23:255–7.

48. D'Acunto C, Gurioli C, Neri I. Plaque stage mycosis fungoides treated with bexarotene at low dosage and UVB-NB. J Dermatolog Treat 2010;21:45–8.

49. MacKie RM, Fitzsimons CP. Risk of carcinogenicity in patients with psoriasis treated with methotrexate or PUVA singly or in combination. J Am Acad Dermatol 1983;9:467–9.

50. Zanolli MD, Feldman SR, Clark AR, et al. Phototherapy treatment protocols for psoriasis and other phototherapy responsive dermatoses. 2nd edition. Boca Raton (FL): CRC Press; 2000.

51. Menter A, Korman NJ, Elmets CA, et al. Guidelines of care for the management of psoriasis and psoriatic arthritis: section 5. Guidelines of care for the treatment of psoriasis with phototherapy and photochemotherapy. J Am Acad Dermatol 2010;62:114–35.

Creating and Managing a Phototherapy Center

Zizi Yu, BA[a], Kathie P. Huang, MD[b], Elizabeth A. Buzney, MD[b],*

KEYWORDS

• Phototherapy center • Photomedicine • Psoriasis • Management • Operations

KEY POINTS

• Phototherapy is a safe and effective treatment for many dermatoses, but its availability is limited by the lack of geographically convenient phototherapy centers.

• Creating and managing a phototherapy center requires careful consideration of physical setup, finances, operations and personnel, patient education and consent, and patient safety and troubleshooting.

• The modalities of phototherapy offered should depend on patient population served, but 1 recommended model is to start with full-body narrowband UVB (NBUVB), then consider adding excimer laser and hand/foot NBUVB, followed by UVA for UVA with psoralen, UVA-1, and last, broadband UVB.

INTRODUCTION

Phototherapy is a safe and effective treatment for a wide variety of cutaneous diseases, including psoriasis, vitiligo, atopic dermatitis, contact dermatitis, cutaneous T-cell lymphoma (CTCL), chronic pruritus, mastocytosis, and polymorphous light eruption. It is particularly useful for patients who fail topical therapy but who may not be candidates for biologic agents or other systemic therapies. Currently, irradiation with narrowband UVB (NBUVB) (311–313 nm), UVA with psoralen (PUVA), broadband UVB (290–320 nm), 308-nm excimer laser, and UVA-1 (340–400 nm) is used for therapeutic purposes.[1] UVB radiation primarily affects the epidermis and superficial dermis and is the preferred phototherapy modality for treatment of psoriasis, whereas UVA radiation can penetrate the mid and deep dermal components and may be more effective for thicker plaques and nodular lesions, for example, for CTCL or hand-foot dermatitis.[1,2] Excimer laser is a targeted 308-nm UVB radiation system consisting of a noble gas and halide, used to treat more focused areas of severe or recalcitrant disease.[3]

Although protocols may differ according to treatment indication, disease severity, and type of phototherapy prescribed, most regimens require a commitment of 2 to 3 weekly treatments often extending over the course of several months. One of the biggest barriers to accessing phototherapy is the lack of phototherapy center locations across the country. A recent study showed that although there is at least 1 phototherapy center in 46 of the 50 states, most centers are concentrated along the East and West Coasts and in the Midwest region east of the Mississippi River.[4] About 19 million people live in the 89% of all counties in the United States that lack a phototherapy center.[4] Thus, there is a crucial need to expand access to phototherapy across the United States. This review serves as a general guide to

Disclosure Statement: Dr K.P. Huang has received royalty payments from Pfizer for licensing ALTO and consulting fees from Pfizer. She has also participated in clinical trials related to alopecia from Incyte, Aclaris, Concert, and Lily. The other authors have nothing to disclose.
[a] Harvard Medical School, 25 Shattuck Street, Boston, MA 02115, USA; [b] Department of Dermatology, Brigham and Women's Hospital, 221 Longwood Avenue, Boston, MA 02115, USA
* Corresponding author.
E-mail address: EBuzney@BICS.BWH.harvard.edu

Dermatol Clin 38 (2020) 137–143
https://doi.org/10.1016/j.det.2019.08.014
0733-8635/20/© 2019 Elsevier Inc. All rights reserved.

creating and managing a phototherapy center, acknowledging that specific limitations and considerations will differ by practice setting, geographic location, and the patient population served. The major components to consider in creating and managing a phototherapy center are outlined, including physical setup of the center, financial considerations, the operational details and personnel needed to run the center, the patient education and consent process, and issues surrounding patient safety and troubleshooting (**Fig. 1**).

PHYSICAL SETUP

The first thing to consider when starting a new phototherapy center is the physical space: the location of the space, the amount of space necessary, and the layout or setup of the space. The importance of the design and layout of the phototherapy center cannot be understated. In one study of health care environments, visibility, accessibility, and layout design were the most cited aspects of health care facility design to enhance teamwork and communication for the delivery of safe and effective patient care.[5] Phototherapy centers can be stand-alone spaces, or they can be located within or in conjunction with a hospital or academic practice for ease of physician and/or dermatologist access and follow-up. In fact, a study has shown that the limited access to phototherapy centers nationwide is not an isolated pattern and that it parallels the geographic concentration of dermatology providers in urban areas.[4] Regardless of physical proximity to dermatology providers, it is important to place the phototherapy center in a location that is easily accessible with adequate parking for patient convenience.

Importantly, there is evidence that for some patients, process-related attributes of treatment, such as treatment location, frequency, duration, delivery method, and cost, can outweigh the risks of adverse events related to treatment.[6] In a study to assess psoriasis treatment preferences and to identify the effect of demographic and socioeconomic characteristics on these preferences, researchers found that the most highly valued quality was treatment location, followed by probability of treatment benefit and method of treatment delivery.[6] In the patients studied, all process attributes were rated higher in relative importance than adverse effect–related attributes, such as probability, severity, and reversibility of adverse effects. These results suggest that patients with psoriasis may be willing to accept treatment-related adverse effects and other tradeoffs in favor of the convenience of a treatment compatible with their personal and professional lives.[6] When selecting between treatment options, patients may thus be more willing to accept a systemic treatment with greater risk of side effects that they can take at home rather than drive to an inconveniently located phototherapy center multiple times a week. This underscores the importance of designing phototherapy centers with patient convenience in mind, in order to increase utilization and adherence to this safe and effective treatment option.

The amount and layout of the space in a phototherapy center will depend heavily on the patient population treated. Although the general setup of a phototherapy center should likely include a waiting room, check-in area, and lockers and/or cubbies for patients to keep their personal belongings, the space allocated for a certain number and type of phototherapy machines may be more fluid. The decision about which phototherapy modalities to offer and how many of each machine to purchase should be driven by the patient population served, namely the cutaneous conditions most commonly treated, the patient volume expected

1 Consider the physical space.

The location, size, layout, and setup of the phototherapy center should be determined with the patient population and their needs and convenience in mind.

2 Anticipate the finances.

Be aware of issues around billing, insurance, and reimbursement. Anticipate the various costs associated with establishing and running the phototherapy center.

3 Lay the operational groundwork.

Set the hours of operation for the center and hire and train personnel accordingly. Establish protocols for treatment modalities and possible adverse events.

4 Establish a consent & education process.

Create treatment-specific information packets and consent forms to educate patients. Consider holding in-person patient orientations prior to beginning treatment.

Fig. 1. Steps to creating a phototherapy center. The steps to establishing a new phototherapy center include consideration of the physical space, anticipating finances, laying the operational groundwork, and establishing a patient consent and education process.

(which may depend on the number of patients in a practice, local availability of phototherapy, and referral base), as well as financial considerations, such as insurance coverage and reimbursement for various types of phototherapy.

Because full-body NBUVB is the most versatile and forgiving modality, it is a reasonable first device to purchase. Excimer laser and hand/foot NBUVB can later be added to address more focused areas. Last, more specialized choices can be added, such as UVA (for systemic, hand/foot, and topical/bath PUVA), then UVA-1, followed by broadband UVB (**Fig. 2**). As 1 example, the authors' phototherapy center at Brigham and Women's Hospital has 2 NBUVB booths, 1 UVA and NBUVB hand/foot booth, and 1 excimer laser, and 1 UVA/NBUVB combination booth. The most frequently treated diagnoses in their center are psoriasis (49%), eczema (18%), vitiligo (10%), pruritus (9%), and CTCL (6%).

Local regulations may vary significantly depending on the phototherapy center location, and these can significantly affect the setup. In many states, the Department of Public Health has specific requirements for space and setup that apply to hospital-based practices as opposed to private practices. However, regulations may vary widely by state and change over time. Other considerations regarding setup include venting and power requirements for each machine and booth, which

Recommended order of modalities to include

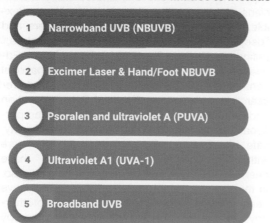

Fig. 2. Recommended order of phototherapy modalities include the following: full-body NBUVB is the most versatile and forgiving modality, so it is a reasonable first device to purchase. Excimer laser and hand/foot NBUVB can later be added to address more focused areas. Last, more specialized choices can be added, such as UVA (for systemic, hand/foot, and topical/bath PUVA), then UVA-1, followed by broadband UVB.

generally will not pose a significant issue with the newer machines. The largest manufacturers of UV phototherapy machines and equipment in the United States are Daavlin, National Biological, Solarc, and UV Biotek. Having a close relationship with the manufacturer of your phototherapy machines, particularly for initial setup and assistance with metering and calibration, bulb replacement, and other general maintenance issues, is very helpful for initiating and maintaining a phototherapy center.

FINANCIAL CONSIDERATIONS

There are several financial considerations in operating and managing a successful new phototherapy center.

Billing and reimbursement may vary depending on whether the phototherapy center is associated with a hospital or private practice. For those phototherapy centers physically located within or otherwise associated with a larger health care organization, there may be separate facility and/or physician fees in addition to fees for the actual treatment itself. As of 2019, the national Medicare reimbursement amounts for common phototherapy treatments are listed as follows:

- 96900: Actinotherapy; UVB: $21.98
- 96910: UVB with mineral oil: $116.77
- 96912: PUVA: $99.11
- 96920: Excimer less than 250 cm^2: $68.47
- 96921: Excimer 250 to 500 cm^2: $77.12
- 96922: Excimer greater than 500 cm^2: $126.61[7]

However, the actual amount paid by the patient and the profits made by the center may be higher or lower than the listed amounts depending on copays, coinsurance, and the aforementioned fees.

The overall costs of running a phototherapy center can be conceptualized in the following 4 categories: initial costs, continued costs, personnel costs, and opportunity costs.[8] Initial costs include those associated with setting up the phototherapy center: establishing and preparing the space, setting up the booths, purchasing the machines and bulbs, and upfront marketing costs.[8] Continued costs include those costs associated with maintenance of the phototherapy center, such as servicing and maintaining the phototherapy machines, changing the bulbs, purchasing supplies, and paying for utilities.[8] Personnel costs include the costs associated with training and employing phototherapy technicians, and opportunity costs refer to the loss of potential gains from other alternative uses for both the personnel and the space dedicated to the phototherapy center.[8] The magnitude of each of these general categories of costs will differ depending on the phototherapy center's location, patient population served, patient volume, and other decisions around personnel and staffing.

Marketing is essential, and ideally, the goal is to open the center on the first day with patients ready to begin treatment. Services can be listed with the American Academy of Dermatology and the National Psoriasis Foundation. Building a local referral base among dermatologists, rheumatologists, allergists, and primary care physicians in the area is also essential. Some phototherapy companies will assist in marketing when new machines are purchased. Last, social media can also be a powerful tool for marketing and advertising.

OPERATIONS AND PERSONNEL

One of the most important decisions, aside from selection of the location, is setting the hours of operation for the phototherapy center. Because patients will often be receiving therapy multiple times a week, it would be ideal for hours to be designed with patient convenience in mind. Depending on the location of the phototherapy center and the target patient population, it may make sense to be accommodating of a standard work schedule, because working patients may prefer to receive treatment in the early morning, around noon, late afternoon, after work, or even on the weekends. For example, the authors' facility is an urban phototherapy center located within a medical area, so there is a large working patient population. Thus, their hours with the highest volume of patients are between 9 and 10 AM and between 4 and 5 PM.[9] Another significant decision is whether to schedule appointments or allow patients to walk in at their convenience, and there are benefits and downsides to each model. Although scheduled appointments may help avoid bottlenecks during popular hours, the flexibility of a walk-in model may actually better facilitate clinic flow for a procedure as quick as most phototherapy treatments. However, it may make sense to schedule appointments for more specific treatments like excimer laser, PUVA, or new patient orientations, all of which are more time and labor intensive for both the patient and the staff.

The next operational issue to consider is human resources, such as how much staff is needed to check patients in and operate the machines, what type of training is required for these roles, and the amount of personnel time required for the various modalities of phototherapy treatment. Phototherapy technicians may be medical/physician assistants, nurses, or other health care professionals, and these qualification requirements may be state and/or hospital dependent. There are specific training courses and workshops dedicated to phototherapy, including one offered by the Dermatology Nurses' Association. Their Fundamentals of Phototherapy course is an intensive 1 day of training for those administering light therapy under a physician's supervision. The workshop covers psoriasis and other photoresponsive skin diseases as well as PUVA, narrow and broadband UVB therapy, equipment operation, metering and calibration, and other responsibilities associated with phototherapy administration.[10] Such additional tasks may include booth cleaning, keeping up a logbook for each phototherapy machine, prior authorizations and referrals, and patient scheduling. Individual centers can consider holding in-person trainings to orient new technicians. Whenever possible, the authors also recommend that new phototherapy technicians starting in a brand-new phototherapy center shadow technicians in an existing facility. In addition, simulations in which health care providers work together to treat a pretend patient have been shown to be beneficial in cultivating a sense of teamwork and improving patient care and safety; this could be a useful exercise for the training of new phototherapy technicians.[11]

In addition to formal training in the technical skills of phototherapy, it has been the authors' experience that successful phototherapy technicians are also detail- and procedure-oriented, flexible, resourceful, team players, good listeners, and "people" people. These "nontechnical skills," defined by The Non-Technical Skills in Medical Education Special Interest Group, an international consortium of clinicians, educators, and researchers, as "a set of social (communication and team work) and cognitive (analytical and personal behavior) skills that support high quality, safe, effective and efficient interprofessional care within the complex healthcare system," have been shown to be just as crucial, if not more so, in the delivery of high-quality, safe, and effective health care.[12] It would be beneficial for phototherapy technicians to be well trained in phototherapy protocols and well supported when there is a question or an issue. Ideally, they would be dedicated to phototherapy rather than rotating between roles, because continuity is the key to patient care. It is helpful for phototherapy technicians to know the patient and treatment regimens well, particularly with complex protocols and medical conditions involved. A new phototherapy center could also consider developing a checklist of site-specific competencies for new technicians, a tool that has been shown to enhance safety and efficiency in health care settings.[12]

Phototherapy treatments should be documented; ideally this would be integrated into the clinic electronic medical record (EMR) or other health record. The order set placed by physicians can be confirmed, carried out, and documented by the technician after each treatment. Each documentation would ideally include at least the following information: patient name/identification, date, outcome/reactions from last treatment, machine used, name of technician providing treatment, topicals applied (ie, petrolatum, sunscreen), dose/time planned, actual dose received, and other special notes, such as planned follow-up or alterations/deviations from protocol, and reason for deviation. A patient registry can be created with an embedded dosimetry calculator, and a database of treatment doses and calculations for each patient can be maintained.

As part of phototherapy center operation, written protocols should be in place to address the following: starting doses, dose escalation, maximum doses before contacting the physician, missed doses, shielding and draping, and emergency situations, including patient concerns regarding burns. Phototherapy technicians would ideally be comfortable navigating these different types of protocols and feel supported in handling unforeseen situations that might arise. Good communication between phototherapy technicians, nurses, and physicians is important to address any questions or concerns that arise. This communication can occur through regular formal meetings with physicians and managers or in more informal settings. With regard to follow-up, the authors recommend regular visits with the dermatologists prescribing phototherapy to manage the treatment course.[13,14] Some centers also follow a 6- to 12-month follow-up schedule after an initial 6-week follow-up after starting phototherapy. To ensure proper follow-up, the authors recommend alerts in the EMR or phototherapy database alerting technicians to an upcoming appointment (or lack thereof).

CONSENT AND EDUCATION PROCESS

Once the phototherapy center is set up and operational details are worked out, educating and consenting patients to phototherapy treatment is the next step. Because each type of phototherapy regimen offered has different protocols, the authors recommend treatment-specific information packets with general information explaining the treatment, details on the indications, risks, and benefits of treatment, as well as what to expect before, during, and after treatment. The authors

also recommend including consent forms for the specific treatment and consent forms for photographs to document treatment response. Information about treatment can also be provided through a variety of creative modalities, including online video platforms, through which a provider can record short videos addressing the most frequently asked questions by new phototherapy patients.

It may also be helpful to include insurance information within the packet, particularly a script for patients to reach out to their insurance companies regarding the details of insurance coverage. This script can provide patient-specific diagnosis codes and procedure codes and prompt patients to ask their insurance companies about the necessity of a primary care physician referral, prior authorization, and specific out-of-pocket responsibility, such as co-pays or deductibles.

Once the patient has been consented, the authors' center provides an in-person orientation at the phototherapy center, during which the phototherapy team can review the center's hours of operation, the patient's specific treatment regimen and follow-up plan, the process of receiving treatment from start to finish, expectations for treatment efficacy, risks and side effects, and specific safety points pertaining to treatment. These safety points include the need for consistency of treatment, the importance of reporting any new medications, the need to avoid applying creams or lotions before treatment, the shielding of particular body areas, and the avoidance of sun exposure outside of treatment. It may be helpful to devise and fill out a checklist for each new patient to the phototherapy center, in order to ensure that all paperwork and tasks have been completed before beginning therapy.

With proper consent, education, and setting of expectations, phototherapy is generally well tolerated with good patient satisfaction ratings. One study found that when considering treatment satisfaction, patients rated treatment efficacy as most important, followed by treatment safety and doctor-patient communication.[15] In a study of treatment satisfaction among patients with moderate to severe psoriasis, mean self-reported global satisfaction for phototherapy treatment was 5.2 out of 6, which was equal to that of systemic treatment.[16] Both phototherapy and systemic treatment outscored topical treatments in global satisfaction.[16] Patients also rated phototherapy higher in safety (5.0/6.0) than systemic (4.9/6.0) or topical treatments (4.5/6.0), but convenience of phototherapy (4.6/6.0) lagged behind systemic treatment (5.1/6.0).[16] Similarly, another study of NBUVB phototherapy treatment in adults with guttate psoriasis found high treatment satisfaction with a mean of 8.75 out of 10 in all patients treated.[17] Patients who achieved a complete response had a higher satisfaction score than patients with an incomplete response (9/10 vs 8.35/10), but the difference was not found to be statistically significant.[17] Nevertheless, 96% of patients would choose to repeat treatment again if necessary, even in the case of a poor response or adverse event.[17]

SAFETY/TROUBLESHOOTING

Patient safety is of utmost importance when establishing and running a new phototherapy center. There are many steps in the process of administering a phototherapy treatment, and some of the most common pitfalls stem from a failure to verify the details of each step of that process. Among the most apparent errors is the failure to confirm patient-specific information, such as the identity of the patient, date and time of the previous treatment, and the most recent dose. It is important to understand how the patient responded to his or her most recent treatment in order to inform how to proceed with the current treatment. In addition, the failure to continually educate and communicate with the patient can have dire consequences. Phototherapy technicians must confirm at each treatment any new medications the patient is taking (prescription, over-the-counter, and herbal/supplements), instruct the patient to maintain consistency of positioning and draping, verbally communicate the UV dose administered, and closely track the timing of UV administration. Another common pitfall is calculation error; even when the proper dose and timing are communicated with the patient, there may be math errors or a failure to correctly follow protocol following a burn or a lapse in treatment. Some patients may press for higher doses or longer treatment times hoping for a quicker response, but there should ideally be no deviations from protocol without physician approval. The authors recommend multiple layers of safety checks and double checks to help avoid these types of errors, which in turn require staff education and periodic oversight and retraining.

A further category of error is a failure to properly maintain the equipment. The authors recommend calibrating each phototherapy machine frequently and regularly with a radiometer as well as measuring and recording output on a regular basis to ensure that output falls within an adequate targeted range. Tsui and Levitt[18] recommend calibration every 2 weeks and bulb output measurement monthly or bimonthly. Bulbs will need to be changed depending on the center's usage and the manufacturer's recommendations, which may be as often as every 8 to 10 months for regularly used machines.[18] UV lamps generally have a lifespan of about 800 to 1000 hours, and a meter that tracks total hours of use can serve as an indicator for when the change the bulbs.[18] The authors recommend logging measurements of the bulbs both before and after a bulb change for comparison.

Despite taking precautions, unforeseen situations are inevitable, and there should be a specific protocol in place to address errors and emergencies. In the case of erythema or burns, phototherapy technicians will need to meticulously document and photograph the details of the burn, including onset, location, grade of severity, duration, level of discomfort, and possible reasons or explanations for the burn. As appropriate, the physician should be alerted, and the authors recommend establishing specific criteria for when the patient should be urgently evaluated in the clinic. In the authors' center, they recommend that the patient be seen urgently if there is presence of blistering, moderate to severe pain, swelling, evidence of infection at sites of broken skin, any question as to diagnosis, or in the event of patient upset or concern. Treatments for a burn can include topical steroids (under occlusion if severe), petrolatum, aloe, ice, or nonsteroidal anti-inflammatory drugs.[13,19,20]

Regardless of the underlying reason for the situation that has arisen, honesty, flexibility, and resourcefulness are key. It is important to stress a culture of open communication between all providers, such that staff feels comfortable reporting errors and working together to come up with solutions and ways to prevent future incidents. One study on medical error revealed 4 main themes preventing reporting of medical errors among physicians and nurses: fear of consequences, attitude of the administration, system-related barriers, and differing perceptions about the error.[21] Studies have also shown negative physical, occupational, and mental health outcomes among health care providers involved in medical error, such as increased rates of depression and burnout as well as lack of concentration and poor work performance.[22] Thus, it is of utmost importance to cultivate a proactive, collaborative, and nonpunitive work environment to promote provider well-being and resilience and ensure patient safety. Organizational context influences team processes and outcomes, and organizational culture provides the operating conditions necessary to promote effective teamwork toward accomplishing a common goal.[12,23]

SUMMARY

Phototherapy is a safe and effective treatment for a wide variety of benign and malignant inflammatory cutaneous diseases. Access to this powerful treatment can be expanded by creating new phototherapy centers in areas of need around the country. Creating and managing a phototherapy center requires careful research and planning to achieve a nuanced understanding of the medical and social needs of the targeted patient population as well as the financial and operational principles behind running a health care facility. The specific steps involved include physical setup, patient education and consent, operations and personnel, finances, and patient safety and troubleshooting. Successful expansion of phototherapy centers to previously underserved areas will be crucial in reducing burden of disease, improving patient care, and fighting health care inequity in this country.

REFERENCES

1. Situm M, Dediol I. The mechanisms of action of phototherapy in the treatment of the most common dermatoses. Coll Antropol 2011;35 Suppl 2:147–51.

2. Vieyra-garcia PA, Wolf P. From early immunomodulatory triggers to immunosuppressive outcome: therapeutic implications of the complex interplay between the wavebands of sunlight and the skin. Front Med (Lausanne) 2018;5:1–9.

3. Mehraban S, Feily A. 308nm excimer laser in dermatology. J Lasers Med Sci 2014;5(1):8–12.

4. Tan SY, Buzney E, Mostaghimi A. Trends in phototherapy utilization among Medicare beneficiaries in the United States, 2000 to 2015. J Am Acad Dermatol 2018;79(4):672–9.

5. Gharaveis A, Hamilton DK, Pati D. The impact of environmental design on teamwork and communication in healthcare facilities: a systematic literature review. HERD 2018;11(1):119–37.

6. Schaarschmidt ML, Schmieder A, Umar N, et al. Patient preferences for psoriasis treatments: process characteristics can outweigh outcome attributes. Arch Dermatol 2011. https://doi.org/10.1001/archdermatol.2011.309.

7. CY 2019 Physician Fee Schedule. Centers for Medicare & Medicaid Services. 2019. Available at: https://www.cms.gov/medicare/medicare-fee-for-service-payment/physicianfeesched/. Accessed May 4, 2019.

8. Evans CC. Establishing and operating a phototherapy clinic. Annual Meeting of the Photomedicine Society. Orlando, FL, 2017.

9. Buzney EA. Practical tips: establishing and running a phototherapy center. Annual Meeting of the American Academy of Dermatology. Washington, DC, 2019.

10. The Joan Shelk Fundamentals of Phototherapy Workshop. Dermatology Nurses' Association. Available at: https://www.dnanurse.org/dnaeducation/phototherapy-workshop/. Accessed May 4, 2019.

11. Freytag J, Stroben F, Hautz WE, et al. Improving patient safety through better teamwork: how effective are different methods of simulation debriefing? Protocol for a pragmatic, prospective and randomised study. BMJ Open 2017;7(6):1–9.

12. Rosen MA, DiazGranados D, Dietz AS, et al. Teamwork in healthcare: key discoveries enabling safer, high-quality care. Am Psychol 2018. https://doi.org/10.1037/amp0000298.

13. Menter A, Korman NJ, Elmets CA, et al. Guidelines of care for the management of psoriasis and psoriatic arthritis. Section 5. Guidelines of care for the treatment of psoriasis with phototherapy and photochemotherapy. J Am Acad Dermatol 2010. https://doi.org/10.1016/j.jaad.2009.08.026.

14. Mehta D, Lim HW. Ultraviolet B phototherapy for psoriasis: review of practical guidelines. Am J Clin Dermatol 2016;17(2):125–33.

15. Sylwestrzak G, Liu J, Stephenson JJ, et al. Considering patient preferences when selecting anti-tumor necrosis factor therapeutic options. Am Health Drug Benefits 2014;7(2):71–81.

16. Finch T, Shim TN, Roberts L, et al. Treatment satisfaction among patients with moderate-to-severe psoriasis. J Clin Aesthet Dermatol 2015;8(4):26–30.

17. Fernández-Guarino M, Aboín-González S, Velázquez D, et al. Phototherapy with narrow-band UVB in adult guttate psoriasis: results and patient assessment. Dermatology 2017;232(5):626–32.

18. Tsui CL, Levitt J. Practical Pearls in Phototherapy. International Journal of Dermatology 2013;52(11):1395–7.

19. Jeon C, Nakamura M. Recognizing and overcoming phototherapy-induced initiation burn. J Am Acad Dermatol 2017;77(4):e103.

20. Singh RK, Lee KM, Jose MV, et al. The patient's guide to psoriasis treatment. Part 1: UVB phototherapy. Dermatol Ther (Heidelb) 2016;6(3):307–13.

21. Soydemir D, Seren Intepeler S, Mert H. Barriers to medical error reporting for physicians and nurses. West J Nurs Res 2017;39(10):1348–63.

22. Robertson JJ, Long B. Suffering in silence: medical error and its impact on health care providers. J Emerg Med 2018;54(4):402–9.

23. Tawfik DS, Sexton JB, Adair KC, et al. Context in quality of care: improving teamwork and resilience. Clin Perinatol 2017;44(3):541–52.

Phototherapy for Itch

Connie S. Zhong, MSc[a], Sarina B. Elmariah, MD, PhD[a,b],*

KEYWORDS

• Phototherapy • PUVA • UVA • UVB • Itch • Pruritus • Prurigo

KEY POINTS

- Phototherapy reduces itch by suppressing the immune system, decreasing key cytokines that may contribute to itch and skin inflammation, and modulating neural signaling.
- Phototherapy is effective at reducing itch severity in inflammatory and noninflammatory skin conditions.
- In general, narrowband ultraviolet B and ultraviolet A are the preferred modalities for the management of chronic pruritic conditions. Which therapy is optimal between these two options depends on the type of disease being managed.
- Before initiating phototherapy, it is critical that physicians consider the patient's medical comorbidities, as phototherapy may exacerbate some types of skin disease and concurrent medications may result in patient photosensitivity.

INTRODUCTION

Itch, medically termed pruritus, is a frustrating symptom that affects many individuals and is associated with numerous dermatologic and systemic medical conditions. First-line therapy for pruritus includes application of moisturizers and emollients to hydrate and seal the skin barrier, topical corticosteroids, topical immunomodulators, and oral antihistamines in the appropriate scenarios. However, for many patients with pruritus who fail to respond to these interventions, phototherapy has emerged as an effective treatment. Phototherapy has long been used to treat inflammatory conditions, such as psoriasis and atopic dermatitis (AD); in many cases, pruritus improves before resolution of skin lesions.[1] Phototherapy has also been beneficial in controlling itch in patients with systemic disease who do not have apparent cutaneous inflammation, for example, end-stage renal, cholestatic liver and hematologic diseases.

Phototherapy is a popular therapeutic modality for the management of generalized or chronic pruritus for several reasons. Phototherapy can be used with relative ease in patients when large body surface areas are affected, making topical therapy unfeasible and inconvenient. Because phototherapy is a skin-directed therapy, it also does not pose systemic side effects that could compromise immune function, as may be the case with many biological or other systemic therapies.

Despite its benefits, phototherapy also poses several challenges. Accessibility to physician offices with phototherapy units may be a barrier for many patients. In addition, patients typically require the flexibility to pursue treatment 2 to 3 times weekly for many months to years. Common side effects are generally mild, including erythema, edema, pruritus, and blistering.[2] However, more severe side effects, such as pigmentary disorders, photoaging, cataracts, and carcinogenesis, may also occur.[2]

A wide range of phototherapy modalities including ultraviolet A (UVA), UVA with psoralen (PUVA), broad-band ultraviolet B (BB-UVB), and narrowband UVB (NBUVB) have been used to treat chronic pruritus. Of these options, NBUVB is usually preferred over BB-UVB or UVA because it is

a Harvard Medical School, 25 Shattuck Street, Boston, MA, 02115, USA; b Department of Dermatology, Massachusetts General Hospital, 50 Staniford Street, Boston, MA, 02114, USA
* Corresponding author. Department of Dermatology, Massachusetts General Hospital, Boston, MA.
E-mail address: SBELMARIAH@mgh.harvard.edu

Dermatol Clin 38 (2020) 145–155
https://doi.org/10.1016/j.det.2019.08.008

derm.theclinics.com

typically as effective as other modalities, widely available, and less erythemogenic.[1] UVA and UVA1 are effective in conditions that require deeper penetration and may be coupled with oral or topical psoralen when managing more aggressive inflammatory skin disease.[2] The excimer laser has the advantage of delivering UVB to discrete areas using a wand, which may be helpful in areas of localized disease (eg, lichen simplex chronicus or individual refractory prurigo nodularis lesions). In general, choosing the optimal type of phototherapy will be based on the disease entity and the availability of the specific modality.

This review explores what is known about the pathophysiology of phototherapy in treating pruritus and discusses the evidence supporting phototherapy in a wide variety of pruritic skin conditions.

Phototherapy and Itch Pathophysiology

Because the pathophysiology of itch is poorly understood in most conditions, the exact mechanisms by which phototherapy alleviates itch are also not fully understood. Evidence suggests that phototherapy has both anti-inflammatory and neuromodulatory effects, either of which may influence the sensation of pruritus.[3]

Phototherapy induces immunosuppression in the skin via multiple mechanisms. Both UVA and UVB have been shown to induce apoptosis in multiple cell types in the skin including keratinocytes, effector T-cell populations, and Langerhans cells (LCs).[4] Apoptosis may result from increased reactive oxygen species that damage the cellular and nuclear membranes, direct DNA damage, and upregulation of various cell surface markers that are associated with programmed cell death such as Fas ligand.[5] Studies demonstrate that natural sunlight, as well as UVA or UVB, are capable of reducing LCs in healthy human skin after exposure.[6]

UV radiation may also evoke immunosuppression by increasing tolerance through modulating regulatory T cells.[7] For example, in patients with psoriasis, irradiation with natural sunlight led to recruitment of FOXP3+ regulatory T cells into the dermis.[8] UV exposure also decreased expression of human leukocyte antigen-DR, interleukin (IL)-2 receptor, and CD30 on skin-homing T cells.[9] In vitro studies demonstrated that low-dose UVB irradiation of healthy human skin decreases dendritic cell expression of B7 costimulatory signals, which normally bind to CD28 and CTLA-4 on T lymphocytes.[10] UV may also reduce immunoglobulin E (IgE) binding, mast cell degranulation, and histamine release in the dermis, and inhibit the migration of LCs out of the epidermis, resulting in relative immune suppression and thereby relieving inflammatory pruritus.[11]

Phototherapy may exert part of its effects by reducing cytokines that have been implicated in provoking pruritus in common inflammatory skin conditions. For example, PUVA downregulates IL-17 and IL-23, cytokines important in psoriatic pruritus,[12] and UVA1 reduces IL-4 and IL-13, cytokines elevated in subsets of patients with AD.[13] The relationship between UV dosage and individual cytokine levels may vary greatly and is not necessarily inversely proportional, such that higher UV doses do not always lead to lower cytokine levels. For example, repeated delivery of low doses of UVA1 and NBUVB reduces IL-31, a cytokine that binds to receptors on sensory nerves to induce itch and growth of new nerves.[14] In contrast, acute, high doses of UVB increase IL-31 and may trigger pruritus.[15] This suggests that repeated suberythemogenic doses of UV light induce the antipruritic effect of phototherapy, whereas high doses of UV, particularly UVB, induces skin inflammation and exacerbates pruritus.

In addition to having immunosuppressive effects, UV phototherapy directly influences neural signaling. In some cases, UV may actually induce inflammation and itch via modulation of the TRPV1 receptor, an ion channel that regulates the effects of the aforementioned cytokines. When TRPV1 receptors are inhibited by 5′-iodoresiniferatoxin, the proinflammatory effects of acute high-dose UV radiation are attenuated.[16] UV may also reduce pruritus through modulation of signaling via the endogenous opioid system. Increased μ-opioidergic tone results in reduced pain but may increase pruritus[17]; as such, μ-opioid receptor (MOR) antagonists, such as naloxone and naltrexone, have been reported to ameliorate itch in certain conditions. In contrast, activation of κ-opioid receptors (KORs) reduces itch, and KOR agonists including nalfurafine have been used successfully to manage uremic pruritus (UP).[18,19] In patients with AD, PUVA decreases MORs without altering the number of KORs, presumably restoring the balance of the opioid system and relieving itch.[19]

Finally, phototherapy may influence nerve fiber density in the skin. In mice, UV increases the number of calcitonin gene-related peptide (CGRP)-positive cutaneous nerve fibers,[20,21] which in turn reduces the number of epidermal LCs.[22] In contrast, in humans, various forms of UV radiation including BB, NBUVB, and UVA with or without psoralen, have been reported to decrease the number of CGRP-positive nerve fibers.[23] It is still unclear as to why the discrepancy between mice and human studies exists, but it likely reflects the complex interplay between immune cells and sensory nerves that varies with different disease states.

PHOTOTHERAPY IN SPECIFIC PRURITIC SKIN CONDITIONS

Psoriasis

Psoriasis is a chronic, inflammatory skin disease that affects up to 2% to 3% of the world's population.[2] Phototherapy is a safe and effective treatment that can easily be combined with other modalities for the treatment of refractory psoriasis.[24]

UVB therapy is generally used to treat psoriatic lesions or associated itch covering at least 10% body surface area.[25] NBUVB reduces psoriatic lesions quickly and induces longer remissions than BB-UVB.[2] Typical dosing of NBUVB is 3 times per week for at least 3 months starting at 50% minimal erythema dose (MED).[26] A randomized double-blind trial found that high- and low-dose NBUVB radiation have comparable clearance rates, but high-dose radiation induces prolonged remission within fewer treatment sessions.[27] Combining NBUVB and oral retinoids reduces treatment time, recovery time, and dose-limiting side effects.[28]

With respect to psoriatic pruritus, UVB was shown to decrease the mean numerical rating itch score in 59 psoriasis patients from 7 to 1.05,[29] which is consistent with a previous study, in which 70% of 98 patients had pruritus improvement or complete resolution.[30] The severity of itch is predictive of the number of irradiation sessions needed to clear the psoriatic lesions.[31] In a study comparing UVB phototherapy and visible light, there was an improvement in the itch visual analogue scale (VAS) at week 12 in 62% of patients treated with UVB versus 27% of patients treated with visible light, although the difference failed to reach statistical significance.[32] Although phototherapy has emerged as an effective treatment of both the pruritus and lesions of psoriasis, the potential side effects of burning, stinging, erythema, and itch in the first two weeks may limit its use in any individual patient.[33]

Atopic Dermatitis

Pruritus is a central feature of AD, with approximately 87% to 100% of patients with AD suffering from chronic pruritus.[34] Pruritus in AD is thought to arise due to a variety of factors, including barrier dysfunction, neural hypersensitization, and immune dysregulation.[35] Phototherapy is a safe and effective treatment of AD and is often combined with topical corticosteroids especially in the initial phase of treatment. Although the mechanisms by which phototherapy reduces atopic

itch has not be thoroughly investigated, some studies demonstrate that UV treatment induces thickening of the stratum corneum and stratum spinosum, which prevents penetration of antigens and inhibits *Malassezia furfur* and *Staphylococcus aureus* colonization. Phototherapy also suppresses excess ICAM-1 expression, alters LC function, and reduces immune cell infiltration.[36,37] The effects of phototherapy are limited to areas of skin undergoing irradiation because untreated areas do not show reduction of itch.[38]

Although pruritus from AD has been shown to respond to a variety of phototherapy wavelengths, including UVB, combined UVA and UVB, and UVA alone,[39] medium-dose UVA1 and NBUVB are the preferred modalities for AD.[40] A randomized controlled trial found that UVA was superior to UVB in reducing total eczema severity, but no significant difference was observed between the two wavelengths in degree of pruritus reduction.[41] Similar findings that NBUVB and UVA1 are equally as effective in reducing pruritus in patients with moderate to severe AD have been reported by others.[42,43] In contrast, some studies have found that NBUVB is more effective than UVA treatment in reducing atopic itch, as 90% of patients reported decreased itch severity with NBUVB compared with 63% of patients receiving UVA.[44] In general, UVA1 is thought to be more effective for controlling acute flares of AD, whereas NBUVB is more often used to manage chronic disease.[45–47] PUVA is also an option, and although superior to BB-UVB,[48] it is comparable to NBUVB.[49]

No clear differences have been demonstrated in efficacy of reducing AD severity and itch burden between high-dose and medium-dose UVA1 in light skin types.[43,50] In darker skin types (III or higher), high-dose UVA1 was significantly more effective than medium-dose UVA1 at reducing AD symptoms.[51] Both high and medium dosages are more effective than low-dose UVA1 at reducing AD severity and itch burden, as measured by SCORAD, but recurrence within 3 months is often observed.[52]

In the pediatric population (ages 4–14 years), NBUVB has been shown to be an efficacious and safe modality in reducing the lesions and pruritus of AD with minimal side effects, and improvement may be maintained for up to 2 years.[47,53] In general, children with MEDs greater than 390 mJ/cm^2 are more likely to clear.[54]

Prurigo Nodularis

Prurigo nodularis (PN) is a debilitating disease characterized by intensely pruritic nodules commonly on the extensor surfaces of the extremities. Phototherapy has been shown to be a safe and efficacious treatment of PN, particularly when generalized. Phototherapy has been hypothesized to work in this condition by decreasing the number of epidermal and dermal nerve fibers and neuropeptide expression in the skin.[1]

Several phototherapy modalities have been shown to be effective in the management of PN, including UVA, PUVA, BB-UVB, NBUVB, and excimer laser.[55,56] There is no clear evidence as to which phototherapy method is best, although excimer may be preferred when treating resistant nodules because it can be delivered locally.[55] Combination therapies including BB-UVB and PUVA,[57] bath PUVA and excimer,[58] excimer and potent topical steroid,[59] and Goeckerman therapy (BB-UVB, coal tar, and topical steroid) all seem to be safe and effective for management of PN.[60] Specifically, in patients with recalcitrant PN, the combination of UVB 308nm-excimer light with bath PUVA results in greater complete remission rates after a mean of 9.8 treatments compared with PUVA alone.[58]

Relapse rates were noted in a handful of studies, mostly using NBUVB and BB-UVB. The range of time of relapse was 2.5 to 12 months after discontinuation of therapy.[55] Side effects of UV therapy reported in patients with PN include erythema, increased pruritus, hyperpigmentation, vesicles, and edema in up to 40% of patients.[56,58]

Pretreatment of Polymorphic Light Eruption

Polymorphic light eruption (PMLE) is a common photosensitivity disorder in which patients develop pruritic papules, vesicles, or plaques within hours of UV radiation exposure. First-line treatment includes sun avoidance, use of sunscreen, and topical steroids. In moderate to severe cases, PUVA, NBUVB, or BB-UVB administered in the early spring may be effective for PMLE prophylaxis.[61] Phototherapy is thought to modulate adhesion molecule expression and induce antiinflammatory cytokines, which in turn promotes LC migration from the epidermis to skin-draining lymph nodes and suppresses cutaneous immune responses.[62,63] Vitamin D may also play a role as topical treatment with calcipotriol diminishes PMLE symptoms, and murine studies have shown that 1,25-dihydroxyvitamin D has comparable immunosuppressive effects as UV.[64]

In general, UVA irradiation provokes PMLE more often than UVB.[65] As such, fewer studies have examined the efficacy of UVA phototherapy for its management. One small, randomized controlled trial found that UVA alone is as effective

prophylactic therapy as PUVA, but because of the high incidence of provoked reactions with UVA, the treatment may be difficult to tolerate.[66]

NBUVB is usually preferred over PUVA because of the lower risks of carcinogenesis and nausea and the lack of need for posttreatment eye protection. However, PUVA can be considered before other systemic treatments if patients with PMLE have either failed NBUVB or if NBUVB has triggered the eruption in the past.[67] A randomized controlled trial between PUVA and NBUVB plus placebo tablets, 3 times weekly for 5 weeks, found no significant difference in efficacy between the 2 treatments.[68] A 10-year retrospective review of 170 patients with moderate-to-severe PMLE also reported similar results in efficacy between PUVA and UVB.[69] In contrast, a retrospective study examining long-term remission rates in 79 patients followed for more than 14-years found that 65% of patients had complete or partial remission with PUVA, 82% with BB-UVB, and 83% with UVA alone.[70] These results must be interpreted with caution, as the patients treated with PUVA may have had more severe forms of PMLE.

Common side effects of NBUVB reported in patients with PMLE include worsening erythema and pruritus.[62] To maintain the benefit of prophylactic phototherapy, regular sun exposure throughout the summer is encouraged.

Mycosis Fungoides/Sezary Syndrome

Mycosis fungoides (MF) and Sezary syndrome (SS) are cutaneous T-cell lymphomas characterized by pruritic, erythematous patches or plaques of the skin. In conjunction with topical corticosteroids or topical and systemic retinoids, phototherapy may be considered a first-line therapy for management of cutaneous lesions and pruritus. The goal of phototherapy is to induce long-lasting remission off therapy and minimize active disease.[71] Recent findings of UV-induced p53 mutations in advanced MF have raised concerns that phototherapy may contribute to disease progression.[72] However, a retrospective study revealed that patients who received phototherapy had longer median time to tumor progression and longer overall survival than those who did not, suggesting that the therapeutic effects of phototherapy outweigh the potential adverse effects.[72] In general, phototherapy has been shown to be effective in decreasing lymphoma lesions and controlling the associated pruritus.[71]

PUVA, BB and NBUVB, and UVA1 may all be used to treat MF, although PUVA and NBUVB are the most common treatments for early stages of MF (stage IIB or lower).[73,74] In a meta-analysis that compared PUVA with NBUVB in early stage MF, researchers found that PUVA had a significantly higher rate of complete response (73.8% vs 62.2%) and lower rate of failed response than NBUVB.[73] However, the rate of partial responses were similar and there was no difference in side effects.[73] Patients with skin phototypes III or higher were less responsive to PUVA.[75]

In general, thick MF plaques or folliculotropic involvement respond better to PUVA than NBUVB because the former is capable of penetrating deeper into the dermis.[71] Based on this principle, the British Association of Dermatologists guidelines suggest using NBUVB for patch disease and PUVA for plaque disease.[62] UVA1 has been suggested by some to be more beneficial than PUVA because it reaches deeper dermis and broadens T-cell apoptosis[76]; however, its use is limited because it is not widely available, may be expensive, and few comparative studies have focused primarily on UVA1.

When considering which type of treatment to use for patients with MF, risks and benefits must be weighed on an individual basis. In general, NBUVB may be preferred as first-line UV therapy. Although PUVA has a higher complete response rate, the higher risk of cutaneous malignant neoplasms observed with this treatment may preclude its use in higher-risk patients. For others, it may simply be less accessible.[77,78]

In advanced-stage MF or SS (stages IIB–IVB), phototherapy alone is unlikely to achieve full response. Phototherapy in these cases may be combined with interferon-α (IFN-α), systemic retinoids, or more aggressive modalities including chemotherapy, radiotherapy, extracorporeal photopheresis, and allogenic hematopoietic stem cell transplant.[74,79] Caution must be exercised when phototherapy is used in conjunction with photosensitive medications such as retinoids, tetracyclines, and hydrochlorothiazide.[71] These agents should ideally be discontinued before initiating phototherapy, particularly when pursuing PUVA. If this is not possible, the dosage of phototherapy should be reduced and adjusted accordingly.[71] Similarly, lower initial doses and cautious escalation must be used when treating erythrodermic MF because the erythema makes it difficult to assess burning from UV radiation.[71]

Uremic Pruritus

Uremic pruritus (UP) affects more than 40% of patients with chronic kidney disease (CKD), and in most cases, hemodialysis does not provide adequate relief.[80,81] Many factors have been implicated in itch pathogenesis in uremic patients,

including increased parathyroid hormone, histamine, calcium, magnesium, and opioid-receptor imbalances.[80] Several studies have shown that UVB phototherapy reduces pruritus in patients with CKD, whereas UVA does not.[82,83] In contrast, one randomized controlled trial failed to demonstrate a significant difference in the clinical improvement in pruritus following NBUVB as compared with UVA.[84] These antipruritic effects may be observed as early as two weeks after starting phototherapy.[85–87] One study suggested that in UP, phototherapy works on a systemic rather than local level, as BB-UVB exposure to one-half of the body improves pruritus in both the exposed and unexposed sites.[82]

NBUVB may be as effective as BB-UVB with fewer side effects.[87,88] In one study, NBUVB (initial dose, 100 mJ/cm^2; maximum daily dose, 220 mJ/cm^2) reduced pruritus intensity within 6 sessions. In contrast, several case studies reported that patients with UP improved with BB-UVB but not NBUVB.[89] BB-UVB has been shown to reduce phosphorus and mast cells in the skin of uremic patients.[90–92] Although the pathogenesis of UP remains unclear, such effects might contribute to the antipruritic efficacy of phototherapy. The risk for skin malignancies after UVB irradiation, especially in immunocompromised patients suffering from advanced kidney disease or those on immunosuppressive medication after renal transplant, is still unclear, but something that must be taken into special consideration when treating these patients with phototherapy.

Cholestasis-Induced Pruritus

An estimated 25% to 80% of patients with cholestatic liver disease, including those with primary biliary cirrhosis and primary sclerosing cholangitis, experience chronic pruritus.[93,94] The pathophysiology of cholestatic pruritus (CP) is unclear; however, increased serum levels of bile salts, opioids, autotaxin enzyme, and its end product lysophosphatidic acid are all hypothesized to play a role in its pathogenesis.[95]

First-line treatment of CP is cholestyramine, followed by rifampin and opioid antagonists.[96,97] Currently, the European Association of the Study of Liver and American Association for the Study of Liver Diseases guidelines do not mention UVB phototherapy as a treatment of CP due to paucity of evidence.[94,96,98] Small unblinded, nonrandomized pilot studies reported that BB-UVB is effective in reducing CP.[94,99–102] In Decock and colleagues[94] (2012), 10 out of 13 patients with CP had more than 60% reduction in perceived pruritus with BB-UVB, with median VAS scores decreasing from 8.0 before therapy to 2.0 after therapy. The mean number of treatments was 26 performed over an average duration of 8 weeks. There were no significant changes in cholestatic serum markers, suggesting that UVB relieves pruritus by influencing nerve endings or inducing chemical modifications of the pruritogen, rather than influencing the serum parameters of cholestasis.[94] However, it is possible that urinary excretion of bile acids is increased.[101] Four patients in this study needed additional phototherapy due to recurrent symptoms. Side effects of phototherapy in this study included erythema and paresthesia in one case.

Polycythemia Vera

In patients with polycythemia vera (PV), erythryocytosis is often associated with aquagenic pruritus (AP)—itching brought on by the contact of water without any observable skin changes.[103] The exact pathogenesis of AP is unclear; however, increased eicosanoids, mast cell mediators, and serotonin/prostaglandins from platelets have been implicated in itch development.[104] Interestingly, pruritus may be associated with a lower rate of arterial thrombosis and longer survival.[105]

First-line therapy for PV-related pruritus includes antihistamines and selective serotonin reuptake inhibitors, followed by IFN-α therapy and Janus kinase 2 inhibitors for those with IFN-α-resistant pruritus.[106] However, small studies have suggested that NBUVB can effectively treat pruritus in these patients. In a study of 10 patients with PV treated with NBUVB, starting at doses two-thirds of their MED and increasing by 10% to 15% each session, patients reported marked relief of pruritus after an average of 6 treatments.[104] Complete remission occurred in 8 to 10 patients. Case studies have suggested that the combination of UVA and UVB can improve pruritus after one month[107] and that BB-UVB can also be effective, although it has more potential to be erythemogenic.[108] Eleven patients treated with PUVA two to three times a week also showed successful treatment in 10 of the patients with complete resolution of symptoms in 15 treatments.[109] The risks of phototherapy in patients with PV are similar to those patients with other conditions.

Human Immunodeficiency Virus/AIDS

Chronic pruritus affects up to 45% of patients with human immunodeficiency virus (HIV),[110] some of whom may have an apparent primary dermatosis, but many of whom do not.[111] Because of the broad range of associated triggers, the pathogenesis of HIV-associated pruritus is poorly understood. Putative mechanisms that trigger itch in this population include barrier damage, neuropathy, and T-cell imbalance leading to eosinophilia and increased IgE.[110,112,113] As such, various treatments such as oral antihistamines, topical corticosteroids, itraconazole, and phototherapy have been used to reduce pruritus with variable success.

UVB and PUVA phototherapy have both been shown to be effective in decreasing primary HIV pruritus.[40,114,115] UVB may provide significant relief of pruritus in patients with HIV infection with eosinophilic folliculitis as well as those with chronic pruritus without a rash. In one study, 21 male patients with HIV infection with intractable pruritus (14 with eosinophilic folliculitis, 7 with primary pruritus) were treated three times a week with UVB.[111] Pruritus scores decreased from 8.6 to 2.2, with the mean number of treatments to achieve maximum improvement being 20.7. There was no difference between patients with eosinophilic folliculitis and those with primary pruritus.

Another study found that UVB was effective in treating 7 out of 8 patients with pruritic papular eruptions after 1 month.[114] Skin biopsies confirmed that there was less inflammation and reduced T cells following phototherapy. Unfortunately, pruritus recurred in half of the patients after discontinuation of the therapy, with a mean time to recurrence of 8 weeks. Because recurrence is common after phototherapy is stopped, maintenance therapy may be required to continue relief.[40]

One concern of using phototherapy in patients with HIV is the possibility of inducing viral reactivation, as one study found that 12 patients receiving UVB had a decrease in CD4 counts with a corresponding increase in p24 antigen level.[116] However, several other studies found no difference in CD4 counts, β2-microglobulin levels, or HIV-1 viral load with UVB,[111,115,117,118] suggesting that UV radiation is not associated with short-term changes in immune function. Generally, it is thought that UVB modifies local immune cell networks rather than amplifying systemic immunosuppression and thus, should be considered a safe alternative for HIV pruritus.

SUMMARY

Phototherapy has become an important modality for treating a multitude of pruritic conditions. In addition to the conditions discussed earlier, phototherapy has also been shown to be effective in pruritic folliculitis of pregnancy,[119] paraneoplastic itch,[120] and lichen sclerosus.[121] The broad antipruritic effect of phototherapy is thought to work by modulating both the neural and immune systems. Although phototherapy has been shown to work in both inflammatory and noninflammatory skin conditions, from the authors' experience, primary neuropathic itch takes longer to respond than inflammatory dermatoses. In general, NBUVB and UVA are preferred modalities, although some forms of phototherapy work better in some conditions than others. When using phototherapy, it is important to consider the patients' comorbidities, as there are concerns that immunosuppressive effects of phototherapy may exacerbate those conditions or concurrent medications may make skin more sensitive to UV radiation. Although the cost and inconvenience of phototherapy may pose a barrier for some patients, if these barriers can be overcome, phototherapy can offer substantial relief for debilitating pruritus.

REFERENCES

1. Wallengren J, Sundler F. Phototherapy Reduces the Number of Epidermal and CGRP-positive Dermal Nerve Fibres. ActaDerm Venereol 2004;84(2): 111–5.
2. Zhang P, Wu MX. A clinical review of phototherapy for psoriasis. Lasers Med Sci 2018;33(1):173–80.
3. Legat FJ. The Antipruritic Effect of Phototherapy. Front Med 2018;5:333.
4. Krueger JG, Wolfe JT, Nabeya RT, et al. Successful ultraviolet B treatment of psoriasis is accompanied by a reversal of keratinocyte pathology and by selective depletion of intraepidermal T cells. J Exp Med 1995;182(6):2057–68.
5. Wong T, Hsu L, Liao W. Phototherapy in Psoriasis: A Review of Mechanisms of Action. J Cutan Med Surg 2013;17(1):6–12.
6. Seité S, Zucchi H, Moyal D, et al. Alterations in human epidermal Langerhans cells by ultraviolet radiation: quantitative and morphological study. Br J Dermatol 2003;148(2):291–9. Available at: http://www.ncbi.nlm.nih.gov/pubmed/12588382.
7. Schwarz T, Beissert S. Milestones in Photoimmunology. J Invest Dermatol 2013;133(E1):E7–10.
8. Søyland E, Heier I, Rodríguez-Gallego C, et al. Sun exposure induces rapid immunological changes in skin and peripheral blood in patients with psoriasis. Br J Dermatol 2011;164(2):344–55.
9. Piletta PA, Wirth S, Hommel L, et al. Circulating skin-homing T cells in atopic dermatitis. Selective up-regulation of HLA-DR, interleukin-2R, and CD30 and decrease after combined UV-A and UV-B phototherapy. Arch Dermatol 1996;132(10): 1171–6. Available at: http://www.ncbi.nlm.nih.gov/pubmed/8859027. Accessed June 7, 2019.
10. Weiss JM, Renkl AC, Denfeld RW, et al. Low-dose UVB radiation perturbs the functional expression of B7.1 and B7.2 co-stimulatory molecules on human Langerhans cells. Eur J Immunol 1995; 25(10):2858–62.
11. Grabbe J, Welker P, Humke S, et al. High-dose ultraviolet A1 (UVA1), but not UVA/UVB therapy, decreases IgE-binding cells in lesional skin of patients with atopic eczema. J Invest Dermatol 1996;107(3):419–22. Available at: http://www.ncbi.nlm.nih.gov/pubmed/8751980. Accessed June 8, 2019.
12. Hegazy RA, Fawzy MM, Gawdat HI, et al. T helper 17 and Tregs: a novel proposed mechanism for NB-UVB in vitiligo. Exp Dermatol 2014;23(4):283–6.
13. Gambichler T, Kreuter A, Tomi NS, et al. Gene expression of cytokines in atopic eczema before and after ultraviolet A1 phototherapy. Br J Dermatol 2008;158(5):1117–20.
14. Cevikbas F, Wang X, Akiyama T, et al. A sensory neuron-expressed IL-31 receptor mediates T helper cell-dependent itch: Involvement of TRPV1 and TRPA1. J Allergy Clin Immunol 2014;133(2): 448–60.
15. Cornelissen C, Brans R, Czaja K, et al. Ultraviolet B radiation and reactive oxygen species modulate interleukin-31 expression in T lymphocytes, monocytes and dendritic cells. Br J Dermatol 2011; 165(5):966–75.
16. Lee YM, Kang SM, Lee SR, et al. Inhibitory effects of TRPV1 blocker on UV-Induced responses in the hairless mice. Arch Dermatol Res 2011;303(10): 727–36.
17. Ko M-C. Roles of central opioid receptor subtypes in regulating itch sensation. CRC Press/Taylor & Francis; 2014. Available at: http://www.ncbi.nlm.nih.gov/pubmed/24830012. Accessed June 9, 2019.
18. Elliott G, Vanwersch R, Soeberdt M, et al. Topical nalfurafine exhibits anti-inflammatory and anti-pruritic effects in a murine model of AD. J Dermatol Sci 2016;84(3):351–4.
19. Tominaga M, Ogawa H, Takamori K. Possible Roles of Epidermal Opioid Systems in Pruritus of Atopic Dermatitis. J Invest Dermatol 2007;127(9): 2228–35.
20. Benrath J, Eschenfelder C, Zimmerman M, et al. Calcitonin gene-related peptide, substance P and nitric oxide are involved in cutaneous inflammation following ultraviolet irradiation. Eur J Pharmacol 1995;293(1):87–96. Available at: http://www.ncbi.nlm.nih.gov/pubmed/7545583.
21. Legat FJ, Jaiani LT, Wolf P, et al. The role of calcitonin gene-related peptide in cutaneous immunosuppression induced by repeated subinflammatory ultraviolet irradiation exposure. Exp Dermatol 2004;13(4): 242–50.
22. Hosoi J, Murphy GF, Egan CL, et al. Regulation of Langerhans cell function by nerves containing

calcitonin gene-related peptide. Nature 1993; 363(6425):159–63.

23. Wallengren J, Håkanson R. Effects of substance P, neurokinin A and calcitonin gene-related peptide in human skin and their involvement in sensory nerve-mediated responses. Eur J Pharmacol 1987; 143(2):267–73. Available at: http://www.ncbi.nlm. nih.gov/pubmed/2446892. Accessed June 7, 2019.

24. Calzavara-Pinton PG, Sala R, Arisi M, et al. Synergism between narrowband ultraviolet B phototherapy and etanercept for the treatment of plaque-type psoriasis. Br J Dermatol 2013;169(1):130–6.

25. Théréné C, Brenaut E, Barnetche T, et al. Efficacy of systemic treatments of psoriasis on pruritus: a systemic literature review and meta-analysis. J Invest Dermatol 2018;138(1):38–45.

26. Lapolla W, Yentzer BA, Bagel J, et al. A review of phototherapy protocols for psoriasis treatment. J Am Acad Dermatol 2011;64(5):936–49.

27. Kleinpenning MM, Smits T, Boezeman J, et al. Narrowband ultraviolet B therapy in psoriasis: randomized double-blind comparison of high-dose and low-dose irradiation regimens. Br J Dermatol 2009;161(6):1351–6.

28. Mehta D, Lim HW. Ultraviolet B phototherapy for psoriasis: review of practical guidelines. Am J Clin Dermatol 2016;17(2):125–33.

29. Narbutt J, Olejniczak I, Sobolewska-Sztychny D, et al. Narrow band ultraviolet B irradiations cause alteration in interleukin-31 serum level in psoriatic patients. Arch Dermatol Res 2013;305(3):191–5.

30. Gupta G, Long J, Tillman DM. The efficacy of narrowband ultraviolet B phototherapy in psoriasis using objective and subjective outcome measures. Br J Dermatol 1999;140(5):887–90. Available at: http://www.ncbi.nlm.nih.gov/pubmed/10354027.

31. Evers AWM, Kleinpenning MM, Smits T, et al. Itch and scratching as predictors of time to clearance of psoriasis with narrow-band ultraviolet B therapy. Br J Dermatol 2009;161(3):542–6.

32. Levin AA, Aleissa S, Dumont N, et al. A randomized, prospective, sham-controlled study of localized narrow-band UVB phototherapy in the treatment of plaque psoriasis. J Drugs Dermatol 2014;13(8):922–6. Available at: http://www.ncbi. nlm.nih.gov/pubmed/25116969.

33. Menter A, Korman NJ, Elmets CA, et al. Guidelines of care for the management of psoriasis and psoriatic arthritis. J Am Acad Dermatol 2010;62(1): 114–35.

34. Dawn A, Papoiu ADP, Chan YH, et al. Itch characteristics in atopic dermatitis: results of a web-based questionnaire. Br J Dermatol 2009;160(3):642–4.

35. Pavlis J, Yosipovitch G. Management of Itch in Atopic Dermatitis. Am J Clin Dermatol 2018;19(3): 319–32.

36. Valkova S, Velkova A. UVA/UVB phototherapy for atopic dermatitis revisited. J Dermatolog Treat 2004;15(4):239–44.

37. Clowry J, Molloy K, Nestor L, et al. Narrow-band ultraviolet B phototherapy outcomes in atopic dermatitis-A single-centre retrospective review. Photodermatol Photoimmunol Photomed 2018; 34(3):217–9.

38. Jekler J, Larkö O. UVB phototherapy of atopic dermatitis. Br J Dermatol 1988;119(6):697–705. Available at: http://www.ncbi.nlm.nih.gov/pubmed/ 3203067.

39. Elmariah SB. Adjunctive management of itch in atopic dermatitis. Dermatol Clin 2017;35(3): 373–94.

40. Rivard J, Lim HW. Ultraviolet phototherapy for pruritus. Dermatol Ther 2005;18(4):344–54.

41. Jekler J, Larkö O. UVA solarium versus UVB phototherapy of atopic dermatitis: a paired-comparison study. Br J Dermatol 1991;125(6): 569–72. Available at: http://www.ncbi.nlm.nih.gov/ pubmed/1760362. Accessed June 7, 2019.

42. Majoie IML, Oldhoff JM, van Weelden H, et al. Narrowband ultraviolet B and medium-dose ultraviolet A1 are equally effective in the treatment of moderate to severe atopic dermatitis. J Am Acad Dermatol 2009;60(1):77–84.

43. Garritsen FM, Brouwer MWD, Limpens J, et al. Photo(chemo)therapy in the management of atopic dermatitis: an updated systematic review with implications for practice and research. Br J Dermatol 2014;170(3):501–13.

44. Reynolds NJ, Franklin V, Gray JC, et al. Narrowband ultraviolet B and broad-band ultraviolet A phototherapy in adult atopic eczema: a randomised controlled trial. Lancet 2001;357(9273): 2012–6.

45. Ring J, Alomar A, Bieber T, et al. Guidelines for treatment of atopic eczema (atopic dermatitis) part II. J Eur Acad Dermatol Venereol 2012;26(9): 1176–93.

46. Krutmann J, Diepgen TL, Luger TA, et al. High-dose UVA1 therapy for atopic dermatitis: results of a multicenter trial. J Am Acad Dermatol 1998;38(4): 589–93. Available at: http://www.ncbi.nlm.nih.gov/ pubmed/9555799.

47. Dayal S, Pathak K, Sahu P, et al. Narrowband UV-B phototherapy in childhood atopic dermatitis: efficacy and safety. An Bras Dermatol 2017;92(6): 801–6.

48. Morison WL, Parrish J, Fitzpatrick TB. Oral psoralen photochemotherapy of atopic eczema. Br J Dermatol 1978;98(1):25–30. Available at: http:// www.ncbi.nlm.nih.gov/pubmed/626712.

49. Der-Petrossian M, Seeber A, Hönigsmann H, et al. Half-side comparison study on the efficacy of 8-methoxypsoralen bath-PUVA versus narrow-band

ultraviolet B phototherapy in patients with severe chronic atopic dermatitis. Br J Dermatol 2000; 142(1):39–43. Available at: http://www.ncbi.nlm.nih.gov/pubmed/10651692.

50. Tzaneva S, Seeber A, Schwaiger M, et al. High-dose versus medium-dose UVA1 phototherapy for patients with severe generalized atopic dermatitis. J Am Acad Dermatol 2001;45(4):503–7.

51. Pacifico A, Iacovelli P, Damiani G, et al. 'High dose' vs. 'medium dose' UVA1 phototherapy in italian patients with severe atopic dermatitis. J Eur Acad Dermatol Venereol 2019;33(4):718–24.

52. Abeck D, Schmidt T, Fesq H, et al. Long-term efficacy of medium-dose UVA1 phototherapy in atopic dermatitis. J Am Acad Dermatol 2000;42(2):254–7.

53. Darné S, Leech SN, Taylor AEM. Narrowband ultraviolet B phototherapy in children with moderate-to-severe eczema: a comparative cohort study. Br J Dermatol 2014;170(1):150–6.

54. Clayton TH, Clark SM, Turner D, et al. The treatment of severe atopic dermatitis in childhood with narrowband ultraviolet B phototherapy. Clin Exp Dermatol 2006. https://doi.org/10.1111/j.1365-2230.2006.02292.x.

55. Nakamura M, Koo JY. Phototherapy for the treatment of prurigo nodularis: a review. Dermatol Online J 2016;22(4) [pii:13030/qt4b07778z]. Available at: http://www.ncbi.nlm.nih.gov/pubmed/27617458.

56. Qureshi AA, Abate LE, Yosipovitch G, et al. A systematic review of evidence-based treatments for prurigo nodularis. J Am Acad Dermatol 2019; 80(3):756–64.

57. Hann SK, Cho MY, Park YK. UV treatment of generalized prurigo nodularis. Int J Dermatol 1990; 29(6):436–7. Available at: http://www.ncbi.nlm.nlh.gov/pubmed/2397971.

58. Hammes S, Hermann J, Roos S, et al. UVB 308-nm excimer light and bath PUVA: combination therapy is very effective in the treatment of prurigo nodularis. J Eur Acad Dermatol Venereol 2011;25(7): 799–803.

59. Nakashima C, Tanizaki H, Otsuka A, et al. Intractable prurigo nodularis successfully treated with combination therapy with a newly developed excimer laser and topical steroids. Dermatol Online J 2014;20(6) [pii:13030/qt9xp4640d]. Available at: http://www.ncbi.nlm.nih.gov/pubmed/24945654.

60. Sorenson E, Levin E, Koo J, et al. Successful use of a modified Goeckerman regimen in the treatment of generalized prurigo nodularis. J Am Acad Dermatol 2015;72(1):e40–2.

61. Ling TC, Gibbs NK, Rhodes LE. Treatment of polymorphic light eruption. Photodermatol Photoimmunol Photomed 2003;19(5):217–27. Available at: http://www.ncbi.nlm.nih.gov/pubmed/14535892. Accessed June 7, 2019.

62. Ling TC, Clayton TH, Crawley J, et al. British Association of Dermatologists and British Photodermatology Group guidelines for the safe and effective use of psoralen-ultraviolet A therapy 2015. Br J Dermatol 2016;174(1):24–55.

63. Janssens AS, Pavel S, Out-Luiting JJ, et al. Normalized ultraviolet (UV) induction of Langerhans cell depletion and neutrophil infiltrates after artificial UVB hardening of patients with polymorphic light eruption. Br J Dermatol 2005;152(6):1268–74.

64. Gruber-Wackernagel A, Bambach I, Legat FJ, et al. Randomized double-blinded placebo-controlled intra-individual trial on topical treatment with a 1,25-dihydroxyvitamin D3 analogue in polymorphic light eruption. Br J Dermatol 2011;165(1):152–63.

65. Hönigsmann H. Polymorphous light eruption. Photodermatol Photoimmunol Photomed 2008;24(3): 155–61.

66. Berg M, Ros AM, Berne B. Ultraviolet A phototherapy and trimethylpsoralen UVA photochemotherapy in polymorphous light eruption–a controlled study. Photodermatol Photoimmunol Photomed 1994;10(4):139–43. Available at: http://www.ncbi.nlm.nih.gov/pubmed/7803223.

67. Lembo S, Raimondo A. Polymorphic Light Eruption: What's New in Pathogenesis and Management. Front Med 2018;5.

68. Bilsland D, George SA, Gibbs NK, et al. A comparison of narrow band phototherapy (TL-01) and photochemotherapy (PUVA) in the management of polymorphic light eruption. Br J Dermatol 1993;129(6):708–12. Available at: http://www.ncbi.nlm.nih.gov/pubmed/8286256.

69. Man I, Dawe RS, Ferguson J. Artificial hardening for polymorphic light eruption: practical points from ten years' experience. Photodermatol Photoimmunol Photomed 1999;15(3–4):96–9. Available at: http://www.ncbi.nlm.nih.gov/pubmed/10404717.

70. Mastalier U, Kerl H, Wolf P. Clinical, laboratory, phototest and phototherapy findings in polymorphic light eruptions: a retrospective study of 133 patients. Eur J Dermatol 1998;8(8):554–9. Available at: http://www.ncbi.nlm.nih.gov/pubmed/9889427.

71. Olsen EA, Hodak E, Anderson T, et al. Guidelines for phototherapy of mycosis fungoides and Sézary syndrome: a consensus statement of the United States Cutaneous Lymphoma Consortium. J Am Acad Dermatol 2016;74(1):27–58.

72. Hoot JW, Wang L, Kho T, et al. The effect of phototherapy on progression to tumors in patients with patch and plaque stage of mycosis fungoides. J Dermatolog Treat 2018;29(3):272–6.

73. Phan K, Ramachandran V, Fassihi H, et al. Comparison of Narrowband UV-B With Psoralen-UV-A Phototherapy for Patients With Early-Stage Mycosis

Fungoides: A Systematic Review and Meta-analysis. JAMA Dermatol 2019;155(3):335.

74. Jawed SI, Myskowski PL, Horwitz S, et al. Primary cutaneous T-cell lymphoma (mycosis fungoides and Sézary syndrome): part I. Diagnosis: clinical and histopathologic features and new molecular and biologic markers. J Am Acad Dermatol 2014;70(2):205.e1-16.

75. Nikolaou V, Sachlas A, Papadavid E, et al. Phototherapy as a first-line treatment for early-stage mycosis fungoides: The results of a large retrospective analysis. Photodermatol Photoimmunol Photomed 2018;34(5):307–13.

76. Plettenberg H, Stege H, Megahed M, et al. Ultraviolet A1 (340-400 nm) phototherapy for cutaneous T-cell lymphoma. J Am Acad Dermatol 1999;41(1):47–50. Available at: http://www.ncbi.nlm.nih.gov/pubmed/10411410.

77. Martin JA, Laube S, Edwards C, et al. Rate of acute adverse events for narrow-band UVB and Psoralen-UVA phototherapy. Photodermatol Photoimmunol Photomed 2007;23(2–3):68–72.

78. Sidbury R, Davis DM, Cohen DE, et al. Guidelines of care for the management of atopic dermatitis. J Am Acad Dermatol 2014;71(2):327–49.

79. Jawed SI, Myskowski PL, Horwitz S, et al. Primary cutaneous T-cell lymphoma (mycosis fungoides and Sézary syndrome): part II. Prognosis, management, and future directions. J Am Acad Dermatol 2014;70(2):223.e1-17 [quiz: 240–2].

80. Mettang T, Kremer AE. Uremic pruritus. Kidney Int 2015;87(4):685–91.

81. Murphy M, Carmichael AJ. Renal itch. Clin Exp Dermatol 2000;25(2):103–6. Available at: http://www.ncbi.nlm.nih.gov/pubmed/10733630.

82. Gilchrest BA, Rowe JW, Brown RS, et al. Ultraviolet phototherapy of uremic pruritus.Long-term results and possible mechanism of action. Ann Intern Med 1979;91(1):17–21. Available at: http://www.ncbi.nlm.nih.gov/pubmed/464448.

83. Tan JK, Haberman HF, Coldman AJ. Identifying effective treatments for uremic pruritus. J Am Acad Dermatol 1991;25(5 Pt 1):811–8. Available at: http://www.ncbi.nlm.nih.gov/pubmed/1839393.

84. Ko M-J, Yang J-Y, Wu H-Y, et al. Narrowband ultraviolet B phototherapy for patients with refractory uraemic pruritus: a randomized controlled trial. Br J Dermatol 2011;165(3):633–9.

85. Ada S, Seçkin D, Budakoğlu I, et al. Treatment of uremic pruritus with narrowband ultraviolet B phototherapy: an open pilot study. J Am Acad Dermatol 2005;53(1):149–51.

86. Seckin D, Demircay Z, Akin O. Generalized pruritus treated with narrowband UVB. Int J Dermatol 2007;46(4):367–70.

87. Wang T-J, Lan L-C, Lu C-S, et al. Efficacy of narrowband ultraviolet phototherapy on renal pruritus. J Clin Nurs 2014;23(11–12):1593–602.

88. Sherjeena PB, Binitha MP, Rajan U, et al. A controlled trial of narrowband ultraviolet B phototherapy for the treatment of uremic pruritus. Indian J Dermatol Venereol Leprol 2017;83(2):247–9.

89. Hsu MM-L, Yang CC. Uraemic pruritus responsive to broadband ultraviolet (UV) B therapy does not readily respond to narrowband UVB therapy. Br J Dermatol 2003;149(4):888–9. Available at: http://www.ncbi.nlm.nih.gov/pubmed/14616389.

90. Blachley JD, Blankenship DM, Menter A, et al. Uremic pruritus: skin divalent ion content and response to ultraviolet phototherapy. Am J Kidney Dis 1985;5(5):237–41. Available at: http://www.ncbi.nlm.nih.gov/pubmed/4003393.

91. Cohen EP, Russell TJ, Garancis JC. Mast cells and calcium in severe uremic itching. Am J Med Sci 1992;303(6):360–5. Available at: http://www.ncbi.nlm.nih.gov/pubmed/1605164.

92. Szepietowski J. Selected elements of the pathogenesis of pruritus in hemodialysis patients: My own study. Med Sci Monti 1996;2:343–7.

93. Bergasa NV. The pruritus of cholestasis. J Hepatol 2005;43(6):1078–88.

94. Decock S, Roelandts R, Van Steenbergen W, et al. Cholestasis-induced pruritus treated with ultraviolet B phototherapy: An observational case series study. J Hepatol 2012;57(3):637–41.

95. Kremer AE, Martens JJWW, Kulik W, et al. Lysophosphatidic Acid Is a Potential Mediator of Cholestatic Pruritus. Gastroenterology 2010;139(3):1008–18.e1.

96. European Association for the Study of the Liver. EASL Clinical Practice Guidelines: Management of cholestatic liver diseases. J Hepatol 2009;51(2):237–67.

97. Pinheiro NC, Marinho RT, Ramalho F, et al. Refractory pruritus in primary biliary cirrhosis. BMJCase Rep 2013;2013. https://doi.org/10.1136/bcr-2013-200634.

98. Lindor KD, Bowlus CL, Boyer J, et al. EASL clinical practice guidelines: management of cholestatic liver diseases. Hepatol 2018;0:237–67.

99. Hanid MA, Levi AJ. Phototherapy for pruritus in primary biliary cirrhosis. Lancet 1980;2(8193):530. Available at: http://www.ncbi.nlm.nih.gov/pubmed/6105574.

100. Cerio R, Murphy GM, Sladen GE, et al. A combination of phototherapy and cholestyramine for the relief of pruritus in primary biliary cirrhosis. Br J Dermatol 1987;116(2):265–7. Available at: http://www.ncbi.nlm.nih.gov/pubmed/3828220.

101. Rosenthal E, Diamond E, Benderly A, et al. Cholestatic pruritus: effect of phototherapy on pruritus and excretion of bile acids in urine. Acta Paediatr 1994;83(8):888–91. Available at: http://www.ncbi.nlm.nih.gov/pubmed/7981571.

102. Perlstein SM. Phototherapy for primary biliary cirrhosis. Arch Dermatol 1981;117(10):608. Available at: http://www.ncbi.nlm.nih.gov/pubmed/7283453.

103. Lelonek E, Matusiak Ł, Wróbel T, et al. Aquagenic pruritus in polycythemia vera: a cross-sectional study. J Am Acad Dermatol 2017. https://doi.org/10.1016/j.jaad.2017.10.021.

104. Baldo A, Sammarco E, Plaitano R, et al. Narrow-band (TL-01) ultraviolet B phototherapy for pruritus in polycythaemia vera. Br J Dermatol 2002;147(5):979–81. Available at: http://www.ncbi.nlm.nih.gov/pubmed/12410710.

105. Tefferi A, Rumi E, Finazzi G, et al. Survival and prognosis among 1545 patients with contemporary polycythemia vera: an international study. Leukemia 2013;27(9):1874–81.

106. Tefferi A, Vannucchi AM, Barbui T. Polycythemia vera treatment algorithm 2018. BloodCancer J 2018;8(1):3.

107. Hernández-Núñez A, Daudén E, Córdob S, et al. Water-induced pruritus in haematologically controlled polycythaemia vera: response to phototherapy. J Dermatolog Treat 2001;12(2):107–9.

108. Baldo A, Sammarco E, Martinelli V, et al. UVB phototherapy for pruritus in polycythaemia vera. J Dermatolog Treat 1996;7(4):245–6.

109. Jeanmougin M, Rain JD, Najean Y. Efficacy of photochemotherapy on severe pruritus in polycythemia vera. Ann Hematol 1996;73(2):91–3. Available at: http://www.ncbi.nlm.nih.gov/pubmed/8774618.

110. Kaushik SB, Cerci FB, Miracle J, et al. Chronic pruritus in HIV-positive patients in the southeastern United States: Its prevalence and effect on quality of life. J Am Acad Dermatol 2014;70(4):659–64.

111. Lim HW, Vallurupalli S, Meola T, et al. UVB phototherapy is an effective treatment for pruritus in patients infected with HIV. J Am Acad Dermatol 1997;37(3 Pt 1):414–7. Available at: http://www.ncbi.nlm.nih.gov/pubmed/9308556.

112. Serling SLC, Leslie K, Maurer T. Approach to Pruritus in the Adult HIV-Positive Patient. Semin Cutan Med Surg 2011;30(2):101–6.

113. Yokobayashi H, Sugaya M, Miyagaki T, et al. Analysis of serum chemokine levels in patients with HIV-associated eosinophilic folliculitis. J Eur Acad Dermatol Venereol 2013;27(2):e212–6.

114. Pardo RJ, Bogaert MA, Penneys NS, et al. UVB phototherapy of the pruritic papular eruption of the acquired immunodeficiency syndrome. J Am Acad Dermatol 1992;26(3 Pt 2):423–8. Available at: http://www.ncbi.nlm.nih.gov/pubmed/1564149. Accessed June 7, 2019.

115. Ranki A, Puska P, Mattinen S, et al. Effect of PUVA on immunologic and virologic findings in HIV-infected patients. J Am Acad Dermatol 1991;24(3):404–10. Available at: http://www.ncbi.nlm.nih.gov/pubmed/2061436.

116. Duvic M, Ulmer R, Crane M, et al. Treatment of HIV+ patients with UVB is associated with a significant increase in p24 antigen levels. J Invest Dermatol 1995;104:581.

117. Fotiades J, Lim HW, Jiang SB, et al. Efficacy of ultraviolet B phototherapy for psoriasis in patients infected with human immunodeficiency virus. Photodermatol Photoimmunol Photomed 1995;11(3):107–11. Available at: http://www.ncbi.nlm.nih.gov/pubmed/8555008.

118. Meola T, Soter NA, Ostreicher R, et al. The safety of UVB phototherapy in patients with HIV infection. J Am Acad Dermatol 1993;29(2 Pt 1):216–20. Available at: http://www.ncbi.nlm.nih.gov/pubmed/8335741.

119. Reed J, George S. Pruritic folliculitis of pregnancy treated with narrowband (TL-01) ultraviolet B phototherapy. Br J Dermatol 1999;141(1):177–9. Available at: http://www.ncbi.nlm.nih.gov/pubmed/10417550.

120. Kaptanoglu AF, Oskay T. Ultraviolet B treatment for pruritus in Hodgkin's lymphoma. J Eur Acad Dermatol Venereol 2003;17(4):489–90. Available at: http://www.ncbi.nlm.nih.gov/pubmed/12834480.

121. Kreuter A, Gambichler T, Avermaete A, et al. Low-dose ultraviolet A1 phototherapy for extragenital lichen sclerosus: results of a preliminary study. J Am Acad Dermatol 2002;46(2):251–5. Available at: http://www.ncbi.nlm.nih.gov/pubmed/11807437.

Beyond the Booth
Excimer Laser for Cutaneous Conditions

Karen Ly, BA, Mary P. Smith, BS, Quinn G. Thibodeaux, MD,
Kristen M. Beck, MD, Wilson Liao, MD, Tina Bhutani, MD*

KEYWORDS

- Excimer laser • Phototherapy • UV therapy • UVB

KEY POINTS

- The dermatologic excimer laser emits a 308 nm wavelength that can provide targeted ultraviolet B (UVB) treatment.
- The excimer laser is most appropriate for patients with limited skin disease.
- It offers the advantage of limiting UVB exposure to affected skin, can be used in difficult to reach sites, allows for site-specific dosing, and requires a lower cumulative UVB dose to achieve treatment efficacy.
- It has demonstrated efficacy in many dermatologic diseases, including psoriasis, vitiligo, atopic dermatitis, hypopigmented disorders, alopecia areata, and cutaneous T-cell lymphoma.

INTRODUCTION

Since its introduction in 1997,[1] the excimer laser has emerged as an efficacious treatment modality for many dermatologic diseases. Using energy created by "excited dimers" (excimer) of xenon and chloride gases, the dermatologic excimer laser emits a 308 nanometer (nm) wavelength that can provide targeted ultraviolet B (UVB) treatment.[2] Although conventional narrowband UVB (NBUVB) phototherapy is an appropriate treatment of patients with extensive disease, the excimer laser provides an alternative therapy that can limit UV exposure to affected skin, while sparing healthy skin.[2]

The excimer laser delivers UV light via a hand piece with a spot diameter of 14 to 30 mm. As such, the excimer laser is most appropriate for localized lesions and limited disease. It can also be used in difficult to reach sites, such as the scalp, palms, and soles that would have limited UV exposure with conventional phototherapy. In addition, the excimer laser allows for region-specific dosing, which is important in the treatment of recalcitrant lesions. In comparison to standard NBUVB, the excimer laser requires fewer treatment sessions, has reduced treatment duration, and requires a lower cumulative UVB dose, thus reducing the possible side effects associated with UV therapy.[2–6]

Given these many advantages, the excimer laser has emerged as a widely used modality for the treatment of several dermatologic conditions. It is currently approved by the Food and Drugs Administration (FDA) for the treatment of psoriasis, vitiligo, atopic dermatitis (AD), and leukoderma.[7] In addition to these diseases, the excimer laser has also demonstrated efficacy in the treatment of other hypopigmented disorders, alopecia areata, and cutaneous T-cell lymphoma.[3,4] This review addresses the mechanism, safety, application, and efficacy of the excimer laser for the treatment of these conditions.

Disclosure Statement: The authors have nothing to disclose.
Department of Dermatology, University of California San Francisco, 515 Spruce Street, San Francisco, CA 94118, USA
* Corresponding author.
E-mail address: tina.bhutani@ucsf.edu

Dermatol Clin 38 (2020) 157–163
https://doi.org/10.1016/j.det.2019.08.009
0733-8635/20/© 2019 Elsevier Inc. All rights reserved.

MECHANISM OF ACTION

The dermatologic excimer laser uses a gas mixture of xenon and chloride to form unstable dimers on exposure to a high-energy electric current. These "excited dimers" will dissociate and emit a 308 nm monochromatic, coherent wavelength laser beam.[2,8] The absorption of 308 nm light by keratinocytes and T lymphocytes induces DNA damage,[9] leading to a reduction in T-lymphocyte inflammation and keratinocyte proliferation. This leads to the upregulation of the p53 tumor suppressor pathway and downregulation of the Bcl-2 proto-oncogene, contributing to cell cycle arrest and apoptosis.[3,10,11] The increased efficacy observed in the excimer laser compared with NBUVB may be due to the deeper penetration and higher irradiance of the excimer laser.[8,11,12]

In disorders of depigmentation and hypopigmentation, the excimer laser is theorized to promote repigmentation through melanocyte migration, activation, and production of melanin. UVB stimulates the proliferation of melanocytes and migration of melanocytes from the hair follicles to the epidermis. Irradiation leads to apoptosis of inflammatory cells and the reduction of inflammatory mediators and cytokines.[8] It also increases the secretion of endothelin 1 from keratinocytes, which increases melanocyte migration, proliferation, and melanogenesis.[13,14]

SAFETY

The excimer laser has a favorable safety profile and is typically well tolerated by patients. The most common side effects include erythema, blistering, hyperpigmentation, hypopigmentation, and pruritus. These side effects are localized to the area treated in contrast to the larger areas observed with full-body phototherapy treatment. The long-term effects of UVB phototherapy include photodamage and photoaging, which are likely reduced with the excimer laser due to the reduced cumulative dose required for treatment efficacy. The risk of malignancy from UVB is unclear; however, long-term UVB studies have not demonstrated an increased risk of cutaneous malignancy.[2–4,15] There is no published evidence that therapeutic use of the excimer laser increases the risk of skin cancer.

APPLICATIONS AND EFFICACY IN DERMATOLOGIC CONDITIONS
Psoriasis

The excimer laser was first studied and proved to be effective in patients with chronic plaque psoriasis.[1] It has emerged as a treatment option in patients with mild to moderate, localized, refractory plaque psoriasis, who have had a suboptimal response or contraindication to alternative treatments. Because of the limited spot size, the excimer laser is most appropriate for patients with psoriasis with a body surface area (BSA) of less than 10% and for plaques located in sites that are difficult to access with conventional phototherapy, such as the scalp and genitals.

Excimer laser treatments typically occur 2 to 3 times a week, with a minimum of 48 hours between treatments, for 3 to 6 weeks.[16] Clearance typically occurs within 8 to 10 treatment sessions, and maintenance therapy can be considered in patients with extensive disease.[16–18] Excimer laser dosing initially used the minimal erythema dose protocol, which tested the minimal dose that would cause an erythematous macule on normal skin.[19] Current protocols have evolved to include induration and anatomic location of the lesion, as sites like the hands and feet can withstand a higher energy dose than the face.[3]

Bonis and colleagues[1] were the first to report the efficacy of the excimer laser in patients with plaque psoriasis in a study comparing NBUVB therapy and the excimer laser. This study reported that NBUVB required an average of 30.1 treatment sessions to achieve clearance, compared with an average of 8.33 treatment sessions in patients treated with the excimer laser. The cumulative dose of radiation was also found to be 6.47 times less with the excimer laser.[20] Feldman and colleagues[5] supported these findings in a large, multicenter study, which reported 72% of patients achieving a 75% improvement with a mean of 6.2 treatments.[5] This supported the earlier finding by Bonis and colleagues that the excimer laser required fewer treatment sessions than conventional phototherapy. The safety and efficacy of the excimer laser in patients with plaque psoriasis have been reported in multiple subsequent studies.[18,21–26]

This difference in treatment efficacy between standard phototherapy and the excimer laser is likely due to the higher fluence of the excimer laser, which leads to deeper UVB penetration and increase in the induction of apoptosis. Furthermore, psoriatic plaques have been shown to tolerate higher doses of UVB than healthy skin, allowing for greater irradiance.[27]

The excimer laser can be used as monotherapy or in combination with other treatments. Adjuvant topical treatments can augment treatment results, with flumetasone ointment,[28] clobetasol propionate spray,[29] calcipotriol ointment,[29,30] dithranol ointment,[30] tacrolimus ointment,[31] and 8-methoxypsoralen[32] demonstrating increased efficacy when used with the excimer laser. Trott and colleagues[33] reported that although psoralen ul-traviolet A (PUVA) monotherapy and PUVA in combination with the excimer laser demonstrated similar efficacy, patients treated with combination therapy went into remission with half the number of treatments and with half the cumulative UVA dose.[17,33]

The excimer laser can also be used to treat psoriasis that is refractory to other treatments and has even demonstrated efficacy in patients who have failed biological agents.[34,35] In addition to the treatment of refractory disease, the excimer laser is also effective in difficult-to-treat psoriasis subtypes, such as palmoplantar psoriasis,[36] palmoplantar pustular psoriasis,[37] nail psoriasis,[38] and scalp psoriasis.[20,39,40] The excimer laser can be used to treat mild to moderate chronic plaque psoriasis in children. A study comparing the safety and efficacy of the excimer laser in adults versus children reported that 12.5 treatments were needed for children compared with 9.7 needed in adults.[41]

Vitiligo

Excimer lasers are also indicated for the treatment of localized vitiligo in patients with less than 10% BSA and have been found to be effective in patients of all skin types.[7,42,43] Because of the smaller spot size, the excimer laser is often preferred by patients, as it can better target depigmented skin, reducing the adverse event of hyperpigmentation of healthy skin.

Currently, there is limited evidence on the optimal dosing, frequency, and duration of excimer laser treatments for vitiligo. Treatment typically involves 2 to 3 sessions weekly, with a minimum of 48 hours between treatments, for a treatment duration of 4 to 36 weeks.[7] Although increased frequency may result in earlier onset of repigmentation, it was discovered that the total number of treatments is the more important predictor of response.[44,45]

The excimer laser response depends on age, lesion location, disease duration, and treatment duration.[46–48] Treatment response is mostly depends on the location of lesions,[44] with lesions on the face, neck, trunk, and proximal extremities having a better outcome than UV-resistant sites, such as the distal extremities.[49] In a controlled study by Hofer and colleagues,[44] repigmentation was noted after 13 treatments for lesions located on the face, trunk, arm, and leg. In contrast, lesions on the elbow, wrist, knee, and dorsum of the hands and feet responded after a mean of 22 treatments.[44] In addition, several studies reported that repigmentation outcomes were better in patients with Fitzpatrick skin type III and above

than in patients with skin types I and II.[50,51] Repigmentation initially occurs in a perifollicular distribution, followed by the margins, with eventual coalescence of pigment.[52]

Multiple trials have compared the efficacy of the excimer laser versus NBUVB. Although some studies found the excimer laser to be more effective with a more rapid induction of repigmentation, in addition to requiring fewer treatments,[53–59] a 2016 meta-analysis comparing the excimer laser, lamp, and NBUVB found no significant difference in efficacy between these treatment modalities.[49]

Combination therapy has significantly higher rates of repigmentation in comparison to excimer laser monotherapy. Topical calcineurin inhibitors, such as tacrolimus[60–63] and pimecrolimus,[64] khellin 4% ointment,[65] hydrocortisone 17-butyrate cream,[66] and tetrahydrocurcuminoid cream,[67] have demonstrated improved efficacy when used in combination with excimer laser therapy. A study combining NBUVB with excimer laser reported an increase in treatment response in patients who were previously resistant to conventional NBUVB monotherapy.[68]

Hypopigmented Conditions

In addition to vitiligo, the excimer laser can also be used to treat hypopigmented diseases. It has demonstrated efficacy in diseases including nevus depigmentosus,[46,69] idiopathic guttate hypomelanosis,[70] lichen striatus,[71] and pityriasis alba.[72] Nevus depigmentosus is a rare disease with few treatment options. A case report of an infant with facial nevus depigmentosus reported repigmentation of the lesion after 10 treatments.[46] Although studied in striae distensae, the excimer laser was not found to improve the texture or erythema associated with the disease. It was also found to require regular treatment sessions to maintain treatment response.[73,74]

Atopic Dermatitis

The excimer laser is FDA-approved for the treatment of AD and can be used in both adults and children. Baltas and colleagues[75] reported that excimer laser therapy significantly reduced clinical scores and improved quality of life and pruritus in patients with AD. A subsequent study evaluating the efficacy of the excimer laser in adults and children with AD reported that 66.7% of patients achieved complete remission with 6 to 12 treatments, and 44% of patients maintained results at 16 weeks.[76] A study investigating the prurigo form of AD compared the excimer laser with clobetasol propionate 0.05% ointment. Both treatments demonstrated efficacy, but the excimer laser showed more improvement at follow-up. This study concluded that the excimer laser is an effective alternative to topical corticosteroids and can be used in patients with recalcitrant disease.[77]

Alopecia Areata

The excimer laser has also demonstrated efficacy in treating AA, with clinical trials reporting between 36.9% and 100% of patients experiencing hair regrowth of 50% or greater.[78] Most of these patients had previously failed standard treatment, indicating the excimer laser's utility in recalcitrant disease. A controlled clinical trial by Al-Mutairi and colleages[79] reported that the excimer laser was most efficacious on the scalp and beard, with poorer outcomes observed on the extremities. Notably, the excimer laser has not demonstrated efficacy in alopecia universalis or alopecia totalis.[79] The excimer laser was found to be an effective treatment in the pediatric population.[80] Although the mechanism of action in AA is not fully understood, it is proposed that the induction of apoptosis of T lymphocytes results in reduced perifollicular inflammation and damage to the hair follicle.[81]

Cutaneous T-Cell Lymphoma

The excimer laser has demonstrated efficacy in early stage mycosis fungoides (MF). Multiple studies evaluated the excimer laser as a treatment in patients with stage IA MF and found the excimer laser to be safe and effective.[82–84] In a study by Nistico and colleagues,[82] all 5 patients treated with the excimer laser achieved remission with less than 10 treatment sessions. The excimer laser was also found to be effective in the treatment of mycosis fungoides palmaris et plantaris, a rare variant of MF limited to the palms and soles.[85]

Other Conditions

The excimer laser has been reported to be an effective treatment of oral lichen planus, especially in patients with erosive disease.[86–88] In a report evaluating a patient with a 40-year history of granuloma annulare, complete remission was achieved with 15 treatments with the excimer laser.[89] The excimer laser was used as an adjuvant therapy in adult cutaneous Langerhans cell histiocytosis and was found to significantly improve symptoms, although a cure was not achieved.[90] In a study of 5 patients with localized scleroderma, 3 patients experienced significant improvement in skin texture with 7 treatment sessions.[15]

SUMMARY

The excimer laser is an excellent treatment modality and has demonstrated efficacy in many dermatologic diseases. It offers the advantage of limiting treatment to affected skin, can be used in difficult to reach sites, allows for site specific dosing, and requires a lower cumulative UVB dose to achieve treatment efficacy. However, when considering treatment with the excimer laser, the appropriate patient selection must be made. Because of the limited treatment field, the excimer laser is most practical for patients with localized and limited disease. In those with extensive lesions, the excimer laser would be time consuming and labor intensive. In addition, the excimer laser is a well-tolerated treatment option for patients. Although further studies are needed to evaluate the long-term safety of the excimer laser, current studies suggest that the safety profile is more favorable than conventional phototherapy due to less cumulative exposure to UV light. Because of these distinct advantages, the excimer laser is an increasingly popular treatment modality and an important tool for dermatologists. The role of the excimer laser in dermatology will continue to expand as more studies investigate its application in different diseases.

REFERENCES

1. Bonis B, Kemeny L, Dobozy A, et al. 308 nm UVB excimer laser for psoriasis. Lancet 1997;350:1522.
2. Spencer JM, Hadi SM. The excimer lasers. J Drugs Dermatol 2004;3(5):522–5.
3. Beggs S, Short J, Rengifo-Pardo M, et al. Applications of the excimer laser: a review. Dermatol Surg 2015;41(11):1201–11.
4. Mehraban S, Feily A. 308nm excimer laser in dermatology. J Lasers Med Sci 2014;5(1):8–12.
5. Feldman SR, Mellen BG, Housman TS, et al. Efficacy of the 308-nm excimer laser for treatment of psoriasis: results of a multicenter study. J Am Acad Dermatol 2002;46(6):900–6.
6. Trehan M, Taylor CR. Medium-dose 308-nm excimer laser for the treatment of psoriasis. J Am Acad Dermatol 2002;47(5):701–8.
7. Park KK, Liao W, Murase JE. A review of monochromatic excimer light in vitiligo. Br J Dermatol 2012; 167(3):468–78.
8. Novak Z, Bonis B, Baltas E, et al. Xenon chloride ultraviolet B laser is more effective in treating psoriasis and in inducing T cell apoptosis than narrow-band ultraviolet B. J Photochem Photobiol B 2002;67(1):32–8.
9. Wong T, Hsu L, Liao W. Phototherapy in psoriasis: a review of mechanisms of action. J Cutan Med Surg 2013;17(1):6–12.

10. Bulat V, Situm M, Dediol I, et al. The mechanisms of action of phototherapy in the treatment of the most common dermatoses. Coll Antropol 2011;35(Suppl 2):147–51.

11. Bianchi B, Campolmi P, Mavilia L, et al. Monochromatic excimer light (308 nm): an immunohistochemical study of cutaneous T cells and apoptosis-related molecules in psoriasis. J Eur Acad Dermatol Venereol 2003;17(4):408–13.

12. Novak Z, Berces A, Ronto G, et al. Efficacy of different UV-emitting light sources in the induction of T-cell apoptosis. Photochem Photobiol 2004; 79(5):434–9.

13. Noborio R, Morita A. Preferential induction of endothelin-1 in a human epidermal equivalent model by narrow-band ultraviolet B light sources. Photodermatol Photoimmunol Photomed 2010;26(3):159–61.

14. Hara M, Yaar M, Gilchrest BA. Endothelin-1 of keratinocyte origin is a mediator of melanocyte dendricity. J Invest Dermatol 1995;105(6):744–8.

15. Nistico SP, Saraceno R, Schipani C, et al. Different applications of monochromatic excimer light in skin diseases. Photomed Laser Surg 2009;27(4):647–54.

16. Totonchy MB, Chiu MW. UV-based therapy. Dermatol Clin 2014;32(3):399–413. ix–x.

17. Matos TR, Ling TC, Sheth V. Ultraviolet B radiation therapy for psoriasis: pursuing the optimal regime. Clin Dermatol 2016;34(5):587–93.

18. Housman TS, Pearce DJ, Feldman SR. A maintenance protocol for psoriasis plaques cleared by the 308 nm excimer laser. J Dermatolog Treat 2004;15(2):94–7.

19. Mudigonda T, Dabade TS, Feldman SR. A review of protocols for 308 nm excimer laser phototherapy in psoriasis. J Drugs Dermatol 2012;11(1):92–7.

20. Gattu S, Rashid RM, Wu JJ. 308-nm excimer laser in psoriasis vulgaris, scalp psoriasis, and palmoplantar psoriasis. J Eur Acad Dermatol Venereol 2009; 23(1):36–41.

21. Hsu S, Papp KA, Lebwohl MG, et al. Consensus guidelines for the management of plaque psoriasis. Arch Dermatol 2012;148(1):95–102.

22. Hadi SM, Al-Quran H, de Sa Earp AP, et al. The use of the 308-nm excimer laser for the treatment of psoriasis. Photomed Laser Surg 2010;28(5):693–5.

23. Han L, Somani AK, Huang Q, et al. Evaluation of 308-nm monochromatic excimer light in the treatment of psoriasis vulgaris and palmoplantar psoriasis. Photodermatol Photoimmunol Photomed 2008; 24(5):231–6.

24. Nistico SP, Saraceno R, Stefanescu S, et al. 308-nm monochromatic excimer light in the treatment of palmoplantar psoriasis. J Eur Acad Dermatol Venereol 2006;20(5):523–6.

25. Gerber W, Arheilger B, Ha TA, et al. Ultraviolet B 308-nm excimer laser treatment of psoriasis: a new phototherapeutic approach. Br J Dermatol 2003; 149(6):1250–8.

26. Kollner K, Wimmershoff MB, Hintz C, et al. Comparison of the 308-nm excimer laser and a 308-nm excimer lamp with 311-nm narrowband ultraviolet B in the treatment of psoriasis. Br J Dermatol 2005; 152(4):750–4.

27. Alshiyab D, Edwards C, Chin MF, et al. Targeted ultraviolet B phototherapy: definition, clinical indications and limitations. Clin Exp Dermatol 2015;40(1):1–5.

28. Dong J, He Y, Zhang X, et al. Clinical efficacy of flumetasone/salicylic acid ointment combined with 308-nm excimer laser for treatment of psoriasis vulgaris. Photodermatol Photoimmunol Photomed 2012;28(3):133–6.

29. Levin E, Debbaneh M, Malakouti M, et al. Supraerythemogenic excimer laser in combination with clobetasol spray and calcitriol ointment for the treatment of generalized plaque psoriasis: interim results of an open label pilot study. J Dermatolog Treat 2015;26(1):16–8.

30. Rogalski C, Grunewald S, Schetschorke M, et al. Treatment of plaque-type psoriasis with the 308 nm excimer laser in combination with dithranol or calcipotriol. Int J Hyperthermia 2012;28(2):184–90.

31. Carrascosa JM, Soria X, Domingo H, et al. Treatment of inverse psoriasis with excimer therapy and tacrolimus ointment. Dermatol Surg 2007;33(3):361–3.

32. Asawanonda P, Amornpinyokeit N, Nimnuan C. Topical 8-methoxypsoralen enhances the therapeutic results of targeted narrowband ultraviolet B phototherapy for plaque-type psoriasis. J Eur Acad Dermatol Venereol 2008;22(1):50–5.

33. Trott J, Gerber W, Hammes S, et al. The effectiveness of PUVA treatment in severe psoriasis is significantly increased by additional UV 308-nm excimer laser sessions. Eur J Dermatol 2008;18(1):55–60.

34. Malakouti M, Brown GE, Sorenson E, et al. Successful use of the excimer laser for generalized psoriasis in an ustekinumab non-responder. Dermatol Online J 2014;21(3) [pii:13030/qt76m221mt].

35. Park KK, Swan J, Koo J. Effective treatment of etanercept and phototherapy-resistant psoriasis using the excimer laser. Dermatol Online J 2012;18(3):2.

36. Goldberg DJ, Chwalek J, Hussain M. 308-nm Excimer laser treatment of palmoplantar psoriasis. J Cosmet Laser Ther 2011;13(2):47–9.

37. Sevrain M, Richard MA, Barnetche T, et al. Treatment for palmoplantar pustular psoriasis: systematic literature review, evidence-based recommendations and expert opinion. J Eur Acad Dermatol Venereol 2014;28(Suppl 5):13–6.

38. Al-Mutairi N, Noor T, Al-Haddad A. Single blinded left-to-right comparison study of excimer laser versus pulsed dye laser for the treatment of nail psoriasis. Dermatol Ther (Heidelb) 2014;4(2):197–205.

39. Taylor CR, Racette AL. A 308-nm excimer laser for the treatment of scalp psoriasis. Lasers Surg Med 2004;34(2):136–40.

40. Guenther L. Current management of scalp psoriasis. Skin Therapy Lett 2015;20(3):5–7.

41. Pahlajani N, Katz BJ, Lozano AM, et al. Comparison of the efficacy and safety of the 308 nm excimer laser for the treatment of localized psoriasis in adults and in children: a pilot study. Pediatr Dermatol 2005; 22(2):161–5.

42. Baltas E, Csoma Z, Ignacz F, et al. Treatment of vitiligo with the 308-nm xenon chloride excimer laser. Arch Dermatol 2002;138:1619–20.

43. Spencer JM, Nossa R, Ajmeri J. Treatment of vitiligo with the 308-nm excimer laser: a pilot study. J Am Acad Dermatol 2002;46(5):727–31.

44. Hofer A, Hassan AS, Legat FJ, et al. The efficacy of excimer laser (308 nm) for vitiligo at different body sites. J Eur Acad Dermatol Venereol 2006;20(5): 558–64.

45. Shen Z, Gao TW, Chen L, et al. Optimal frequency of treatment with the 308-nm excimer laser for vitiligo on the face and neck. Photomed Laser Surg 2007; 25(5):418–27.

46. Zeng Q, Shi Q, Huang J, et al. Facial nevus depigmentosus getting remarkable repigmentation by treatment with a 308-nm excimer laser: a case report. Dermatol Ther 2018;31(5):e12662.

47. Fa Y, Lin Y, Chi XJ, et al. Treatment of vitiligo with 308-nm excimer laser: our experience from a 2-year follow-up of 979 Chinese patients. J Eur Acad Dermatol Venereol 2017;31(2):337–40.

48. Al-Shobaili HA. Correlation of clinical efficacy and psychosocial impact on vitiligo patients by excimer laser treatment. Ann Saudi Med 2014;34(2):115–21.

49. Lopes C, Trevisani VF, Melnik T. Efficacy and safety of 308-nm monochromatic excimer lamp versus other phototherapy devices for vitiligo: a systematic review with meta-analysis. Am J Clin Dermatol 2016; 17(1):23–32.

50. Kawalek AZ, Spencer JM, Phelps RG. Combined excimer laser and topical tacrolimus for the treatment of vitiligo: a pilot study. Dermatol Surg 2004;30(2 Pt 1):130–5.

51. Hadi SM, Spencer JM, Lebwohl M. The use of the 308-nm excimer laser for the treatment of vitiligo. Dermatol Surg 2004;30(7):983–6.

52. Patel NS, Paghdal KV, Cohen GF. Advanced treatment modalities for vitiligo. Dermatol Surg 2012; 38(3):381–91.

53. Casacci M, Thomas P, Pacifico A, et al. Comparison between 308-nm monochromatic excimer light and narrowband UVB phototherapy (311-313 nm) in the treatment of vitiligo–a multicentre controlled study. J Eur Acad Dermatol Venereol 2007;21(7):956–63.

54. Hong SB, Park HH, Lee MH. Short-term effects of 308-nm xenon-chloride excimer laser and narrow-band ultraviolet B in the treatment of vitiligo: a comparative study. J Korean Med Sci 2005;20(2): 273–8.

55. Sun Y, Wu Y, Xiao B, et al. Treatment of 308-nm excimer laser on vitiligo: a systemic review of randomized controlled trials. J Dermatolog Treat 2015;26(4): 347–53.

56. Xiao BH, Wu Y, Sun Y, et al. Treatment of vitiligo with NB-UVB: a systematic review. J Dermatolog Treat 2015;26(4):340–6.

57. Shi Q, Li K, Fu J, et al. Comparison of the 308-nm excimer laser with the 308-nm excimer lamp in the treatment of vitiligo–a randomized bilateral comparison study. Photodermatol Photoimmunol Photomed 2013;29(1):27–33.

58. Linthorst Homan MW, Spuls PI, Nieuweboer-Krobotova L, et al. A randomized comparison of excimer laser versus narrow-band ultraviolet B phototherapy after punch grafting in stable vitiligo patients. J Eur Acad Dermatol Venereol 2012; 26(6):690–5.

59. Le Duff F, Fontas E, Giacchero D, et al. 308-nm excimer lamp vs. 308-nm excimer laser for treating vitiligo: a randomized study. Br J Dermatol 2010; 163(1):188–92.

60. Lin AN. Innovative use of topical calcineurin inhibitors. Dermatol Clin 2010;28(3):535–45.

61. Park OJ, Park GH, Choi JR, et al. A combination of excimer laser treatment and topical tacrolimus is more effective in treating vitiligo than either therapy alone for the initial 6 months, but not thereafter. Clin Exp Dermatol 2016;41(3):236–41.

62. Nistico S, Chiricozzi A, Saraceno R, et al. Vitiligo treatment with monochromatic excimer light and tacrolimus: results of an open randomized controlled study. Photomed Laser Surg 2012;30(1):26–30.

63. Passeron T, Ostovari N, Zakaria W, et al. Topical tacrolimus and the 308-nm excimer laser: a synergistic combination for the treatment of vitiligo. Arch Dermatol 2004;140(9):1065–9.

64. Hui-Lan Y, Xiao-Yan H, Jian-Yong F, et al. Combination of 308-nm excimer laser with topical pimecrolimus for the treatment of childhood vitiligo. Pediatr Dermatol 2009;26(3):354–6.

65. Saraceno R, Nistico SP, Capriotti E, et al. Monochromatic excimer light 308 nm in monotherapy and combined with topical khellin 4% in the treatment of vitiligo: a controlled study. Dermatol Ther 2009; 22(4):391–4.

66. Sassi F, Cazzaniga S, Tessari G, et al. Randomized controlled trial comparing the effectiveness of 308-nm excimer laser alone or in combination with topical hydrocortisone 17-butyrate cream in the treatment of vitiligo of the face and neck. Br J Dermatol 2008;159(5):1186–91.

67. Asawanonda P, Klahan SO. Tetrahydrocurcuminoid cream plus targeted narrowband UVB phototherapy for vitiligo: a preliminary randomized controlled study. Photomed Laser Surg 2010; 28(5):679–84.

68. Shin S, Hann SK, Oh SH. Combination treatment with excimer laser and narrowband UVB light in vitiligo patients. Photodermatol Photoimmunol Photomed 2016;32(1):28–33.

69. Bae JM, Jung HM, Chang HS, et al. Treatment of nevus depigmentosus using the 308-nm excimer laser: a retrospective study of 14 patients. J Am Acad Dermatol 2016;75(3):626–7.

70. Gordon JR, Reed KE, Sebastian KR, et al. Excimer Light Treatment for Idiopathic Guttate Hypomelanosis: a Pilot Study. Dermatol Surg 2017;43(4):553–7.

71. Bae JM, Choo JY, Chang HS, et al. Effectiveness of the 308-nm excimer laser on hypopigmentation after lichen striatus: a retrospective study of 12 patients. J Am Acad Dermatol 2016;75(3):637–9.

72. Al-Mutairi N, Hadad AA. Efficacy of 308-nm xenon chloride excimer laser in pityriasis alba. Dermatol Surg 2012;38(4):604–9.

73. Aldahan AS, Shah VV, Mlacker S, et al. Laser and light treatments for striae distensae: a comprehensive review of the literature. Am J Clin Dermatol 2016;17(3):239–56.

74. Ross NA, Ho D, Fisher J, et al. Striae distensae: preventative and therapeutic modalities to improve aesthetic appearance. Dermatol Surg 2017;43(5):635–48.

75. Baltas E, Csoma Z, Bodai L, et al. Treatment of atopic dermatitis with the xenon chloride excimer laser. J Eur Acad Dermatol Venereol 2006;20(6):657–60.

76. Nistico SP, Saraceno R, Capriotti E, et al. Efficacy of monochromatic excimer light (308 nm) in the treatment of atopic dermatitis in adults and children. Photomed Laser Surg 2008;26(1):14–8.

77. Brenninkmeijer EE, Spuls PI, Lindeboom R, et al. Excimer laser vs. clobetasol propionate 0.05% ointment in prurigo form of atopic dermatitis: a randomized controlled trial, a pilot. Br J Dermatol 2010;163(4):823–31.

78. Darwin E, Arora H, Hirt PA, et al. A review of monochromatic light devices for the treatment of alopecia areata. Lasers Med Sci 2018;33(2):435–44.

79. Al-Mutairi N. 308-nm excimer laser for the treatment of alopecia areata. Dermatol Surg 2007;33(12):1483–7.

80. Fenniche S, Hammami H, Zaouak A. Association of khellin and 308-nm excimer lamp in the treatment of severe alopecia areata in a child. J Cosmet Laser Ther 2018;20(3):156–8.

81. Zakaria W, Passeron T, Ostovari N, et al. 308-nm excimer laser therapy in alopecia areata. J Am Acad Dermatol 2004;51:837–8.

82. Nistico S, Costanzo A, Saraceno R, et al. Efficacy of monochromatic excimer laser radiation (308 nm) in the treatment of early stage mycosis fungoides. Br J Dermatol 2004;151(4):877–9.

83. Passeron T, Angeli K, Cardot-Leccia N, et al. Treatment of mycosis fungoides by 308 nm excimer laser: a clinical and histological study in 10 patients. Ann Dermatol Venereol 2007;134(3 Pt 1):225–31 [in French].

84. Mori M, Campolmi P, Mavilia L, et al. Monochromatic excimer light (308 nm) in patch-stage IA mycosis fungoides. J Am Acad Dermatol 2004;50(6):943–5.

85. Nakai N, Hagura A, Yamazato S, et al. Mycosis fungoides palmaris et plantaris successfully treated with radiotherapy: case report and mini-review of the published work. J Dermatol 2014;41(1):63–7.

86. Kollner K, Wimmershoff M, Landthaler M, et al. Treatment of oral lichen planus with the 308-nm UVB excimer laser–early preliminary results in eight patients. Lasers Surg Med 2003;33(3):158–60.

87. Liu WB, Sun LW, Yang H, et al. Treatment of oral lichen planus using 308-nm excimer laser. Dermatol Ther 2017;30(5):1–3.

88. Trehan M, Taylor CR. Low-dose excimer 308-nm laser for the treatment of oral lichen planus. Arch Dermatol 2004;140(4):415–20.

89. Verne SH, Kennedy J, Falto-Aizpurua LA, et al. Laser treatment of granuloma annulare: a review. Int J Dermatol 2016;55(4):376–81.

90. Vogel CA, Aughenbaugh W, Sharata H. Excimer laser as adjuvant therapy for adult cutaneous Langerhans cell histiocytosis. Arch Dermatol 2008;144(10):1287–90.

Feeling the Burn
Phototoxicity and Photoallergy

Andrea N. Hinton, BS[a,1], Ari M. Goldminz, MD[a,b],*

KEYWORDS

- Photoallergy • Phototoxicity • Contact dermatitis • Photopatch testing

KEY POINTS

- Photoallergy and phototoxicity encompass a wide range of clinical presentations and follow varied courses.
- Culprits can be found in different places, from topical medications to ingested ones and from natural compounds to synthetic ones, with many sharing similar chemical structures that predispose to haptenization.
- Several of these same compounds are also used to carefully induce photoreactions for treatment of photoresponsive dermatoses.
- A critical understanding of photoinduced dermatoses and thorough evaluation are required to reach an accurate diagnosis.
- Further research on these entities will enable us to better recognize, diagnose, and treat photoallergy and phototoxicity.

INTRODUCTION/BACKGROUND

An interaction between light's radiation and certain exogenous and endogenous substances can lead to the development of photoallergic and/or phototoxic dermatoses. Clinically, reactions may range from acute and self-limited to chronic and recurrent. Delays in diagnosis are not uncommon due to complex clinical presentations, broad differentials, and limited number of specialists who perform phototesting. Therefore, a critical understanding of these dermatoses is essential for accurate diagnosis and appropriate management.

Thousands of years ago, photosensitizing agents found in nature were combined with light exposure to treat diseases of pigmentation.[1] In modern times, the photosensitizing properties of naturally occurring chemicals, such as psoralens, continue to be used to treat a variety of dermatologic diseases. Photodermatitis can also be an unintended side effect of exposure to certain compounds. Elixir sulfanilamide, introduced in 1937 as a treatment of several medical conditions, was among the first reported culprit of photoallergy in the modern medical literature.[2] Sulfanilamide is an antibiotic that shares structural similarity with another photosensitizer, para-aminobenzoic acid (PABA). Certain medications may also induce clinically unique photoinduced dermatoses, such as the blue-gray dyspigmentation associated with reactions to amiodarone.

The epidemiology, light sources, mechanisms, clinical presentations, evaluation protocols, common culprits, treatments, key challenges, and future directions related to photoallergy and phototoxicity are reviewed herein. Other conditions of photosensitivity, such as connective tissue diseases (ie, lupus erythematosus) and inheritable

Disclosure statement: The authors have nothing to disclose.
[a] Harvard Medical School, Boston, MA, USA; [b] Department of Dermatology, Brigham and Women's Hospital, Boston, MA, USA
[1] Present address: 850 Boylston Street, Chestnut Hill, MA 02467.
* Corresponding author. 850 Boylston Street, Chestnut Hill, MA 02467.
E-mail address: agoldminz@bwh.harvard.edu

Dermatol Clin 38 (2020) 165–175
https://doi.org/10.1016/j.det.2019.08.010
0733-8635/20/© 2019 Elsevier Inc. All rights reserved.

and acquired conditions (ie, porphyrias), are not comprehensively discussed in this article but can be reviewed in other sources.[3–6]

EPIDEMIOLOGY

Among patients who underwent photopatch testing based on clinical suspicion of photoallergy, 5.7% to 49.5% were found to have photoallergic or phototoxic reactions in the larger available studies (**Table 1**).[7–14] It is generally difficult, however, to estimate the true population-wide prevalence of photoallergic and phototoxic reactions. Reactions may have a relatively mild and self-limiting course or patients may simply discontinue the offending agent rather than seek evaluation by a health care provider. When patients do present, clinicians may have a low index of suspicion for the diagnosis. The gold standard methods for diagnosis, including photopatch testing, also have limited availability and in certain cases are an essential part of the work-up.

Epidemiologic research on photoallergic and phototoxic reactions in skin of color also remains scarce.[15] In the United States, only a handful of studies have examined differences in prevalence of photodermatoses between racial and ethnic groups. One study comparing 138 African American and 63 white patients presenting with photodermatoses at an academic institution in the United States between 2004 and 2012 noted a statistically significant difference in the prevalence of phototoxic drug eruptions (0.7% vs 15.9%, respectively) and phytophotodermatitis (0% vs 6.3%, respectively) between the 2 groups; however, the differences in prevalence of all photodermatoses (46.6% vs 42.2%%, respectively),

photoallergic dermatitis (0% vs 1.6%%, respectively), and photosensitivity not-otherwise-specified (9.4% vs 11.1%%, respectively) were not statistically significant.[15]

The prevalence of photoallergic and phototoxic reactions varies not only between racial and ethnic groups but also between geographic locations. Rates of photoallergy among patients in various countries as demonstrated by photopatch testing are shown in **Table 1**. Factors that have an impact on these reported rates may include variations in skin type distribution, sunscreen use, intensity of light exposure, and photopatch testing protocols.

LIGHT SOURCES

The primary light sources that induce photoallergic and phototoxic reactions include those on the UV and visible spectra. The visible spectrum is discernible by the human eye and includes wavelengths between 400 nm and 700 nm. A rainbow, which is composed of colors on the visible spectrum, is a phenomenon created by interactions between visible light and water droplets. These colors include red, orange, yellow, green, cyan, blue, and violet.

The UV spectrum spans wavelengths between 200 nm and 400 nm and is classified as UV-A (315–400 nm), UV-B (290–315 nm), and UV-C (200–290 nm). UV-A is further divided into $UV-A_1$ (340–400 nm) and $UV-A_2$ (315–340 nm). UV radiation-emitting higher energy, including UV-C and the majority of UV-B, is primarily absorbed by the atmosphere and, therefore, earth's inhabitants are mainly exposed to UV-A and some UV-B radiation.[16]

Table 1
Variation in photoallergic reaction frequency between countries

Country	Study	Study Size (n)	Allergens Tested (n)	Patients with Positive Photopatch Testing (%)
Canada	Greenspoon et al,[7] 2013	160	26	33.8
China	Gao et al,[8] 2014	4957	14	49.5
Colombia	Rodríguez et al,[9] 2006	82	19	31.7
Europe	Kerr et al,[10] 2012	1031	24	19.4
Greece	Katsarou et al,[11] 2008	207	29	13.52
Italy	Pigatto et al,[12] 2008	1082	33	21.6[a]
United Kingdom	Bryden et al,[13] 2006	1155	13[b]	5.7
United States	Scalf et al,[14] 2009	182	34	29.7

[a] A total of 290 reactions were demonstrated among 234 patients (21.6%). Of these, 204 (70.3%) were allergic contact and 18 (6.2%) were phototoxic.
[b] Number of agents tested does not include patients' own sunscreen products, which were included in testing as is if there was clinical suspicion of a photosensitivity reaction. Testing in this study was limited to sunscreen agents.

While the sun is nature's source of UV radiation, UV phototherapy booths use bulbs to emit UV radiation. Controlled exposure to these bulbs can be used in the treatment of certain photo-responsive dermatologic conditions, such as psoriasis and atopic dermatitis, and the diagnosis of photoinduced dermatoses, such as photoallergy. Although photosensitizers, such as psoralens, induce phototoxicity, their photosensitizing nature can also be harnessed for therapeutic purposes, as with psoralens plus UV-A (PUVA). Specific wavelengths of light are used to treat cutaneous diseases: blue light for acne vulgaris, red light for skin aging, and excimer laser, narrowband UV-B, and broadband UV-B or PUVA for inflammatory dermatoses, such as psoriasis.

MECHANISMS AND CLINICAL PRESENTATIONS

The overarching mechanisms of photoallergy and phototoxicity in certain aspects parallel those of allergic and irritant contact dermatitis. Photoallergy, as with allergic contact dermatitis, requires sensitization to the offending agent, has a relatively low incidence, often features epidermal spongiosis on histopathology, typically appears hours to days after allergen exposure, and has a dose-dependent response for both the allergen and light (**Table 2**). Conversely, phototoxicity, as with irritant contact dermatitis, can occur in any individual, has a higher incidence, often features keratinocyte necrosis on histopathology, typically has a more rapid clinical onset after exposure to the offending agent, and does not characteristically have a dose-dependent response.

Photoallergy is thought to require sensitization to a hapten.[17] One model of sensitization involves photo-modification of the hapten (prohapten) that subsequently couples with a protein and develops the potential to induce photoallergy. An alternative process first involves hapten-protein binding followed by activation by light (photohapten). Haptens then undergo processing by Langerhans cells, are presented to naïve T cells in the lymph nodes, and lead to differentiation of photoallergen-specific T cells. Re-exposure to the allergen as well as the appropriate light source and radiation dose lead to a photoallergic reaction.

Unlike photoallergy, phototoxicity can occur in any individual exposed to enough of the causative antigen and light source, typically UV-A. Cytotoxic compounds, such as oxygen free radicals, superoxide anions, and singlet oxygen, are generated after interactions between phototoxic substances and light. Other compounds, such as stable photoproducts, photoadducts, and inflammatory mediators, can also be involved in generating phototoxic reactions.[18]

Classically, photoallergy presents as an eczematous dermatitis in a photodistribution. There may be sharp demarcation between photoexposed and photoprotected sites, such as at the border of textiles; naturally shaded areas, such as the philtrum, submandibular, postauricular, and inverse areas, may be spared (**Fig. 1**). Photoxicity is characterized by a sunburn-like reaction and may have associated vesicles and bullae due to direct cellular injury and subsequent epidermal necrosis and edema (**Fig. 2**).

Some agents that cause photoreactions may induce a more unique clinical presentation and recognition can aid in making the diagnosis. Reactions to amiodarone may present with a blue-gray hue,[19] whereas chronic phenothiazine

Table 2
Typical characteristics of photoallergic and phototoxic reactions

Classic Characteristics	Photoallergy	Phototoxicity
Clinical presentation	Dermatitis	Exaggerated sunburn-like reaction
Incidence	Low	High
Sensitization	+	−
Dose response	±	+
Histologic Features	Spongiotic	Necrotic
Clinical onset after exposure	Hours to days	Minutes to days

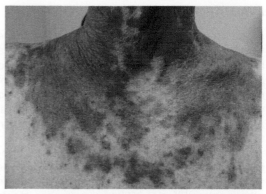

Fig. 1. Erythematous papules and plaques in a photodistribution with relative sparing of the submental area and below the shirt's neck line. A similar distribution can also be seen in cases of airborne allergic contact dermatitis.

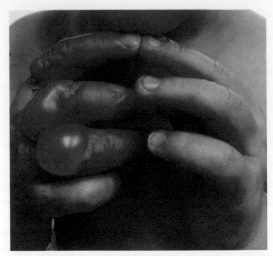

Fig. 2. A phytophoto (phototoxic) reaction in a child after making lime-aid outside in the summertime. Involvement of the right (dominant) hand is observed in this case

antipsychotic use can be associated with a gray-purple pigmentation.[20,21] Calcium channel blockers, such as nifedipine, can induce photoinduced telangiectasia.[22] Erythema multiforme-like reactions also can be seen.[21] Phytophotodermatitis, a type of phototoxic reaction triggered by exposure to certain plant species along with enough UV-A, classically manifests with bullae and/or hyperpigmented patches at the site of contact within 24 hours to 48 hours of exposure (see **Fig. 2**). Classically, a linear configuration may be seen due to smearing or dripping of allergen, such as lime juice.[23] Other atypical clinical presentations of photoreactions are not uncommon, including involvement of photoprotected areas and persistent reactions despite removal of the inciting agent.

EVALUATION

A precise and detailed clinical history is key to the work-up and definitive diagnosis, and, therefore, a high index of suspicion for photoallergic and phototoxic reactions must be maintained. Recent medications or topical product changes, coupled with sun exposure and photodistributed findings, are some factors that might lead to consideration of this diagnosis.

In general, the differential diagnosis for phototoxicity, in particular photoallergy, is wide. The skin findings of a photoallergic reaction can mimic other common dermatoses, such as atopic dermatitis and allergic contact dermatitis. Histologic examination may reveal a spongiotic dermatitis similar to other delayed hypersensitivity reactions.[24] Exacerbation of symptoms with sun

exposure and predominance of skin findings involving sun-exposed areas are suggestive of a photoallergy, but do not confirm the diagnosis.

The differential diagnosis for phototoxic and photoallergic reactions also includes other photo-induced skin sensitivities. The mechanisms underlying polymorphic light eruption may be similar to photoallergic reactions, although the relevant allergens have yet to be identified.[25] Other primary photodermatoses or photo-aggravated dermatoses include solar urticaria, rosacea, systemic lupus erythematous, and the porphyrias. Both the clinical history and examination findings can be particularly helpful in making the accurate diagnosis. Wheals are the primary lesions found in solar urticaria, although they may not be present at the time of evaluation. The systemic involvement and other examination findings of systemic lupus erythematous are not characteristic of photoallergy or phototoxicity, although symptoms, such as fever and rigors, can be uncommonly associated with photocontact dermatitis.[3] Laboratory investigations, including antinuclear antibodies and porphyrins, may also be appropriate in the workup of select cases.

In the pediatric population, additional diagnoses may be considered for patients presenting with photoinduced dermatoses, such as hydroa vacciniforme; juvenile spring eruption; actinic prurigo; connective tissue diseases, such as juvenile dermatomyositis; and other rare genetic conditions, such as xeroderma pigmentosum and Cockayne syndrome (both caused by defects in nucleotide excision repair), Rothmund-Thomson syndrome and Bloom syndrome (both caused by defects in double-stranded break repair), and erythropoietic protoporphyria.[26–28]

Photopatch Testing

In clinical practice, the definitive diagnosis of photoallergic contact dermatitis can be made by examination of the skin after exposure to an allergen and light (photopatch testing). Allergens typically are diluted within a petrolatum or aqueous (eg, alcohol) vehicle and applied in parallel either as a single allergen, when 1 culprit is suspected by clinical history, or more likely as a panel of allergens. The placement of allergens in parallel, with only 1 set exposed to UV radiation, allows differentiation between contact dermatitis reactions that require light (reaction only at the test site exposed to light) and those that do not require light (reactions at both test sites). Because exposure patterns to allergens vary by location, different panels can be ordered by geographic region (**Table 3**). After the placement of allergens,

Table 3
North American Contact Dermatitis Group, European, and Swedish screening allergens for photoallergy

UV Absorbers/Sunscreens	Nonsteroidal Anti-inflammatory Drugs/Medications	Preservatives	Other
North American Contact Dermatitis Group			
Benzophenone-3 10% pet	Bithionol 1% pet	2,2'-thiobis(4-chlorophenol) 1% pet	6-methyl coumarin 1% alc
Benzophenone-4 10% pet	Chlorpromazine hydrochloride 0.1% pet	3,4,5-tribromosalicylanilide 1% pet	Methyl anthranilate 5% pet
Butyl methoxydibenzoylmethane 5% pet	Promethazine hydrochloride 1% pet	Chlorhexidine diacetate 0.5% aq	Petrolatum 100%
Ethylhexyl dimethyl PABA 5% pet & 5% alc		Dichlorophene 1% pet	Sandalwood oil 2% pet
Ethylhexyl methoxycinnamate 7.5% pet		Hexachlorophene 1% pet	Thiourea 0.1% pet
Ethylhexyl salicylate 5% pet		Triclosan 2% pet	
Homosalate 5% pet			
PABA 5.0% alc			
European[a]			
2-(4-diethylamino-2-hydroxybenzoyl)-benzoic acid hexylester 10% pet	Benzydiamine hydrochloride 2% pet	Triclocarban 1% pet[a]	Camphor 10% pet
4-methylbenzylidene camphor 10% pet	Chlopromazine hydrochloride 0.1% pet[a]		Decyl glucoside 5% pet
Benzophenone-3 10% pet	Dexketoprofen 1% pet[a]		Fenofibrate 10% pet[a]
Benzophenone-4 2% pet	Diclofenac sodium salt 5% pet[a]		Olaquindox 1% pet[a]
Benzophenone-10 10% pet[a]	Etofenamate 2% pet		Polysilicone-15 10% pet[a]
Bis-ethylhexylphenol methoxyphenoltriazine 10% pet	Ibuprofen 5% pet[a]		
Butyl methoxydibenzoylmethane 10% pet	Ketoprofen 1% pet		
Diethylhexyl butamido triazone 10% pet	Phenylbenzimidazole sulfonic acid 10% pet[a]		
Diethylhexyl butamido triazone 10% pet[a]	Piroxicam 1% pet		
Disodium phenyl dibenzimidazole tetrasulfonate 10% pet[a]	Promethazone hydrochloride 0.1% pet[a]		

(continued on next page)

Table 3
(continued)

UV Absorbers/Sunscreens	Nonsteroidal Anti-inflammatory Drugs/ Medications	Preservatives	Other
Drometrizole trisiloxane 10% pet			
Ethylhexyl methoxycinnamate 10% pet			
Ethylhexyl triazone 10% pet			
Homosalate 10% pet[a]			
Isoamyl p-methoxycinnamate 10% pet			
Methylene bis-benzotriazolyl tetramethylbutylphenol 10% pet			
Octocrylene 10% pet			
PABA 10% pet			
Swedish			
4-methylbenzylidene camphor 10% pet			Ketoprofen 1% pet
Benzophenone-3 10% pet			Phenylbenzimidazole sulfonic acid 10% pet
Benzophenone-4 10% pet			
Butyl methoxydibenzoylmethane 10% pet			
Drometrizole trisiloxane 10% pet			
Ethylhexyl dimethyl PABA 10% pet			
Ethylhexyl methoxycinnamate 10% pet			
Ethylhexyl salicylate 5% pet			
Ethylhexyl triazone 10% pet			
Homosalate 5% pet			
Isoamyl p-methoxycinnamate 10% pet			
Octocrylene 10% pet			

Bolded allergens present in all 3 screening series.

Abbreviations: alc, alcohol; aq, aqueous; PABA, p-aminobenzoic acid; pet, petrolatum.

[a] Allergens only included in the extended European photoallergy series.

Data from Chemotechnique Diagnostics. Available at: https://www.chemotechnique.se/ Accessed May 4, 2019.

typically on the back, the patches are covered to prevent light exposure. In order to determine the minimum amount of UV exposure required to induce erythema, or the minimal erythema dose (MED), MED assessment can be done before patch testing to determine the appropriate dose of UV-A exposure to use (**Fig. 3**).[29,30] The role of UV-B in photopatch testing is limited, because UV-A exposure induces the vast majority of photoallergic reactions and the amount of energy required to elicit a photoallergic reaction from UV-B typically is greater than what is necessary to induce a sunburn response.[31] After either 24 hours or 48 hours, depending on the protocol used, 1 of the 2 patch series that were placed in parallel is exposed to UV-A radiation, typically at 5 J/cm^2 or 10 J/cm^2. An initial photopatch test read is done at this time and again 24 hours to 48 hours later.

COMMON CULPRITS

Oral and topical medications, sunscreens, and plants are the most common inducers of phototoxic and photoallergic reactions (**Fig. 4**, **Table 4**). Although there are hundreds of compounds

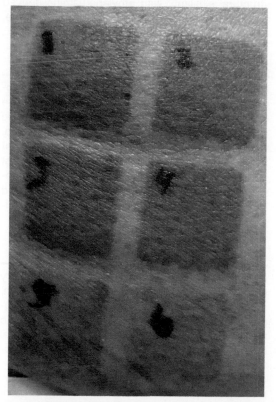

Fig. 3. MED testing (shown here) can be done to assess UV-A sensitivity prior to photopatch testing.

bergamottin (a furanocoumarin)

6-methylcoumarin

chlorpromazine

chlorprothixene

oxybenzone

ketoprofen

vemurafenib

amiodarone

Fig. 4. Several examples of plants, medications, and sunscreens that can induce photoallergy and/or phototoxicity.

reported in the literature as being associated with phototoxic reactions, a systematic review found that many were generally supported with low-quality to mid-quality evidence, including antiarrhythmic drugs, such as amiodarone, antifungals, antipsychotics, nonsteroidal anti-inflammatory drugs (NSAIDs), and angiotensin receptor blockers.[32] Only vemurafenib was associated with high-quality evidence in this study of phototoxic reactions.

Plants

Furanocoumarins, or furocoumarins, refer to numerous compounds commonly found in plants that share an aromatic, polycyclic chemical structure (furan ring fused to a coumarin). The most frequent plant families include *Moraceae* (mulberry), *Rutaceae* (citrus), and *Umbelliferae* (celery and carrots). Phototoxic reactions involving these plants are also referred to as phytophotodermatitis and are triggered in conjunction with UV-A light.[23] Clinically these reactions most often present within 24 hours to 48 hours and appear as vesicles, bullae, and/or hyperpigmentation, often involving the hands (see **Fig. 2**). There is a characteristic linear configuration due to the handling of culprit plants or dripping of citrus extract onto the skin (eg, lime juice).[21,23]

Table 4
Examples of photosensitizing medications, plants, and additives

Category	
Antimicrobials	Azoles (eg, voriconazole) Fluoroquinolones (eg, ciprofloxacin) Sulfonamides (eg, sulfamethoxazole) Tetracyclines (eg, doxycycline)
Antipsychotics	Phenothiazines (eg, chlorpromazine, prochlorperazine) Thioxanthenes (eg, chlorprothixene)
Cardiovascular	Amiodarone Angiotensin receptor blockers Calcium channel blockers (amlodipine, nifedipine) Furosemide Statins (atorvastatin, simvastatin) Thiazides (eg, hydrochlorothiazide)
Dermatologic	5-,8-methoxypsoralen Dapsone Retinoids
Fragrances	Methylcoumarins (6-methylcoumarin) Musk ambrette
NSAIDs	Benzydamine, diclofenac Ibuprofen, naproxen Ketoprofen
Oncologic	5-fluorouracil Imatinib Vemurafenib
Other	Antimalarials (eg, hydroxychloroquine) Furocoumarins (eg, *Moraceae, Rutacea,* and *Umbelliferae)* Oral contraceptives (ethinylestradiol) Sunscreens (eg, oxybenzone and PABA)

This represents a nonexhaustive list of photosensitizing agents. Individual photosensitizers may result in a phototoxic reaction and/or photoallergic reaction.

Fragrances

A derivative of the furanocoumarin family, 6-methylcoumarin was a common fragrance additive in the 1980s; it remains on some standard photopatch test panels given its role as a photosensitizing agent.[41,42] Similarly, musk ambrette was popular in men's fragrances in the 1980s and 1990s but is now less commonly used due to its photosensitizing properties.

Antimicrobials

Several antimicrobial medications are associated with phototoxicity and/or photoallergy, including the tetracycline antibiotics (eg doxycycline and minocycline), fluoroquinolones (eg ciprofloxacin), sulfonamide antibiotics (eg sulfamethoxazole), antifungals (eg voriconazole, itraconazole, ketoconazole, griseofulvin, and terbinafine), and antimalarials (eg hydroxychloroquine and quinidine).[21] Doxycycline is associated with a phototoxic reaction that can manifest as erythema and a sunburn-like eruption within 24 hours. Symptoms are dose dependent and typically triggered with exposure to UV-A light between 340 nm and 400 nm.[33] Photodermatoses associated with antifungals and antimalarials may have more varied clinical morphologies, including lichenoid, purpuric, and vesicular.[21]

Antipsychotics

Numerous antipsychotics, including the phenothiazines (eg chlorpromazine and prochlorperazine) and thioxanthenes (eg chlorprothixene), may induce classic photoallergic and phototoxic reactions[34–36] as well as a gray-purple pigmentation.[20,21] Phenothiazines also share structural similarity with ethylenediamine-derived antihistamines, such as cetirizine and hydroxyzine, which can lead to cross-sensitivity.[36]

Sunscreen Additives/UV Filters

Most commonly, benzophenones, a family of aromatic hydrocarbons that includes oxybenzone (benzophenone-3), are implicated in photoallergic reactions related to sunscreen. Oxybenzone, which serves as an UV filter for light maximally at 290 nm to 340 nm, is considered one of the most prominent contact and photoallergens in sunscreen, based on the larger studies.[37] PABA and its various esters are also common sunscreen culprits of photoallergy.

Nonsteroidal anti-inflammatory Drugs

Examples of offending agents in this category include benzydamine, diclofenac, ketoprofen, and carprofen. For ketoprofen, studies have suggested that a benzophenone moiety similar to that found in sunscreen may serve as a potential hapten or photosensitizer.[38] Conversely, the photoallergic reaction to carprofen is thought to be due to photo-dehalogenation, which leads to formation of an aryl radical.[39] Patients may present with vesicles, bullae, edema, and/or erythema multiforme.[21]

Cardiovascular Medications

Several cardiovascular medications are associated with unique photoinduced-skin eruptions. Along with dysesthesia and erythema, amiodarone may present with a characteristic blue-gray pigmentation, thought to be secondary to metabolite deposition in the skin.[19,40] Calcium channel blockers, such as nifedipine, are associated with photoinduced telangiectasia.[22] Loop diuretics (eg furosemide) and thiazide diuretics (eg hydrochlorothiazide) may elicit photoallergic and/or phototoxic reactions.[19]

Chemotherapeutics

Several classes of chemotherapeutics are associated with photosensitive reactions, such as tyrosine kinase inhibitors (imatinib and vandetinib), pyrimidine analogs (5-fluorouracil), vinca alkaloids (vinblastine), and hydroxyurea.[21] More recently, phototoxic reactions have been reported with newer agents, such as multikinase inhibitors (pazopanib)[43] and antibody-drug conjugate targeting delta-like protein 3 (rovalpituzumab tesirine).[44] Clinicians should maintain a high level of suspicion in order to diagnose photoallergic or phototoxic reactions in patients receiving newer agents because there may be limited literature available.

TREATMENT

For most patients, avoidance of allergens remains the first-line management strategy for photoallergic and phototoxic reactions. This includes photoavoidance and strict photoprotection with sunscreen and sun-protective clothing. In cases when these approaches are ineffective or inadequate or continuation of the culprit agent outweighs the risks of a reaction, other topical and systemic treatment options similar to those for allergic contact dermatitis can be used.[24] Topical steroids, antihistamines for symptomatic treatment of itch, and moisturization are cornerstones of symptomatic treatment. Systemic corticosteroids and other immunosuppressant medications can also be used in severe or recalcitrant cases.[24]

KEY CHALLENGES AND FUTURE DIRECTIONS

A high level of clinical suspicion is required to make the accurate diagnosis of photoallergic and phototoxic reactions. Atypical presentations may be seen, such as persistent dermatitis despite removal of the culprit allergen or involvement of photo-protected areas. These findings may point the clinician away from the diagnosis. Conversely, patient reported history suggesting a photo-aggravated dermatitis does not necessarily confirm an underlying photo-induced mechanism. The development of novel biomarkers for identification of these reactions would be a valuable addition to the field. Additional documentation and classification of photo-induced reactions, such as through large databases with analyses by region, will also improve the ability to recognize, diagnose, and understand trends in photoallergic and phototoxic reactions over time. New photoallergens and phototoxins also continue to emerge as the latest over-the-counter and prescription products are available to patients. Premarket screening measures can assess for potential reactions caused by these new products. New approaches for premarket screening are being investigated for improved sensitivity.[45] Access to experts who perform phototesting is also limited particularly in certain geographic areas. In a 2017 survey of 117 participating members of the American Contact Dermatitis Society, 64 (54.8%) conduct photopatch testing.[46] Increasing the number of physicians who can undertake these evaluations is essential, through increased exposure starting in residency training.

SUMMARY

Photoallergy and phototoxicity encompass a wide range of clinical presentations and follow varied courses. Culprits can be found in different places, from topical medications to ingested ones and natural compounds to synthetic ones, with many sharing similar chemical structures that predispose to haptenization. Several of these same compounds are also used to carefully induce photoreactions for treatment of photoresponsive dermatoses. A critical understanding of photoinduced dermatoses and thorough evaluation are required to reach an accurate diagnosis. Further research on these entities will help better recognize, diagnose, and treat photoallergy and phototoxicity.

REFERENCES

1. Pathak MA, Fitzpatrick TB. The evolution of photochemotherapy with psoralens and UVA (PUVA): 2000 BC to 1992 AD. J Photochem Phtobiol B 1992;14:3–22.
2. Epstein S. Photoallergy and primary photosensitivity to sulfanilamide. J Invest Dermatol 1938;2(2):43–51.
3. Nahhas AF, Oberlin DM, Braunberger TL, et al. Recent developments in the diagnosis and management of photosensitive disorders. Am J Clin Dermatol 2018;19:707–31.

4. Giordano CN, Yew YW, Spivak G, et al. Understanding photodermatoses associated with defective DNA repair: Syndromes with cancer predisposition. J Am Acad Dermatol 2016;75(5):855–70.

5. Yew YW, Giordano CN, Spivak G, et al. Understanding photodermatoses associated with defective DNA repair: photosensitive syndromes without associated cancer predisposition. J Am Acad Dermatol 2016;75(5):873–82.

6. Choi D, Jannan S, Lim HW. Evaluation of patients with photodermatoses. Dermatol Clin 2014;32(3):267–75.

7. Greenspoon J, Ahluwalia R, Juma N, et al. Allergic and photoallergic contact dermatitis: a 10-year experience. Dermatitis 2013;24(1):29–32.

8. Gao L, Hu Y, Ni C, et al. Retrospective study of PhotoPatch testing in a Chinese population during a 7-year period. Dermatitis 2014;25(1):22–6.

9. Rodríguez E, Valbuena MC, Rey M, et al. Causal agents of photoallergic contact dermatitis diagnosed in the National Institute of Dermatology of Colombia. Photodermatol Photoimmunol Photomed 2006;22(4):189–92.

10. Kerr AC, Ferguson J, Haylett AK, et al, The European Multicentre Photopatch Test Study (EMCPPTS) Taskforce. A European multicentre photopatch test study: European photopatch test study. Br J Dermatol 2012;166(5):1002–9.

11. Katsarou A, Makris M, Zarafonitis G, et al. Photoallergic contact dermatitis: the 15-year experience of a tertiary reference center in a sunny Mediterranean city. Int J Immunopathol Pharmacol 2008;21(3):725–7.

12. Pigatto PD, Guzzi G, Schena D, et al. Photopatch tests: an Italian multicenter study from 2004 to 2006. Contact Dermatitis 2008;59:103–8.

13. Bryden AM, Moseley H, Ibbotson SH, et al. Photopatch testing of 1155 patients: results of the U.K. multicentre photopatch study group. Br J Dermatol 2006;155(4):737–47.

14. Scalf LA, Davis MDP, Rohlinger AL, et al. Photopatch testing of 182 patients: a 6 year experience at the Mayo Clinic. Dermatitis 2009;20(1):44–52.

15. Nakamura M, Henderson M, Jacobsen G, et al. Comparison of photodermatoses in African-Americans and Caucasians: a follow-up study: comparison of photodermatoses. Photodermatol Photoimmunol Photomed 2014;30(5):231–6.

16. Honari G. Photoallergy. Rev Environ Health 2014;29(3):233–42.

17. Tokura Y. Drug photoallergy. J Cutan Immunol Allergy 2018;1:48–57.

18. Andreu I, Mayorga C, Miranda MA. Generation of reactive intermediates in photoallergic dermatitis. Curr Opin Allergy Clin Immunol 2010;10:303–8.

19. Drucker AM, Rosen CF. Drug-induced photosensitivity: culprit drugs, management and prevention. Drug Saf 2011;34(10):821–37.

20. Harth Y, Rapoport M. Photosensitivity associated with antipsychotics, antidepressants and anxiolytics. Drug Saf 1996;14:252–9.

21. Monteiro AF, Rato M, Martins C. Drug-induced photosensitivity: photoallergic and phototoxic reactions. Clin Dermatol 2016;34(5):571–81.

22. Collins P, Ferguson J. Photodistributed nifedipine-induced facial telangiectasia. Br J Dermatol 1993;129(5):630–3.

23. Moreau JF, English JC 3rd, Gehris RP. Phytophotodermatitis. J Pediatr Adol Gynec 2014;27(2):93–4.

24. Wilm A, Berenburg M. Photoallergy. J Dtsch Dermatol Ges 2015;13(1):7–13.

25. Snyder M, Turrentine JE, Cruz PD. Photocontact dermatitis and its clinical mimics: an overview for the allergist. Clin Rev Allergy Immunol 2019;56(1):32–40.

26. Chantorn R, Lim HW, Shwayder TA. Photosensitivity disorders in children. J Am Acad Dermatol 2012;67(6):1113.e1–15.

27. Grossberg AL. Update on pediatric photosensitivity disorders. Curr Opin Pediatr 2013;25(4):474–9.

28. Naka F, Shwayder TA, Santoro FA. Photodermatoses: kids are not just little people. Clin Dermatol 2016;34(6):724–35.

29. Deleo VA. Photocontact dermatitis. Dermatol Ther 2004;17(4):279–88.

30. Duguid C, O'Sullivan D, Murphy GM. Determination of threshold UV-A elicitation dose in photopatch testing. Contact Dermatitis 1993;29:192–4.

31. Pollock B, Wilkinson SM. Photopatch test method: influence of type of irradiation and value of day-7 reading. Contact Dermatitis 2001;44(5):270–2.

32. Kim WB, Shelley AJ, Novice K, et al. Drug-induced phototoxicity: a systematic review. J Am Acad Dermatol 2018;79(6):1069–75.

33. Goetze S, Hiernickel C, Elsner P. Phototoxicity of doxycycline: a systematic review on clinical manifestations, frequency, cofactors, and prevention. Skin Pharmacol Physiol 2017;30(2):76–80.

34. Barbaud A, Collet E, Martin S, et al. Contact sensitization to chlorpromethazine can induce persistent light reaction and cross photoreaction to other phenothiazines. Contact Dermatitis 2001;44:373–4.

35. Cardoso JC, Canelas MM, Gonçalo M, et al. Photopatch testing with an extended series of photoallergens: a 5-year study. Contact Dermatitis 2009;60:325–9.

36. Romita P, Foti C, Stingeni L. Photoallergy to promazine hydrochloride. Contact Dermatitis 2017;77(3):182–3.

37. DiNardo JC, Downs CA. Dermatological and environmental toxicological impact of the sunscreen

ingredient oxybenzone/benzophenone-3. J Cosmet Dermatol 2018;17(1):15–9.

38. Loh T, Cohen P. Ketoprofen-induced photoallergic dermatitis. Indian J Med Res 2016;144(6):803.

39. Walker SL, Ead RD, Beck MH. Occupational photoallergic contact dermatitis in a pharmaceutical worker manufacturing carprofen, a canine nonsteroidal anti-inflammatory drug. Br J Dermatol 2006; 154(3):569–70.

40. Ammoury A, Michaud S, Paul C, et al. Photodistribution of blue-gray hyperpigmentation after amiodarone treatment: molecular characterization of amiodarone in the skin. Arch Dermatol 2008; 144(1):92–6.

41. Victor FC, Cohen DE, Soter NA. A 20-year analysis of previous and emerging allergens that elicit photoallergic contact dermatitis. J Am Acad Dermatol 2010;62(4):605–10.

42. Jackson RT, Nesbitt LT, DeLeo VA. 6-Methylcoumarin photocontact dermatitis. J Am Acad Dermatol 1980;2(2):124–7.

43. Udompanich S, Chanprapaph K, Rajatanavin N. Phototoxic reaction induced by Pazopanib. Case Rep Dermatol 2018;10(3):251–6.

44. Hou JL, Bridges AG. Phototoxic drug reaction with the novel agent rovalpituzumab tesirine. Int J Dermatol 2018;57(3):e17–9.

45. Maeda Y, Hirosaki H, Ymanaka H, et al. New approach to predict photoallergic potentials of chemicals based on murine local lymph node assay. J Appl Toxicol 2018;38:1316–22.

46. Asemota E, Crawford G, Kovarik C, et al. A survey examining photopatch test and phototest methodologies of contact dermatologists in the united states: platform for developing a consensus. Dermatitis 2017;28(4):265–9.

Printed and bound by CPI Group (UK) Ltd, Croydon, CR0 4YY

18/10/2024

01775893-0001